Raw + Free

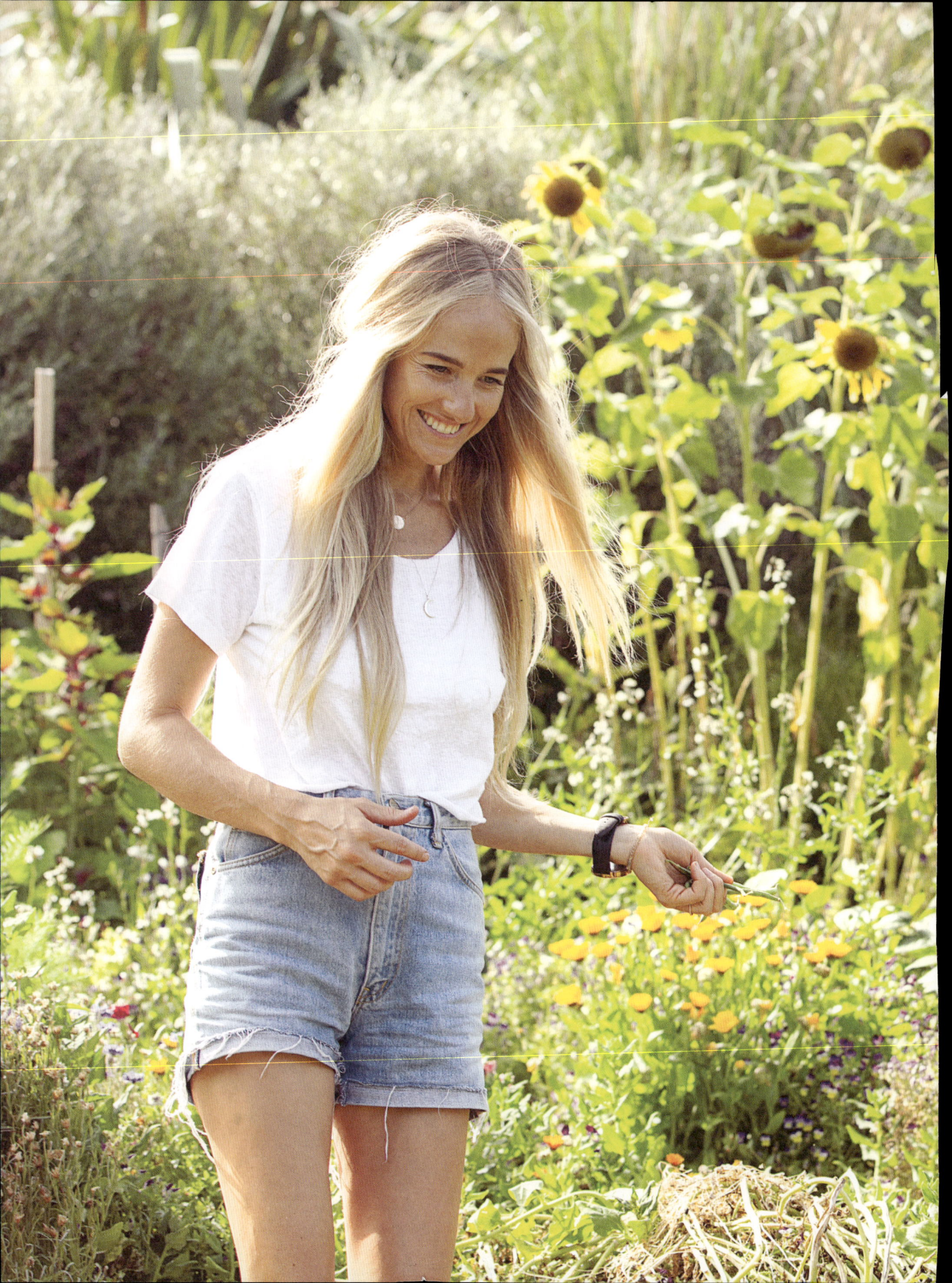

Raw + Free

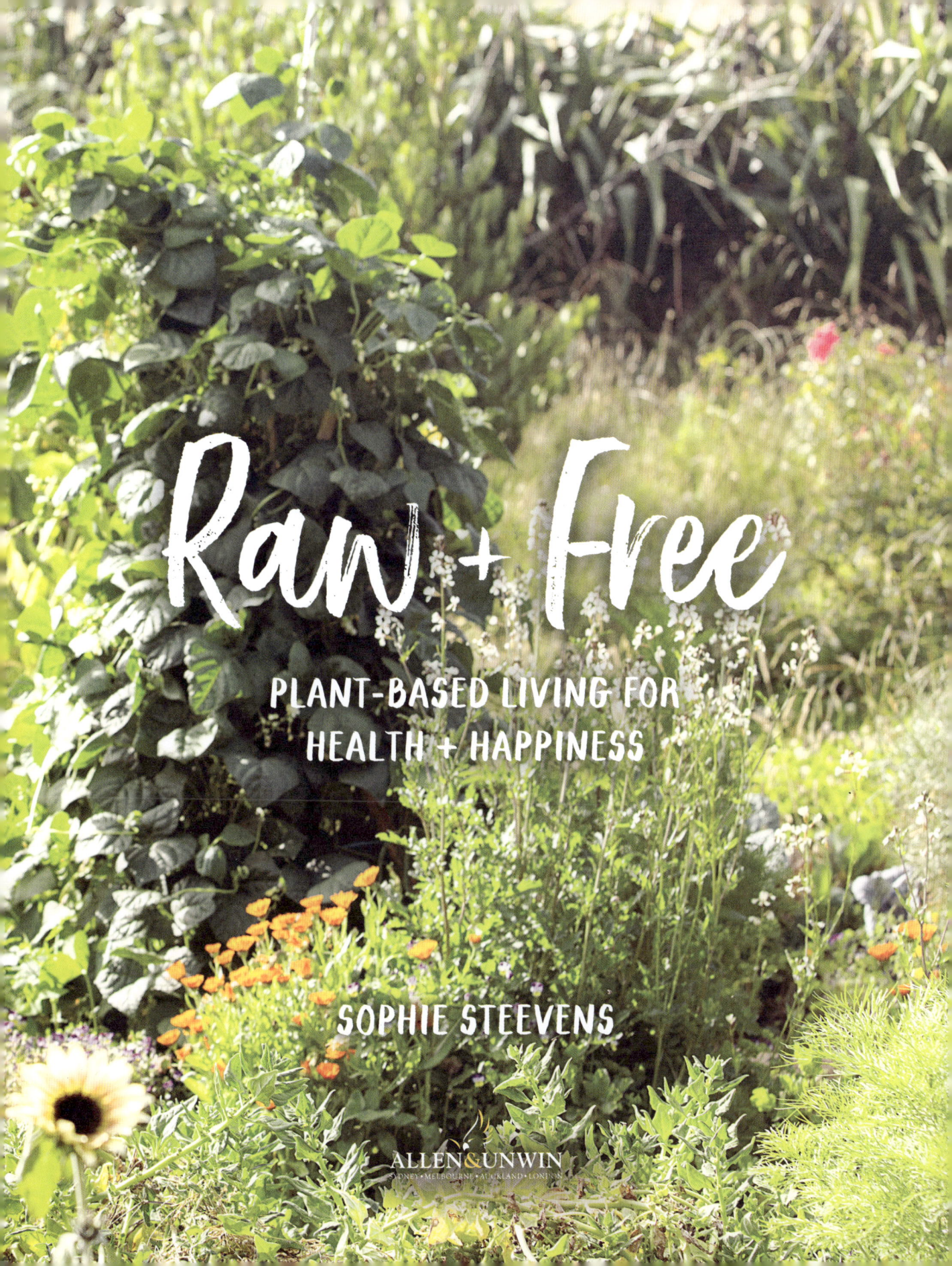

PLANT-BASED LIVING FOR
HEALTH + HAPPINESS

SOPHIE STEEVENS

ALLEN&UNWIN

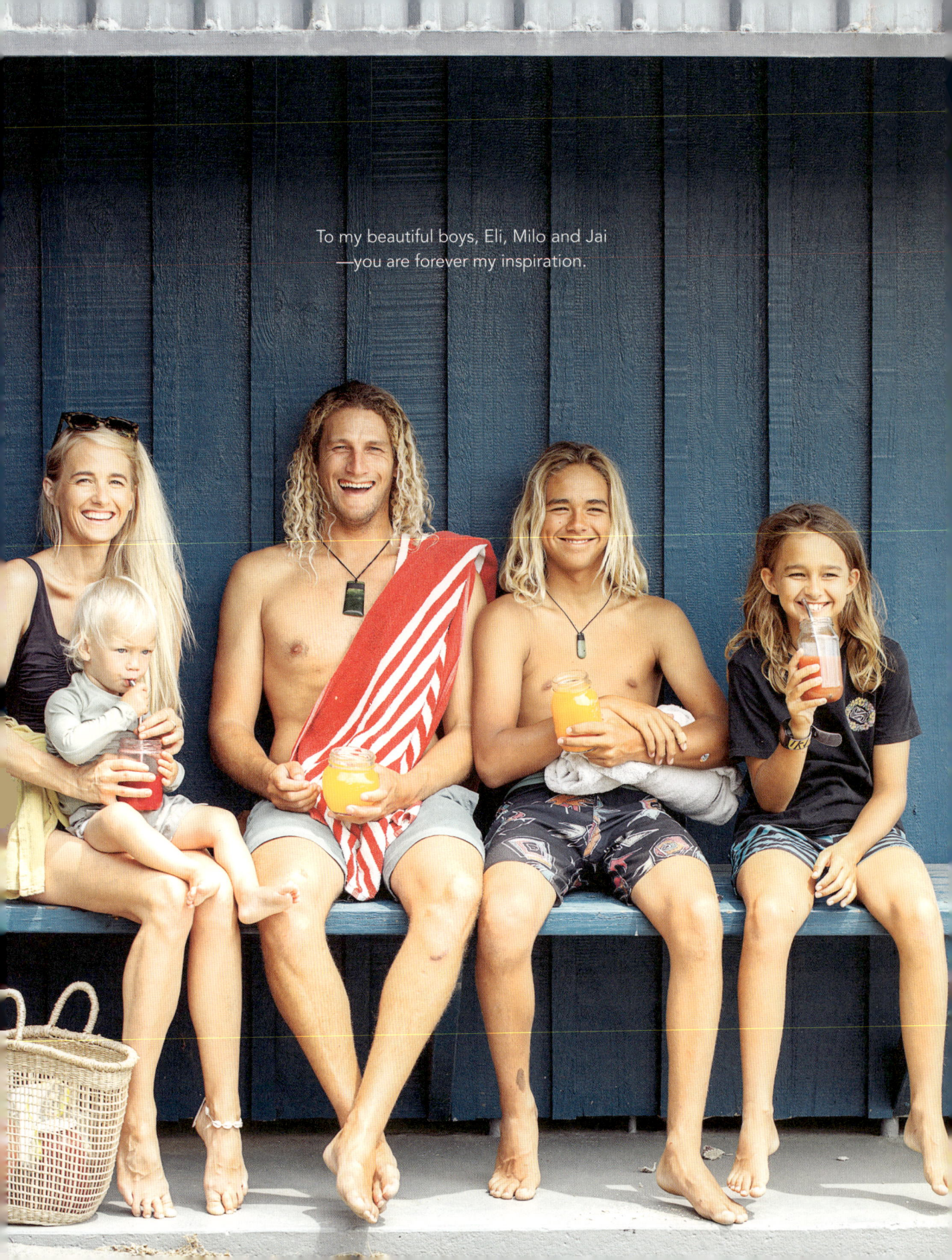

To my beautiful boys, Eli, Milo and Jai
—you are forever my inspiration.

Contents

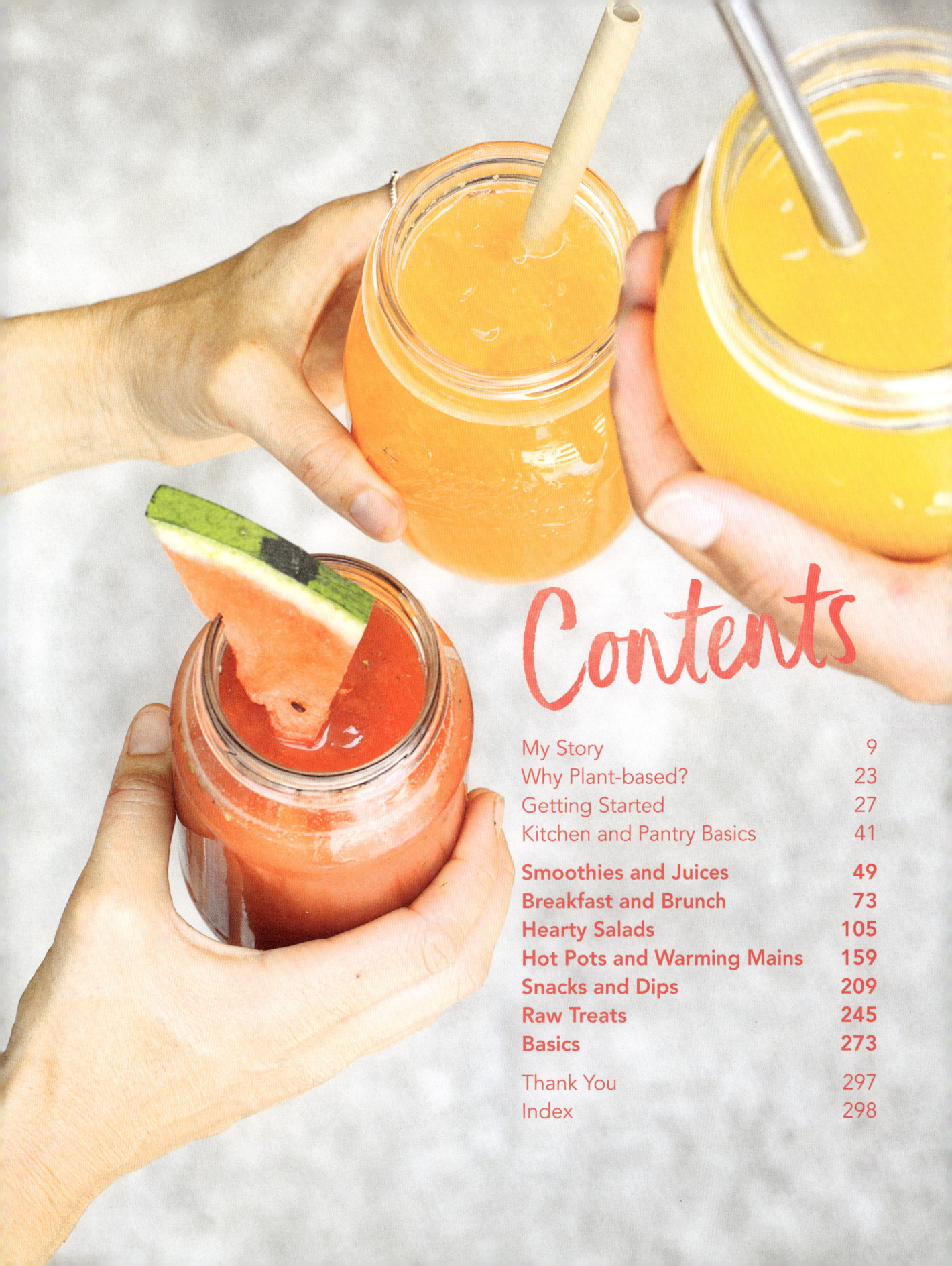

My Story 9
Why Plant-based? 23
Getting Started 27
Kitchen and Pantry Basics 41

Smoothies and Juices 49
Breakfast and Brunch 73
Hearty Salads 105
Hot Pots and Warming Mains 159
Snacks and Dips 209
Raw Treats 245
Basics 273

Thank You 297
Index 298

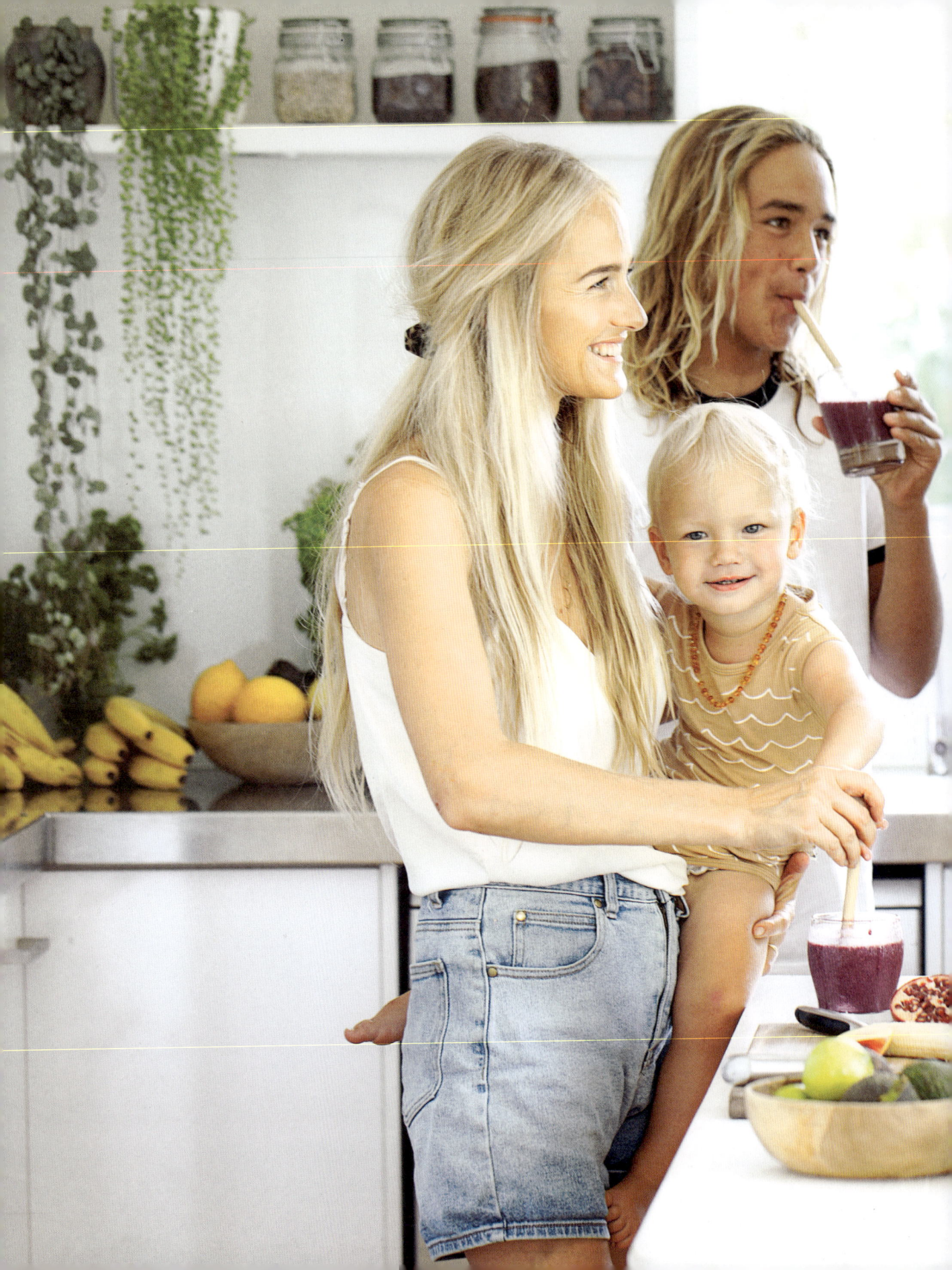

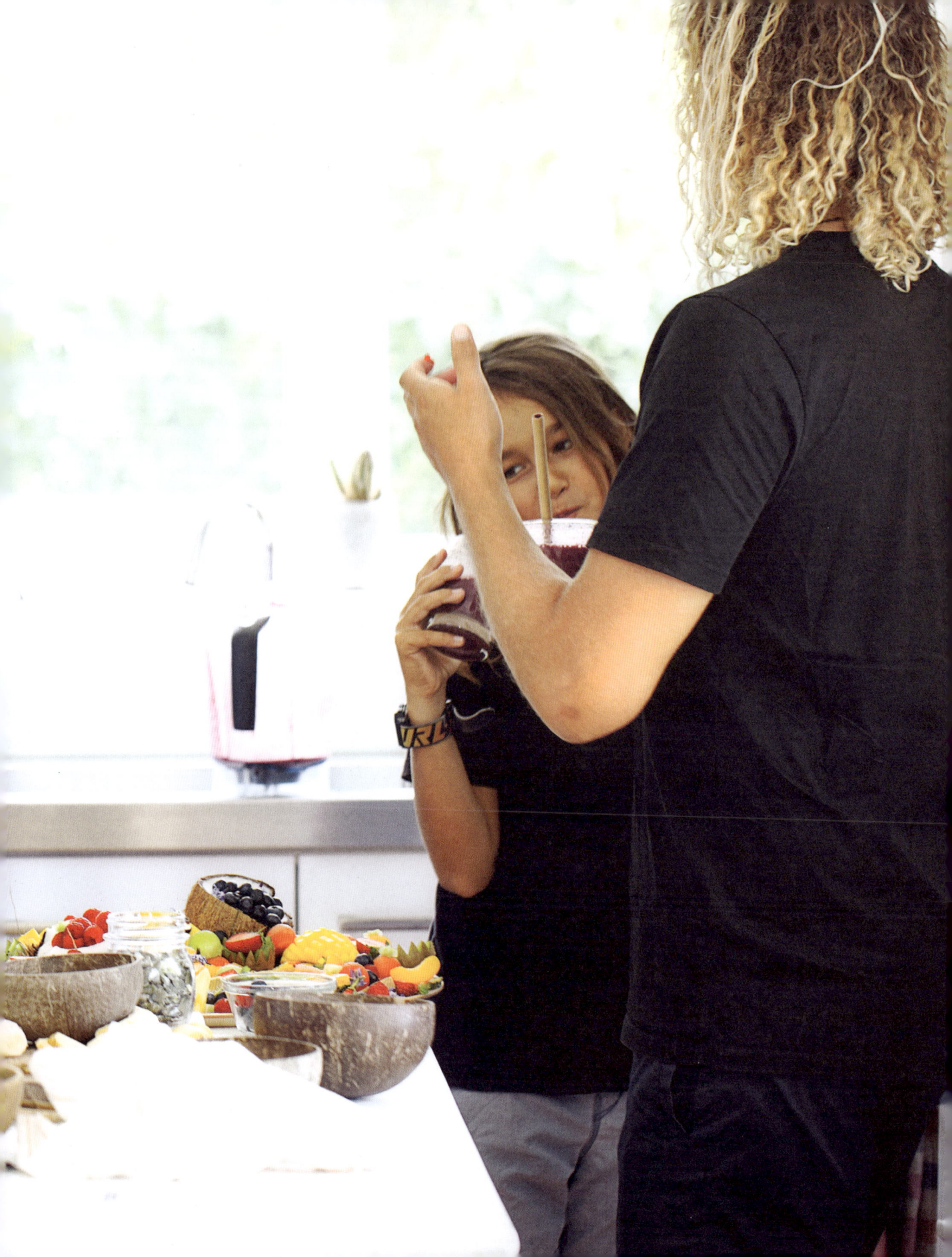

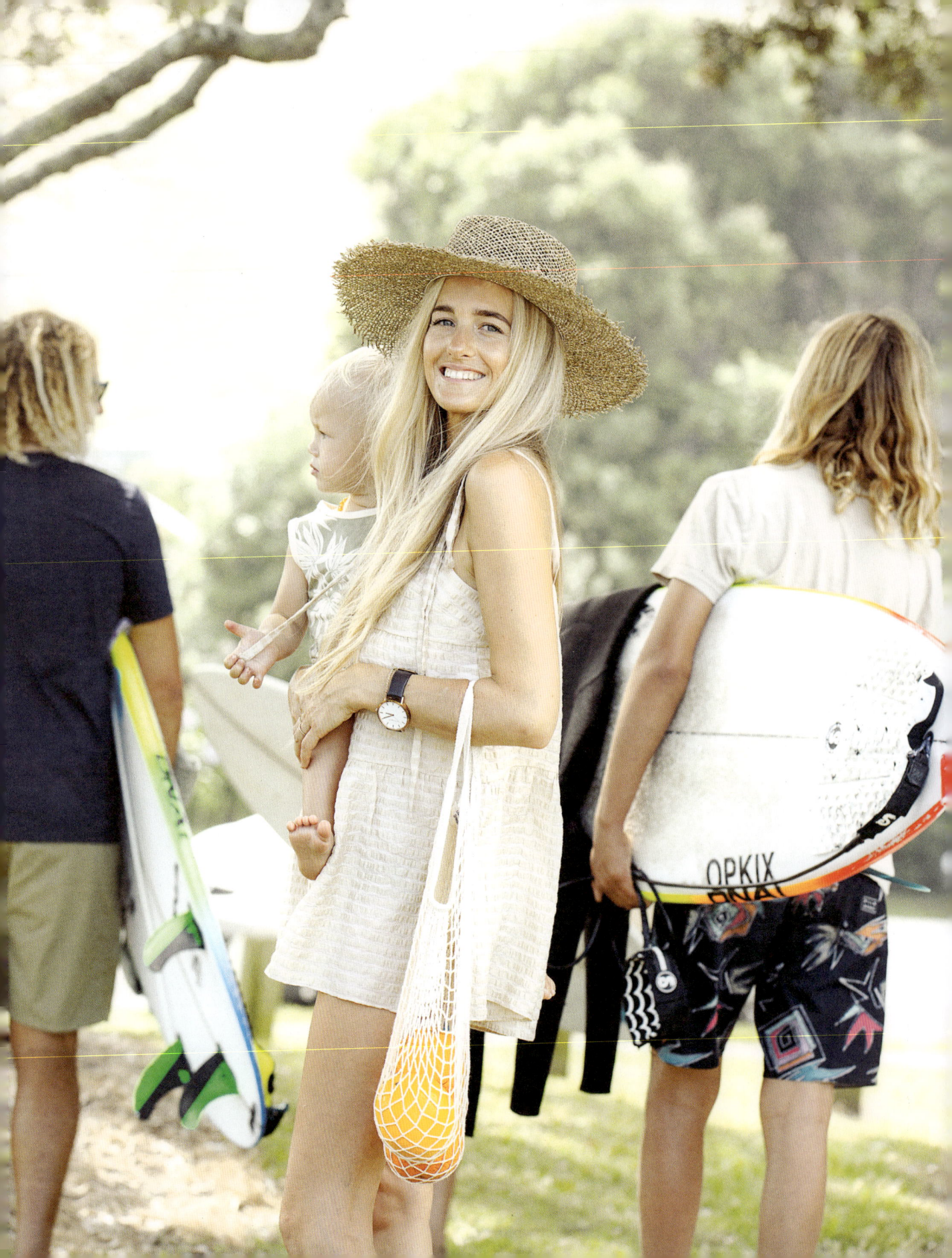

My Story

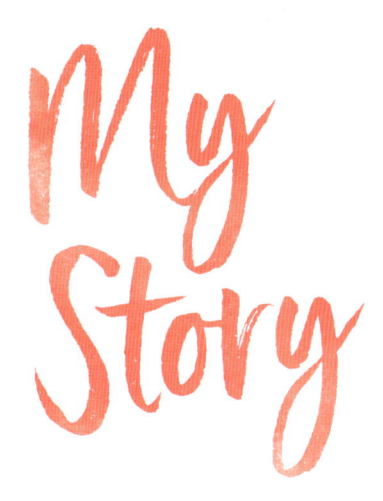

Growing up in New Zealand's largely meat- and dairy-based food culture, I was lucky that both my parents were vegetarians. They also had a great awareness of the health benefits of wholefoods and organic produce, among other things, so I guess the seeds were planted at a young age for the way I eat now. My parents decided to part ways when I was around six years old, which was also around the time that my vegetarianism came to an end. I followed the behaviour of those around me and naïvely began to introduce meat into my diet.

When it came to healthy eating, my teenage years saw a downhill spiral. I became addicted to all things sugar and dairy, and then eventually copious amounts of black tea and coffee. I remember consuming blocks of chocolate as if they were the last food on Earth, completely unaware of the detrimental effects it was having on my body.

I had my first child, Eli, at almost twenty years old, followed by my second, Milo, a few years later, and giving birth to my boys definitely re-ignited some of the health awareness I had as a child—although nothing was going to stop my sugar addiction. I endeavoured to feed my boys the same way my parents had fed me as a young toddler, but I was still neglecting healthy eating myself.

It wasn't until I was about 25 years old that something within me clicked. I vividly remember sitting at the dinner table looking at a freshly cooked chicken, when suddenly the thought of eating a dead bird completely repulsed me. At that moment, I made a conscious choice to never, ever touch meat again—and I haven't since. My partner, Ricardo, was a heavy meat-eater at the time, but not long after he too became vegetarian, along with my boys Eli and Milo.

A year later, our young family decided we would pack our things and move to Bali, Indonesia. Ricardo travels as a professional surfer, and the waves there are some of the best in the world for him to train in, the weather is amazing year-round compared with the chilly New Zealand winters, and we thought it would be a great experience for the boys, aged four and six at the time. For a short time everything was amazing. We were having so much fun adventuring and experiencing life immersed in a completely different culture, but, unbeknown to us at the time, things were about to change.

While Ricardo was overseas competing in South Africa, I suddenly became extremely ill. Initially I self-diagnosed this as a standard Bali bug. But I rapidly took a turn for the worse and was forced to drag myself to the nearest international hospital. After many tests, the doctors diagnosed me with typhoid fever: a life-threatening bacterial infection that's usually spread through contaminated food or water. Without prompt treatment, it can spread throughout the body causing serious complications, and it can be fatal. They also picked up a severe kidney infection, as well as a throat and ear infection. I remember lying on the hospital bed in the emergency ward, barely able to lift my head, with tears rolling down my cheeks and my arms wrapped tightly around my two young boys. In that moment, I felt completely unsure whether or not I was going to be okay. Ricardo was trying to get a flight out of South Africa, and my poor, traumatised mum was stuck on a connection en route to London with my sister. I was alone, incredibly sick, and caring for Eli and Milo in a Balinese hospital. Given the circumstances, my boys were absolutely amazing; they never once left my side. During the daytime we would play games, draw pictures, watch movies, and when I was able to walk around, we would walk back and forth to the hospital shop or café to see what fun we could find— with my intravenous (IV) pole in tow. We would then snuggle into bed together each evening. I managed to convince my mum not to fly over and, after three days, Ricardo finally arrived from South Africa to join in on the hospital sleepover party.

It was on our fourth morning in hospital that something completely unexpected was picked up. My doctor noticed a minute lump on my throat. This immediately sent shivers through my body; after the previous few days, it was hard not to think the worst. After further tests, the doctor felt confident that the lump was only due to an extremely overactive thyroid. She hypothesised that this was due to my severe infection and, eventually, I was discharged from hospital, equipped with the standard thyroid medication. The expectation was that my extreme thyroid levels would soon return to normal as the medication took hold.

Two weeks later, things turned for the worse once again. Ricardo, Milo and I ended up excruciatingly sick with what was later thought to be dengue fever, a mosquito-borne tropical disease. I was admitted back into hospital not only with the dengue fever, but my kidney infection had also returned with a vengeance. It's crazy to think back to how sick I really was, but, understanding what I do now, I can totally see why this was all happening. I stayed for another week, again with my little family by my side. On release, I finally felt like our bad run was over, and that the worst was behind me. I spent the following three months recovering, while enjoying the sun, surf and the beautiful

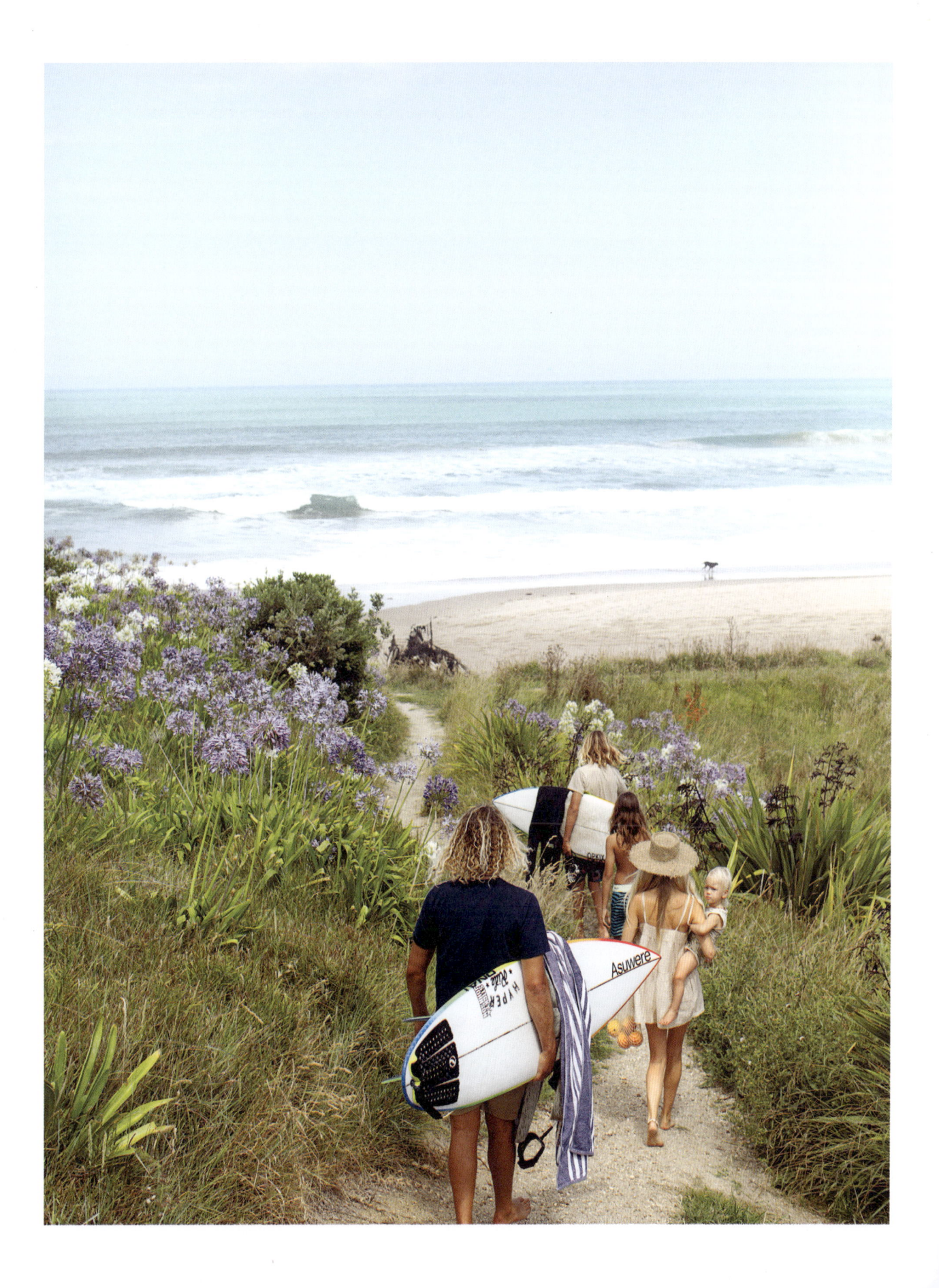

culture Bali has to offer. Deep down, though, I felt toxic. I was experiencing some unusual symptoms and I knew things were not right within my body. It was time we left our Bali bubble and flew home to New Zealand, to find out what was really going on.

In Denpasar airport, while checking into our flight, those underlying symptoms hit me like a ton of bricks. I had a dangerous episode of atrial fibrillation (an extremely rapid heart rate). Ricardo had just left on a flight to Europe to compete, so again it was just my boys and me. It was a complete out-of-body experience; the world was spinning around me and I felt as though I was losing control. I knew I needed to stay calm as I didn't want to let my boys know that something was wrong with me, yet again. They had no idea it was happening and, looking back, I don't know how I did it. I remember feeling insanely thirsty, to the point that there was not one bit of moisture left in my mouth. I managed to purchase five bottles of water before sinking to the ground, depleted. It was at that very moment that a random stranger approached me, completely out of the blue, and engaged in a deep conversation. I flowed with the conversation, trying to take part as it was beginning to take my mind off what was going on. I began to breathe again. I felt my pulse slowing down, and eventually I came back to reality. It was by far the scariest moment of my life. I wish I knew who that person was so I could thank him, even though he had no idea what was going on, or how he had saved me. Luckily, our flight was delayed for several hours, and by the time we had to board I felt strong enough to fly.

Shaken and exhausted, we finally landed at Auckland airport. By this point, I was more than desperate for answers. We left the airport and drove directly to see one of the top endocrinologists in the country. After explaining everything to him in detail, followed by further tests and an ultrasound, he was quick to diagnose me with Graves' disease. All I remember thinking was, *What on earth is that?*

I soon learned that Graves' is an autoimmune disease, where the immune system creates antibodies to attack the thyroid gland, causing it to produce an excessive amount of thyroid hormone and become overactive. This puts the body into overdrive, resulting in a number of symptoms, including a rapid heartbeat, excessive sweating, hand tremors, nervousness, anxiety, weight loss and sleep problems. The scariest aspect of this disease is the risk of experiencing a life-threatening thyroid storm, when the heart rate, blood pressure and body temperature suddenly soar to dangerously high levels. Although the thyroid gland is only a small butterfly-shaped organ located in the front of your neck, it has an enormous role to play in your body and has a big impact on your overall health. In my case, I would later discover that this disease was hereditary, and had passed down to me from my grandmother.

Once again, I was given the standard course of thyroid treatment, as well as cardiac medication to control my rapid heart rate. The standard treatment protocol for Graves' disease means taking thyroid medication to bring down the elevated hormone levels for about one year. In most cases Graves' disease cannot be cured, and eventually radioactive therapy treatment (or surgery) is necessary to kill the overactive thyroid. This effectively causes hypothyroidism (an underactive thyroid, which then causes another set of problems), so you would then need to take another drug for the rest of your life to recreate the function of the destroyed thyroid.

I was 26 years old, and feeling more unhealthy than ever before. Deep down, I knew some big things needed to change if I was going to manage this disease. Looking back, this was the moment when my health journey truly began.

Over the next year, I researched avidly, reading many books and online articles. I cleaned up my diet, cut out most processed foods, worked with both a naturopath and a homeopath (my dad's partner is an amazing naturopath), and fell in love with my blender. I still suffered many symptoms of Graves' including anxiety, irritability, hand tremors, nervousness, weight loss (and gain), extreme fatigue, hair loss, constant achey bones, heart palpitations and a rapid heartbeat—which meant no exercise. I couldn't even walk up a tiny hill without my heart flipping out. On one occasion I ended up back in hospital with a severe allergic reaction to one of the only thyroid medications available in New Zealand. I don't think anyone with Graves' disease can truly explain the feelings you experience, though. It was as if I was an entirely different person. There was such a big hormonal imbalance going on in my body. No one understood how I was feeling, and I couldn't explain it to anyone either. I would never know when a sudden anxiety-type attack would hit me. I could be sitting around with family, reading a book or playing with my children when all of a sudden a rush of something would flood through my body. It was like I could feel the release of excessive hormones, or as if I had just swallowed a psychotropic drug. My head and vision would go fuzzy and my heart rate would accelerate.

Most of the time, no one around me would even know it was happening. There was nothing I could do but breathe through it until it eventually passed. I felt like I had lost myself and it made it hard for me to socialise. I was always living in fear, and I lost my confidence because of that.

But, after fourteen months on the medication, multiple blood tests and back-and-forth visits to my specialist, I was finally in remission. It was the spark of hope I had been so desperate for. That year, my family and I embarked on a six-month trip through Europe and Hawaii to support Ricardo, who was competing in various surf competitions. Throughout this time I tried to be healthy, but at this stage I still didn't entirely know what that meant. When we returned home, on my 29th birthday, I was shocked to discover that my thyroid levels had once again skyrocketed to dangerous heights. This completely threw me; after a year of being in remission, I was once again back in the hot seat.

Upset and disheartened, I returned to my specialist in Auckland to then be given the hard news. I was told that I had no option left but to destroy my thyroid through radioactive iodine treatment (or surgery), and then take thyroxine medication for the rest of my life. He announced that I would never go into remission again, that in my case it was simply not possible to do so. And he was right . . . if I had continued down the same path I was on. I left his office that day with the paperwork for radioactive iodine treatment but, despite what he had said, I was far from ready to give up. I clearly remember thinking that if my body was capable of causing this disease in the state that it was in, then what was next? Something in me knew I needed to dig deeper. The underlying causes of the

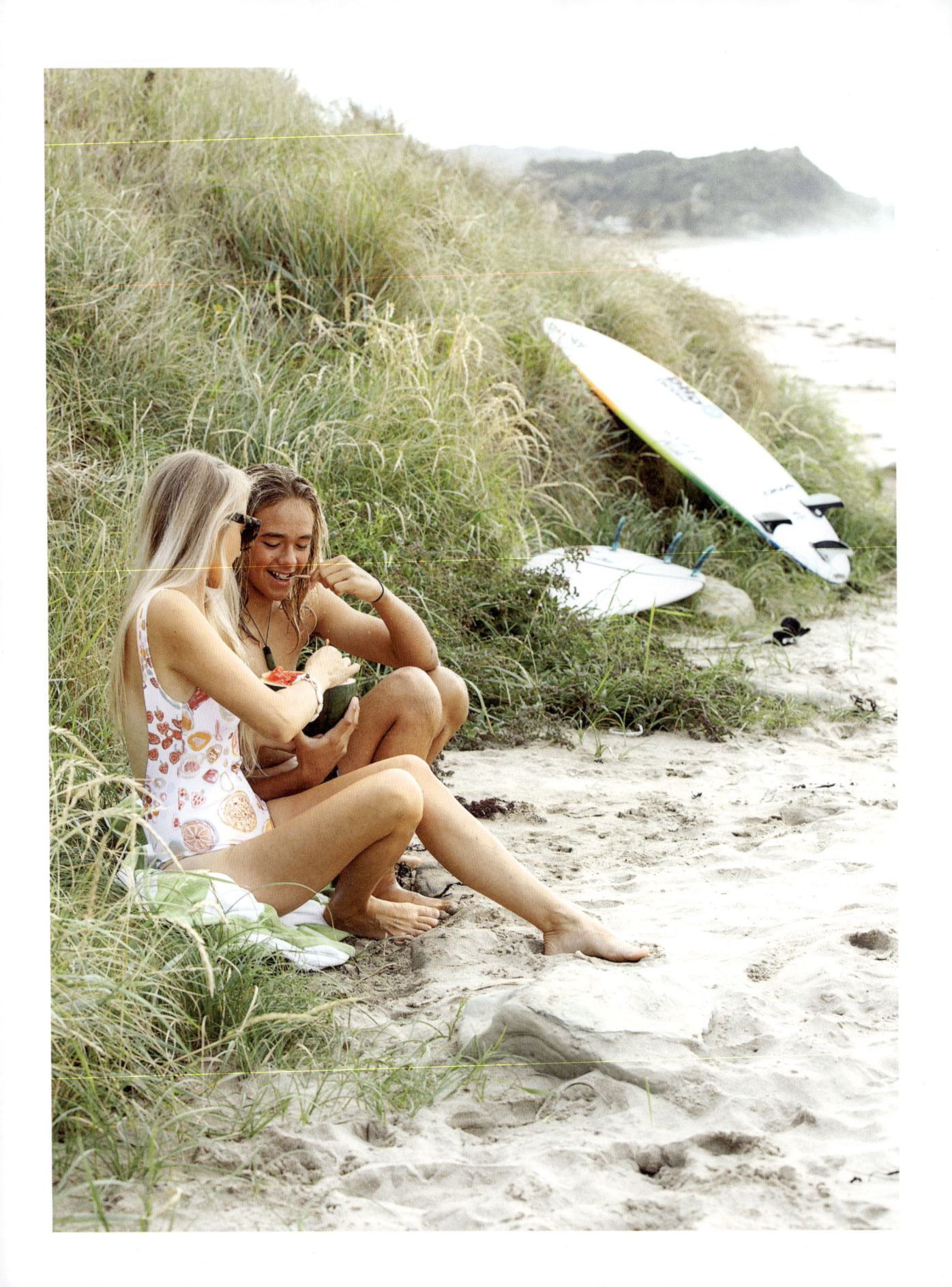

problem were far from being addressed and I felt more determined than ever to heal my body. In fact, I was completely possessed with determination.

That night I went straight home and began my search for answers. For days on end I read and researched, and a recurring theme among all the information I found was this: what we eat, drink, breathe, put on our skin, think and feel affects our health. These are the things that will make us either sick and weak, or experience exceptional and robust health. I also discovered that, simply put, a raw, plant-based diet has the powerful potential to heal. This resonated with me more than anything else and gave me a sense of hope to carry on. I also learnt that just because something may be hereditary, that does not mean it can't be reversed and corrected for the generations to come.

I was on a roll, fuelled with confidence, when I stumbled across a blog post by an incredible woman—Rosanne Calabrese. Rosanne had reversed both her Graves' disease and Hashimoto's (another autoimmune disease) by detoxing her body at a natural clinic in Florida, founded by the incredible Dr Robert Morse.

Morse is regarded as one of the greatest healers of our time, and his incredible work and herbal protocols have helped thousands of people for more than 40 years. His healing philosophy is simple: complete cellular regeneration by alkalising, detoxifying and cleansing the body through eating the foods that are biologically suited to our species—raw, organic fruit and vegetables—and taking powerful herbal formulas that will effectively rebuild and regenerate the entire body, resulting in the reversal of disease.

Morse's theories made sense to me in so many ways, and I knew this was my opportunity to regain control of my health.

The next day, I went completely plant-based. I was already vegetarian, so for me this just meant cutting out dairy and eggs. I also stopped consuming all processed foods, coffee, alcohol and gluten. I wanted to cut out as many toxins from my life as possible, so I also stopped colouring my hair and replaced all of my cosmetics, skin care, nail polish and household cleaners with natural, plant-based alternatives.

I read Dr Robert Morse's book, *The Detox Miracle Sourcebook*, and couldn't wait to book a consultation at his clinic—only to discover it was booked out for months in advance. I was eager to get started, so I began working with a detox specialist who had been trained by Robert Morse and he produced a fourteen-week herbal protocol for me.

Not long after that, I booked my first appointment with Rosanne Calabrese. Rosanne has a clinic in Florida, and works as an acupuncturist and a detoxification specialist, trained and mentored by Dr Robert Morse. Working with Rosanne was the best thing I could have ever done. She is such a wonderful, caring woman full of wisdom, and she gave me so much confidence throughout the entire process of detoxification.

Around this same time, I began a blog on Instagram (@rawandfree) to help encourage myself and anyone else who wanted to follow along. I was learning so much about a wholesome, plant-based lifestyle and I wanted to share my journey, and hopefully help and inspire others along the way. In turn, this helped keep me motivated to discover new food and create new recipes.

In August 2016, I officially embarked on my

detox journey. I was ready to cleanse my body of its built-up toxins and finally correct the underlying causes of my health challenges, including Graves' disease. I was on a mission and it felt amazing.

I also felt extremely prepared; I had read so much about the detox. Detoxification is the process of removing an accumulation of built-up toxins from the body, while cleansing the lymphatic system, eliminating inflammation and regenerating new cells. In turn, this has the potential to correct the many underlying causes of disease, which are often caused by the long-term effects of an extremely acidic diet (see page 24), environmental toxins and chemicals. When the body is overburdened with this acid-forming waste, cells, tissues and organs can become weak and/or damaged, and can eventually begin to break down. I now share the opinion, along with many of the teachers I have learnt from, that this is what we call disease.

Over the next twelve weeks, I ate only raw, organic fruit and vegetables and took herbal formulas. This meant no oil, nuts, seeds, salt, pepper, dressings—nothing but pure fruit and vegetables, as well as baked or steamed kūmara for extra calories. I also practised specific food combining—eating certain foods together for optimum digestion and nutrient absorption. Most days I would have fresh fruit smoothies for breakfast and a large mono meal (see page 74) of fruit for lunch. Dinner would usually consist of an extra-large bowl of salad, filled with a variety of raw vegetables, dark leafy greens, avocado, kūmara and a squeeze of lemon or lime (this is still my favourite meal—one I have all the time). Snacks were fruit, smoothies and fresh fruit and vegetable juices. There were no limits on how much I could eat. I would also take about eight different herbal formulas, three times per day before meals, and would drink powerful herbal teas twice a day.

The first week was the toughest, just taking that first step into the unknown, but it didn't take long to adapt, and then I felt like I was flying through it. This was the moment I was discovering a true understanding of how to feed and nourish my body, and what it meant to eat real food, straight from our earth. I began to crave fruit and veges, and nothing else. I could finally taste their true flavours, and had found a deep respect for the food I was eating, and where it came from. I was 100 per cent committed to this detox, and I made it work around being a busy mum, as well as my other commitments.

After the first two weeks I stopped feeling as hungry, as my body was busy cleansing, and it was at about week five that my detox symptoms crept in. This was a little scary. I had body aches, headaches, skin breakouts, fatigue, weakness, swollen tonsils, swollen glands, weight loss and for a few days I suffered from a sharp pain in my spleen. Because of what I had read and the support from Rosanne, I had enough confidence to welcome these symptoms—which would continue on and off for the next month or so—as signs that the true detoxification and healing process was in full force. I continued to see my GP throughout the entire process and had regular blood tests, including a full blood count and thyroid functions. Although my thyroid levels were initially beginning to climb again, I tried not to let this dishearten me. I continued to have Skype consultations with Rosanne, who gave me incredible support, knowledge and encouragement.

By the end of the fourteen weeks, I was truly feeling better than ever. My digestion

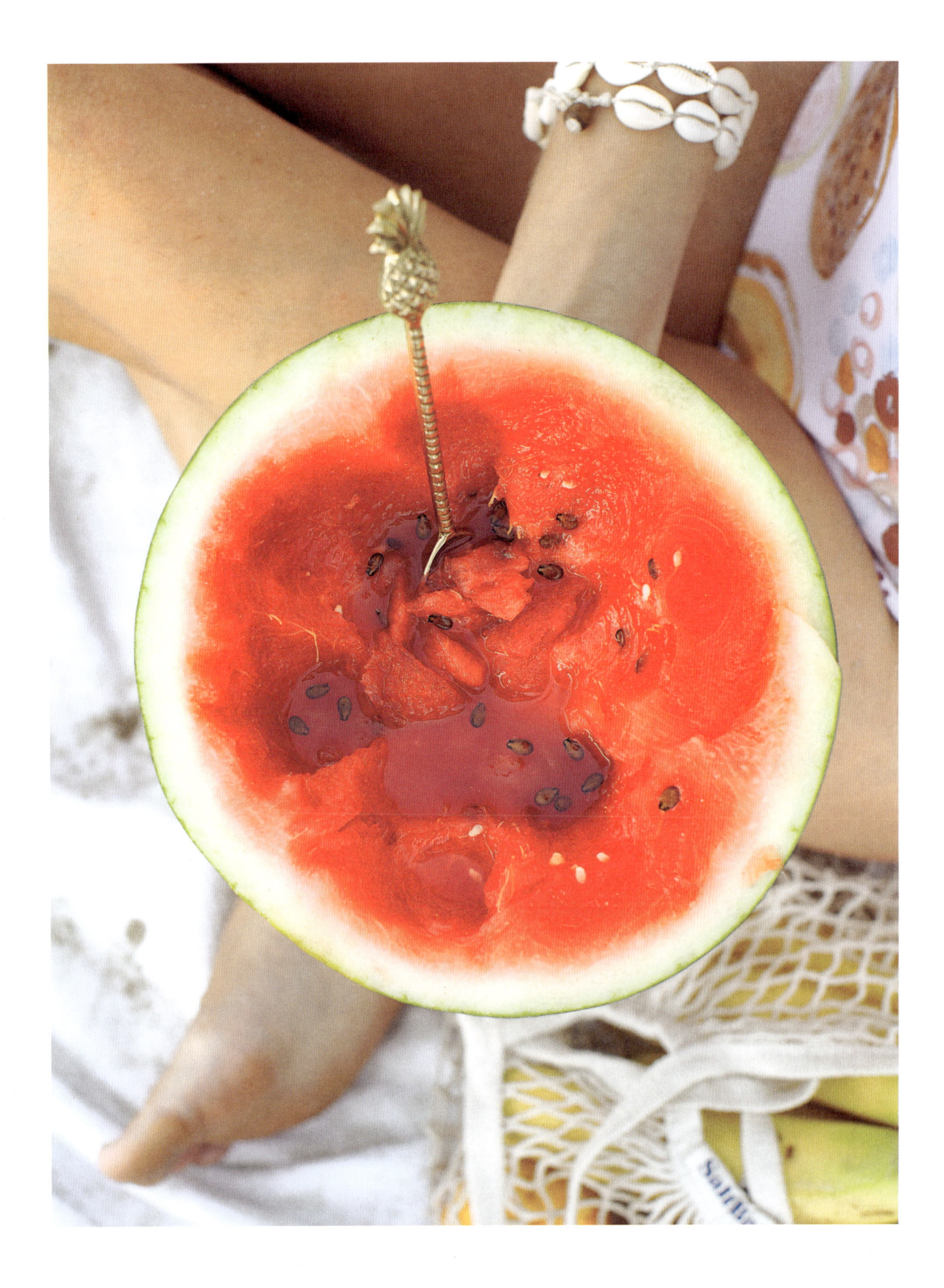

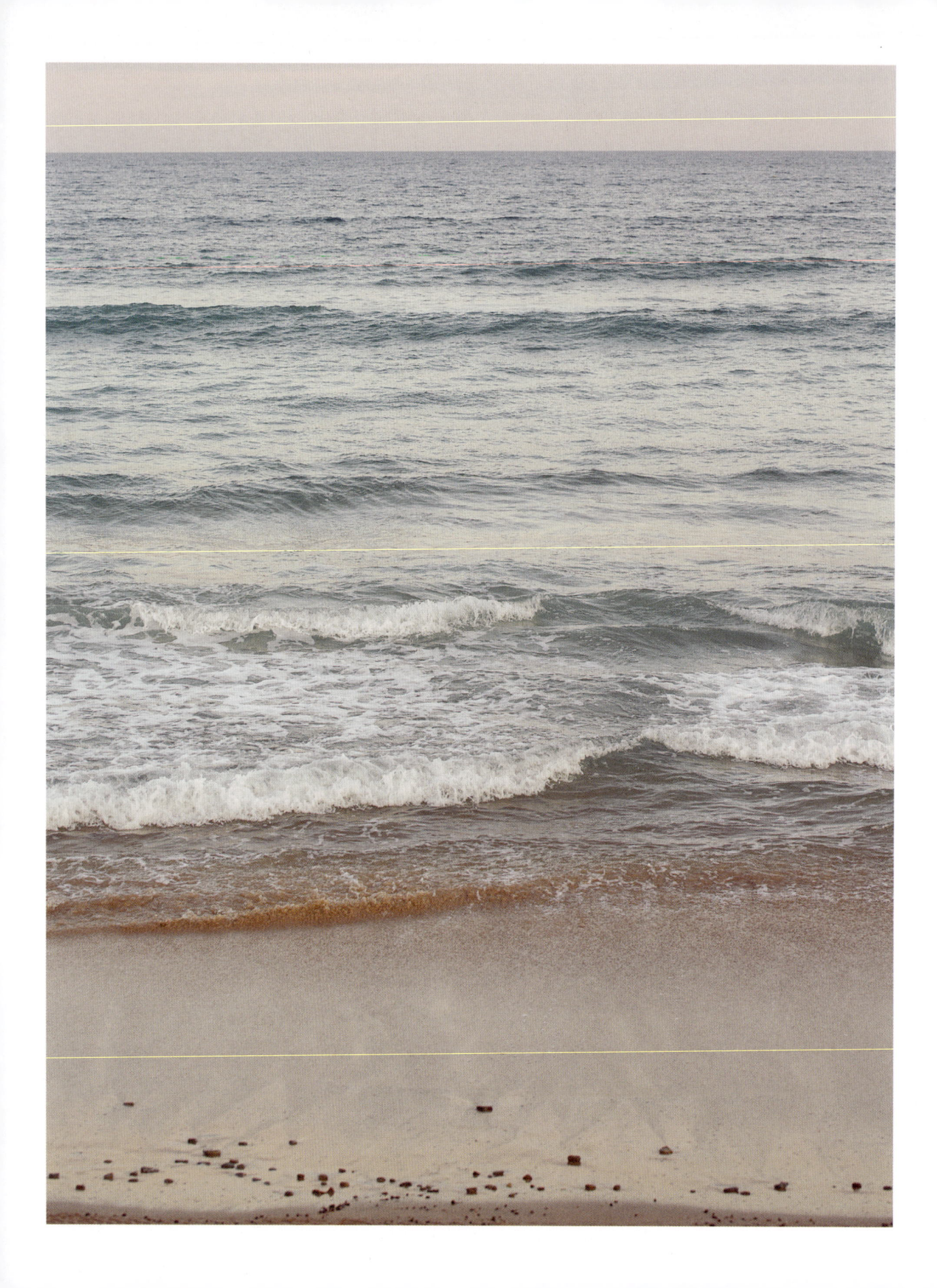

was incredible, my skin was soft and clear, and many things in my body had corrected. At that point, my thyroid levels were starting to improve so I decided to extend the detox for another eight weeks. I knew I had been sick for many years and I felt I needed to keep going for longer. I detoxed for twenty weeks altogether, and as the final week came to an end I was due to check my thyroid levels. It had been eight weeks since my last blood test and 24 weeks without any medication. As I sat in the waiting room with Eli and Milo, who had been by my side every single step of the way, we nervously awaited my results. I felt my heart rate increase, only this time I felt confident it was due to my nerves. I dismissed all doubt and had this strong feeling that everything would be okay. I felt better than ever and I truly believed in this healing process, and the power of pure plants. But who was I to even think this way after my endocrinologist, a highly experienced professor, had told me it was impossible to ever go into remission again?

Well . . . my bloods came back completely normal. My thyroid function was normal and stable, and for the first time ever, my thyroid antibodies were now completely normal.

This was supposed to be impossible! I sat there fighting back tears when all of a sudden, everything hit me. I realised in that moment just how much I had been through to get to this point. I don't think I could ever describe the feeling I had that day, but I was empowered.

I was so lucky to have an extremely supportive family throughout the entire process, especially my partner Ricardo, my mum and my two beautiful boys. I will be forever grateful for their help through it all. Eli and Milo were absolute superstars. They went through the entire three years with me—every setback and every milestone. I was also grateful to the professor I worked with; he definitely had his place in my healing journey. He gave me the diagnosis, followed by the medication I needed to ensure I was safe as I found my feet and truly learnt about the nature of disease, and how to reverse it. I was also grateful for the team in Bali who took such amazing care of me at such a vulnerable time. I was in an outstanding hospital and surrounded by an incredible medical team who impressively picked up my initial diagnosis—something that could easily have been missed.

I've now had a completely normal thyroid function and antibodies for more than three and a half years. I continue to eat raw fruits and vegetables abundantly, as well as nuts, seeds and gluten-free wholegrains. People often ask me if I get bored with the way I eat, but honestly, I absolutely love it. No other food on this planet makes me feel better than this, especially pure raw fruit. I truly believe this is the food that was put on this Earth for humans to eat and I am so grateful I now know how to nourish my body this way, and can teach my children to do the same—including my third beautiful baby, Jai, born in 2018. Despite some concerns of a relapse throughout his pregnancy, I still retained a completely normal thyroid function, as well as antibodies.

It's been amazing to share my journey with my online Raw and Free family. What a wonderful community of the most beautiful and positive people I have been so *blessed* to be involved with, and who have encouraged me more than they will ever know. I love having the opportunity to communicate the importance of eating plants abundantly, as

> 'I deeply, profoundly and personally believe in the endless power and ability of food to heal the human body. More so, the living, energizing, hydrating ability of the most colorful, vibrant food on the planet, fruit! It not only feeds our cells, but nourishes our soul.' —ROSANNE CALABRESE

well as living a wholesome lifestyle with my family.

The opportunity to write this book for you has also been a true blessing. I could definitely fill it with mainly raw fruits and veges (maybe I will for my next book), which continue to make up the basis of my diet, but I chose to write this book for the majority of people as a gentle introduction to a wholesome, plant-based lifestyle, based on many of the (raw and cooked) recipes I create for my family and my Raw and Free blog, as well as my personal favourites.

I also want to emphasise that I'm not a qualified nutritionist nor a professional chef, but a dedicated mother who learnt some big life lessons and was thankfully forced to teach myself the importance of true nourishment and, in turn, how to begin mastering the art of plant-based food.

All of my recipes are from the past four or so years of practising and experimenting in the kitchen, using ingredients as close to Nature as possible. This includes naturally gluten-free and refined-sugar-free ingredients.

In the next chapter, you will find an introduction to a plant-based diet, as well as the tips that helped me to adapt to this lifestyle, including information on essential nutrients and the effects of different foods on the body. Further on I have also included my favourite kitchen equipment and explained the ingredients I commonly use. Then, you'll discover my delicious recipes. I have put so much love into creating these recipes for you, and I hope you enjoy them as much as my family and I do. I also hope that by reading this book, you'll feel inspired to create healthier lifestyle choices. And hopefully you'll fall in love with plants like I did, and feel empowered—and excited—to add more of them into your diet.

I now look at my autoimmune disease as a blessing. It was a massive wake-up call and has taught me how to truly nourish and look after my body, and I will be forever grateful for that. We get one life and one precious vehicle to drive us through it, and one of the biggest lessons I have learnt through this experience is to never take my health for granted again.

I wish you all the love, happiness and good health in the world.

Sophie x

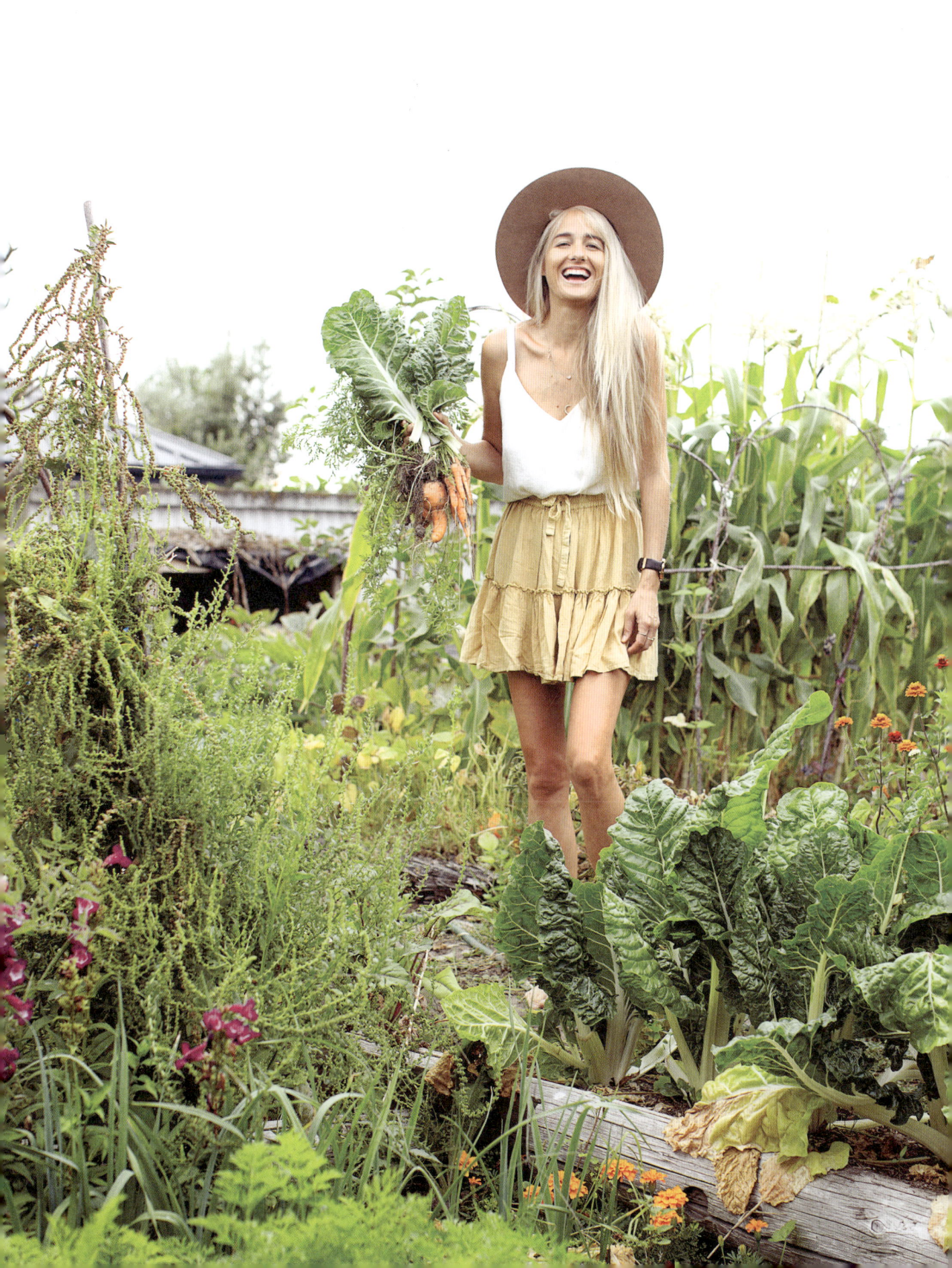

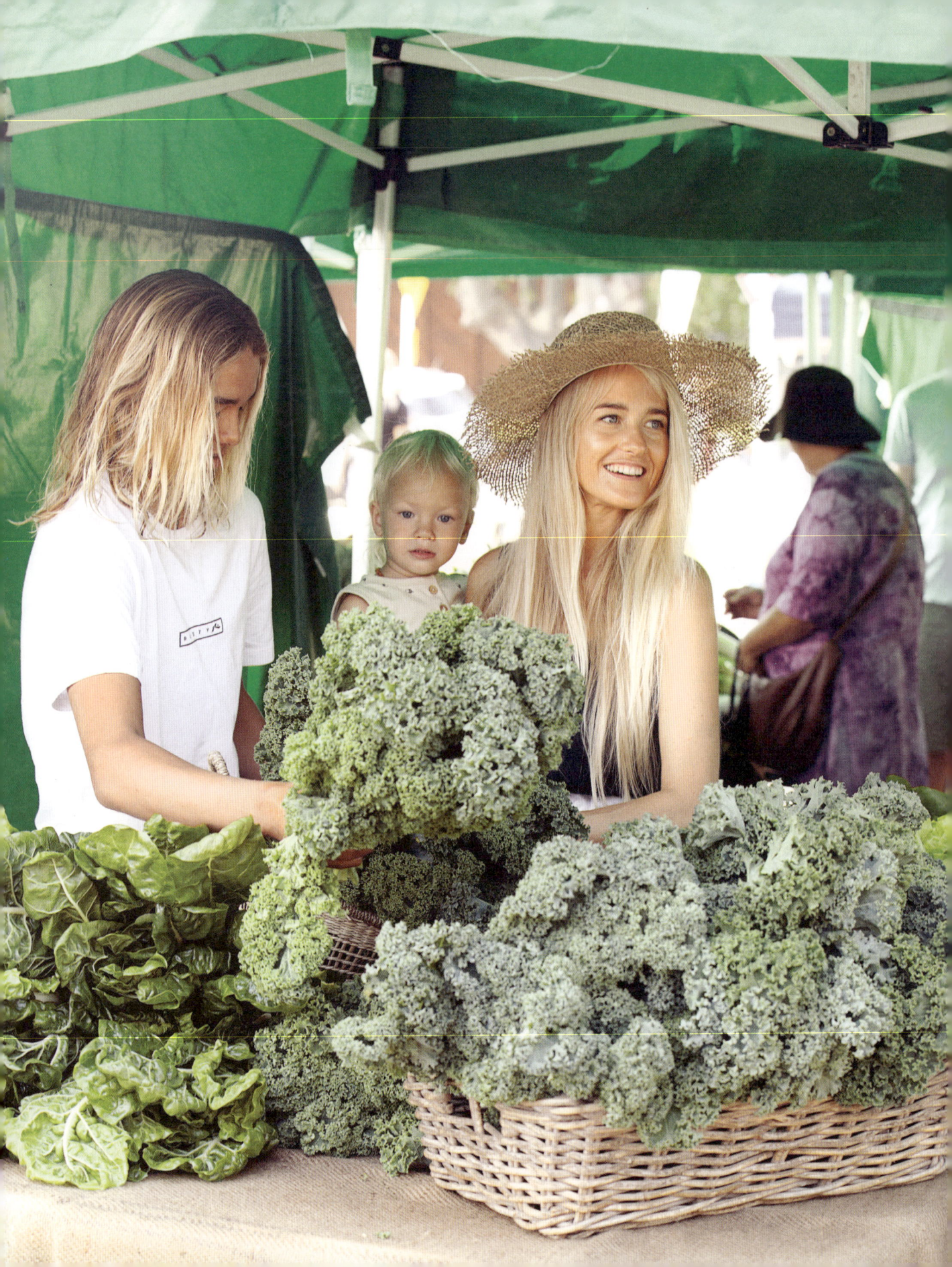

Why Plant-based?

A plant-based diet has the potential to improve our long-term health and well-being, to prevent animal cruelty and to lessen our human footprint on the environment. These are the three main reasons I believe living a plant-based lifestyle is not only a highly beneficial and compassionate choice, but also one that can positively affect the sustainability of our world. Initially health was the main motivation for me and, wow, what a phenomenally positive impact it's had on my life. But as I looked deeper into the effects that animal agriculture is having on our environment—arguably being one of the leading causes of global warming, deforestation, water depletion and pollution—as well as the inhumane treatment of millions of innocent animals, who are unnecessarily consigned to a life of slavery and death, it gave me a much greater purpose in continuing to live this lifestyle.

HEALTH BENEFITS

When I first transitioned into eating only plants (mostly raw), I noticed a remarkable difference within my body. Ideally, a plant-based diet is about eating a variety of foods naturally derived from plants, such as fruits, vegetables, nuts, seeds, wholegrains and legumes. Together, these highly nutritious foods provide the body with everything from simple sugars and carbohydrates to essential amino acids and healthy fats, as well as an abundance of vitamins, minerals, antioxidants, enzymes and fibre.

The extraordinary health benefits associated with eating unprocessed wholefoods continue to astound me, along with an increasing number of people from diverse cultures and backgrounds. Personally, since I transitioned into a mostly raw plant-based diet, the benefits have been astronomical. I went from regularly feeling exhausted and run-down, with skin breakouts and a weak immune system, to an increase in energy, stronger immunity, clearer skin, significantly improved digestion, stronger hair and nails, and an overall feeling of better health than I had ever experienced before—not to mention I reversed my autoimmune disease.

Our bodies are made up of trillions of tiny cells that each require energy from the correct fuel to thrive. Feeding these cells acid-forming or toxic foods, such as highly processed, dead food, can be extremely harmful, destructive and taxing, and can result in an acidic environment in the body. When the body is in this state, it can destroy good healthy cells and tissue, cause malnutrition and inflammation and, eventually, result in an environment vulnerable to illness and disease. Alkalising foods, such as fruits and vegetables, have the completely opposite effect. These are the foods that will strengthen, cleanse, repair, nourish and provide optimal health and vitality in the human body. Some of the most highly nutritional foods on this planet include raw fruits, vegetables, herbs, seaweeds, nuts and seeds, which are all packed with powerful nutrients to support a deep level of vitality in the body. I believe these are the foods that are biologically suited to our species, and they are undoubtably the foods that make me feel the most alive, energised, robust, happiest and healthiest. This is why I choose to live off plants.

EATING AS NATURE INTENDED

All other animals on this planet eat intuitively. They eat the way Nature intended them to eat. They teach their children to do the same, and most of them don't suffer the serious health challenges we're faced with today. As a society, I feel we have lost our own intuitiveness and now eat primarily what we're taught to eat. We follow the trends promoted in the media and support the masses of harmful food sold in supermarkets that is often only produced for financial gain, at the expense of our personal health. The availability of this food makes it difficult for people to avoid overindulging in unhealthy food choices. I believe this is contributing to an epidemic of disease, which is increasing at a scary rate. It's time we made a conscious effort to reduce the toxic foods entering our body. We need to begin eating to live, rather than living to eat. Perhaps in a similar way to our great-grandparents, by consuming more of what they would recognise as wholefood—gathered from the earth, and untampered with.

MY PHILOSOPHY

My philosophy is to create a well-balanced and nourished environment within the body, both physically and mentally, so that you can truly thrive from the inside out. This doesn't necessarily involve eating perfectly 100 per cent of the time, but falling in love with raw fruit and vegetables and incorporating them into your diet will help you tremendously in accomplishing true health and vitality within your body. Taking control of your health is an empowering feeling and, trust me, it becomes highly addictive. Whether you're already living a plant-based lifestyle or simply beginning to include more plants in your diet, any positive change you create, whether small or large, is an amazing step in the right direction.

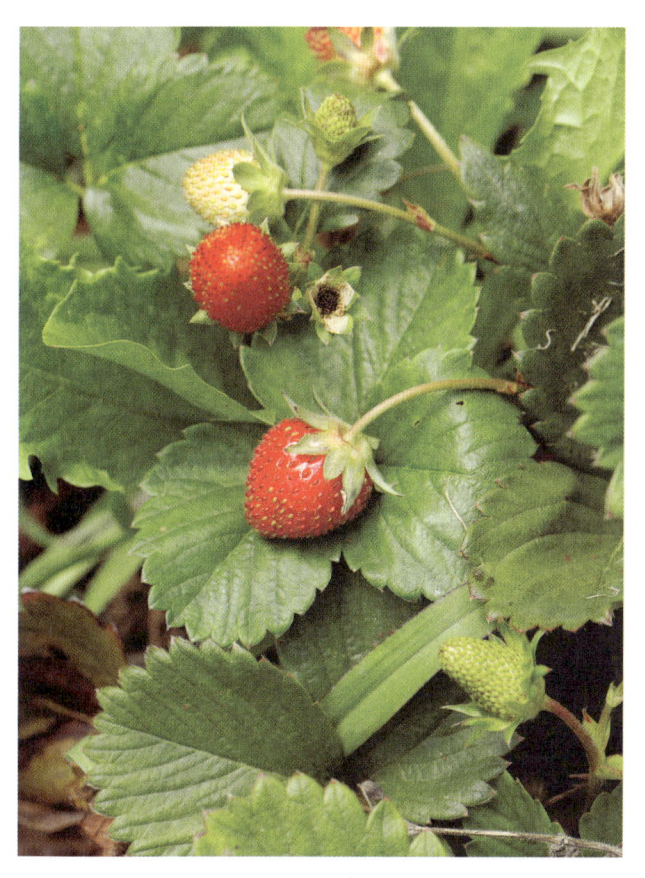

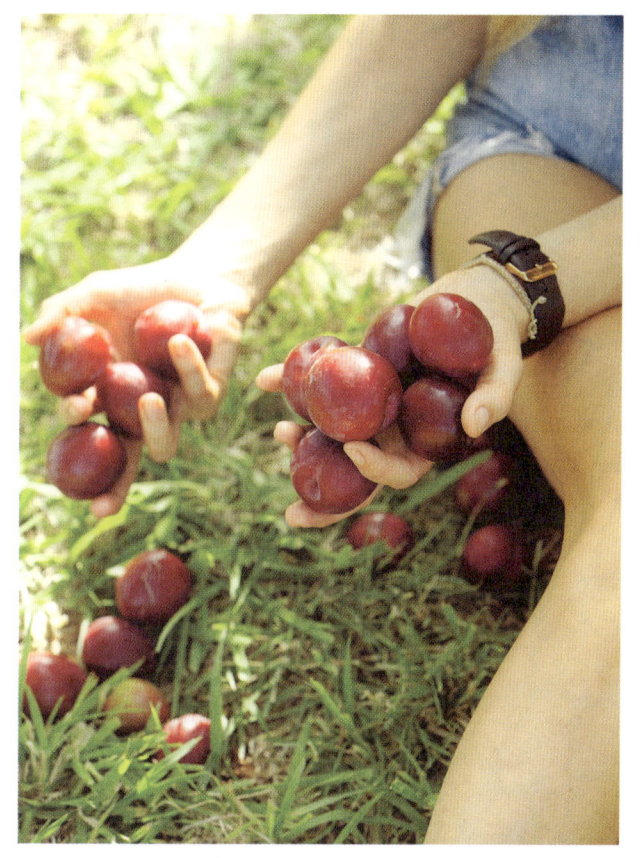

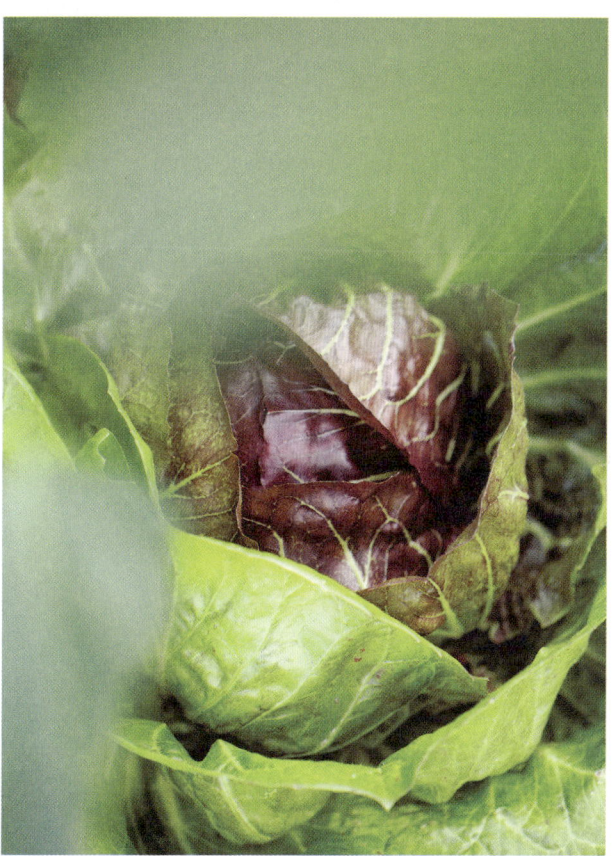

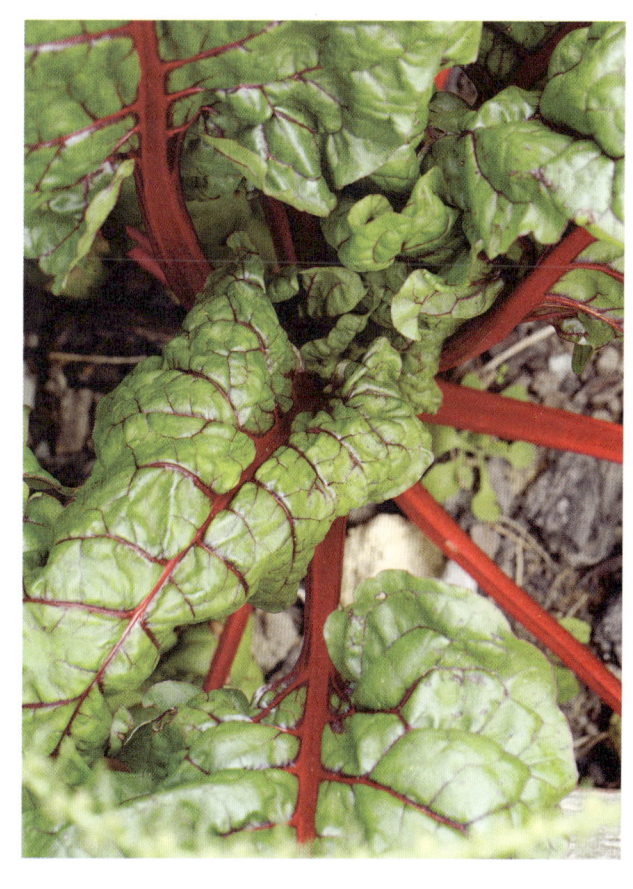

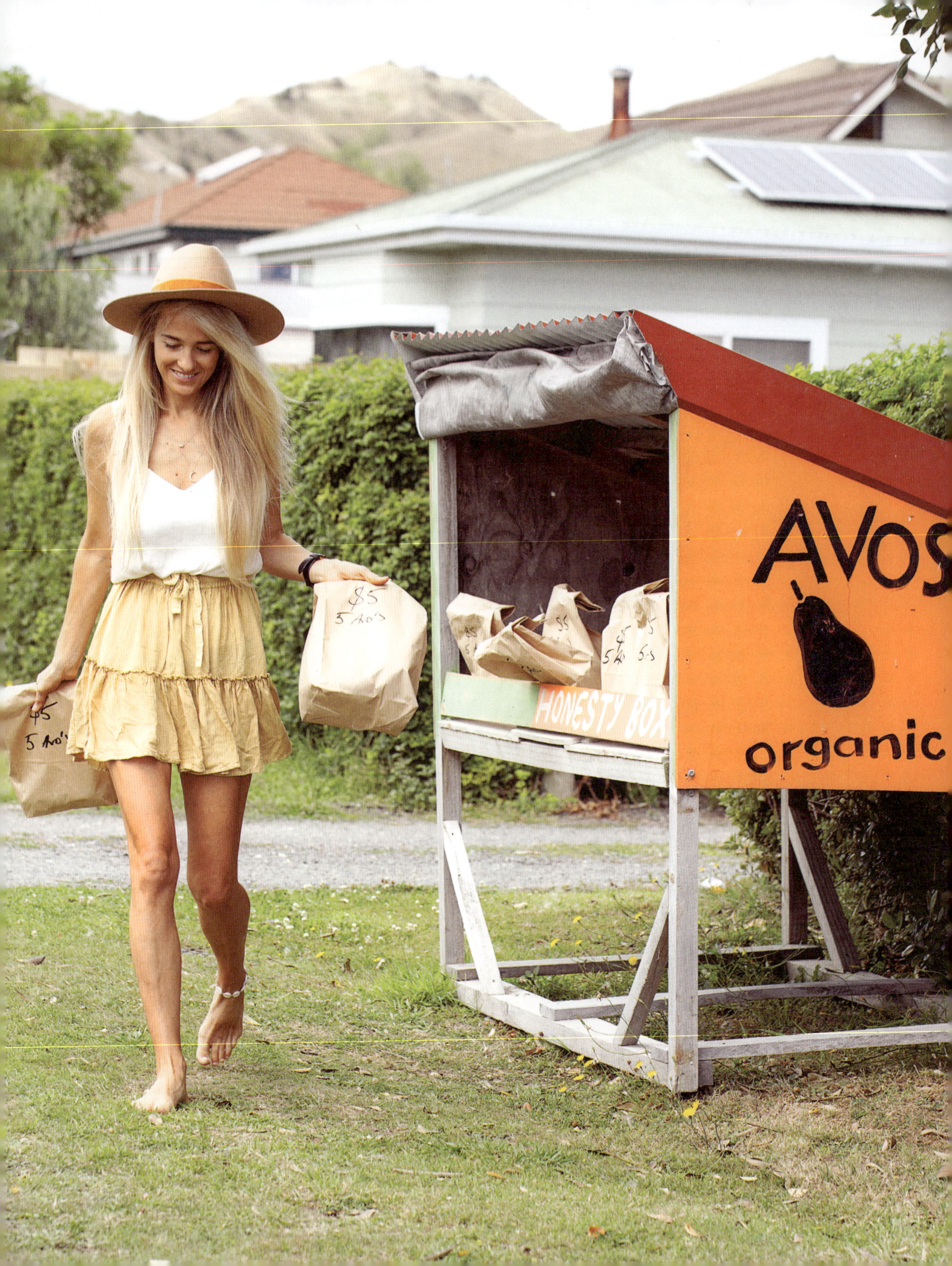
AVOS
organic
HONESTY BOX
$5
5 Avo's

Getting Started

One of the questions I am asked most is how I personally began my health journey, and how I continue to thrive in this lifestyle. I am continuously learning and evolving, but below are the main aspects that really helped me along the way. I hope these tips, along with the healthful recipes in this book, will encourage you to make healthier lifestyle choices, and allow you to discover new and different ways to nourish your body, along with whatever else works best for you.

12 TIPS FOR A WHOLESOME PLANT-BASED LIFESTYLE

1. The first step

Firstly, mindset is everything. When I embarked on a mission to change my health, I felt completely driven. I acknowledged the poor choices I had made that resulted in adverse effects on my health, I accepted the changes that needed to be made and, most importantly, I was fuelled by an intense feeling of determination and desire. I wanted it. For myself and for my children. In the moments before I began my journey, I read something that really hit home: 'You have reached a point in your life where you need to create some big changes in order to survive in this world.' This really stuck with me. The hardest part to any change is always the beginning, taking that very first step. But you are here. Now, you need a realistic goal. Long-term goals are important, but they can initially feel overwhelming, which can often result in reverting back to old habits. Remember, this isn't a 'diet', it is a lifestyle, so I recommend beginning slowly and keeping it simple. This will allow you the time to adjust to a new way of wholesome eating, as well as preparing the corresponding food, until it gradually becomes a sustainable lifestyle. I began my journey simply by making a conscious effort to include more fruit and vegetables into my daily routine. The easiest way to do this was by beginning my morning with a large, wholesome smoothie. One simple, small change gradually changed my perception of food. I began eating not only for pleasure, but also for nourishment. I began eating to live. You deserve to be the best version of you—and you can be. Take it slowly and go with what works for you and your family, and over time, it will become your way of life.

2. Educate yourself

When embarking on any lifestyle change, educating and empowering yourself as much as possible will help you tremendously. The more you learn, the more encouraged and confident you will feel. Plus, the more knowledge you will attain about how best to nourish your individual needs, as well as your daily levels of activity. There are many easily accessible books and documentaries containing a whirlwind of helpful and inspiring information, including the incredible benefits of a plant-based lifestyle. Another idea is to seek the support of a passionate expert, such as a qualified naturopath or nutritionist, for that added level of knowledge and encouragement.

3. Eliminate temptation

Out of sight, out of mind. When you eliminate the unhealthy foods from your home, such as packets of highly processed sugars and carbohydrates, it will help you to avoid using these foods as your primary source of fuel. Over a short period of time, your taste buds will adapt and you'll find you have much fewer cravings for those acidic foods you once thought you could never live a day without—trust me, I've been there. Remember, these highly addictive foods are extremely detrimental to your health; therefore, they do not deserve a place in your home (or your body).

4. Be prepared at home

Now it's time to refill your home with glorious, vibrant and energising wholefoods. Stocking up on fresh produce and plant-based staples is essential in maintaining this lifestyle. However, to be clear, this does *not* mean you need to go out and purchase every single superfood on the market. Keep it simple and remember to make this lifestyle work for you, and within your budget. Focus on seasonal produce; visit your local weekend markets for fresh fruit and vegetables. Buying from a bulk-bin store is a fabulous way to purchase smaller quantities of nuts, seeds, grains and legumes, especially if you're exploring and experimenting with new foods. It's also important to have plentiful healthy snacks on hand, as this will make it easier for you to reach for a wholesome bite, rather than reverting back to old habits. Why not ask for the spare fruit falling from your neighbours' overflowing trees? This gift of Nature is the most wonderful gift. Some of the items I like to have on hand include fresh and frozen fruit, dark leafy greens, seasonal veges, kūmara, bananas, dates, avocados, cashews and hempseeds. In the next chapter (see page 42), I have explained some of the most common plant-based staples that are used to create many of the delicious recipes in this book.

5. Emphasise wholefoods and ensure you eat enough

If the basis of your diet is predominately highly processed foods, it will contribute

tairāwhiti
HEMP CO

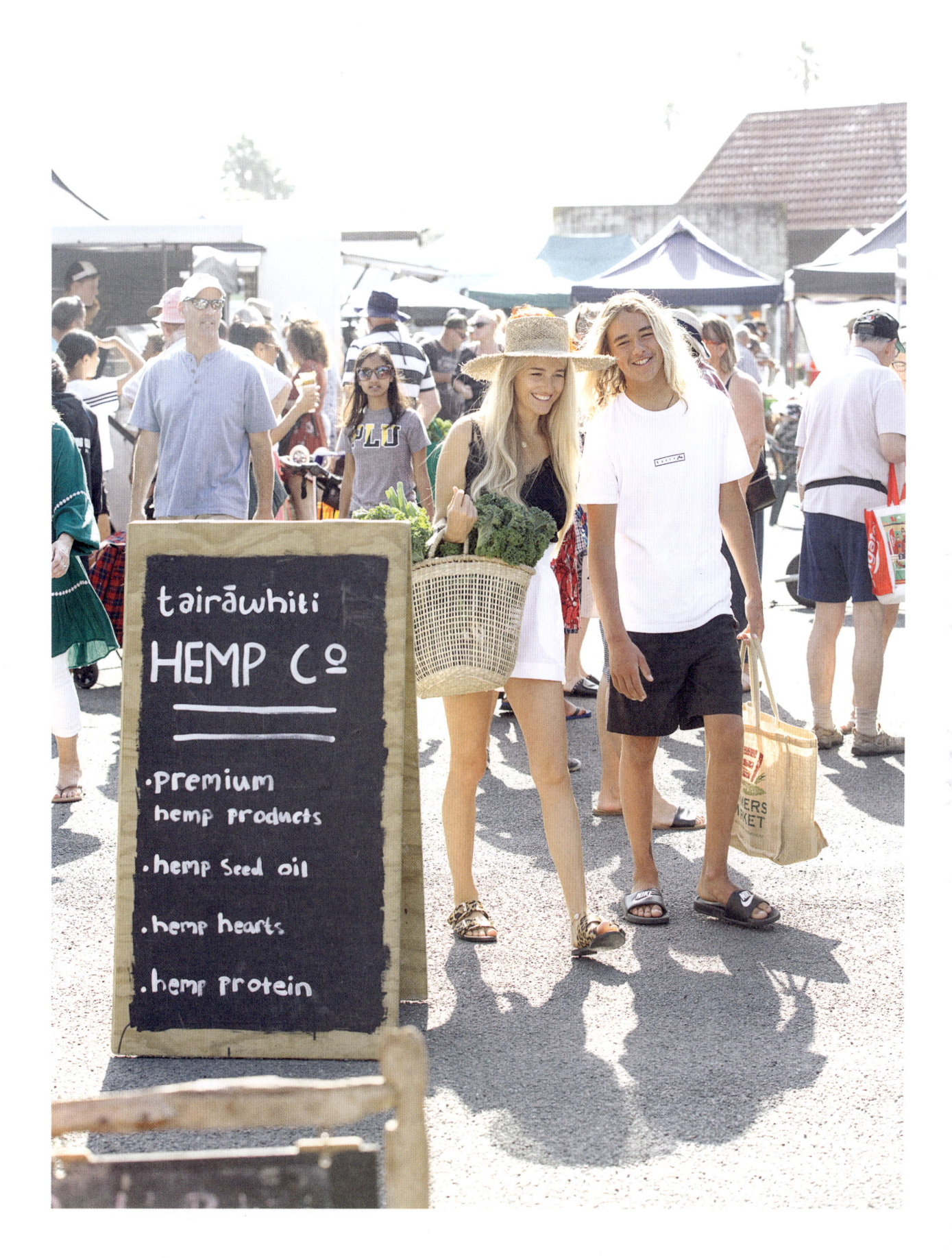

- premium hemp products
- hemp seed oil
- hemp hearts
- hemp protein

to the depletion of many essential vitamins and minerals in your body. This is a common misconception when transitioning into a plant-based diet. Just because you are vegan, it doesn't necessarily mean you are healthy. When you decrease the consumption of animals and their by-products, it is then vital that you 'eat the grass' yourself, so to speak, and in adequate amounts to attain the same level of nutrients and energy that you were receiving second-hand from animals. This is easily obtainable when the emphasis of your diet is on nutrient-dense, wholefoods that are minimally processed, such as fruits, vegetables, nuts, seeds, wholegrains and legumes. Try to ensure at least 80 per cent of your diet is based on nutrient-dense food, including plenty of raw fruits and vegetables. Also, ensure you are eating enough. Generally, plant-based foods are lower in calories than animal-based foods, which means you will likely need to eat more to feel satisfied. It's about listening to your body and eating (wholesomely) when you feel hungry.

6. Recreate your favourite indulgences

We all have our indulgences, the simple pleasures we live for, and I actually believe this is really important. What I found to work wonders in this lifestyle is to recreate the things you love in a healthful way. I have become a master at doing this; it is incredibly easy, can be really fun, and for the most part, the outcome tastes even better than what you were trying to replicate—while also providing nourishment. For example, my Hemp Chocolate Shakes (see page 268)—I'm a little obsessed to say the least.

7. Focus on raw food

Although this book contains both raw and healthy cooked meals, I believe raw food is the key to true health and longevity. The power that raw food has to revitalise the human body is astounding, and something I have personally experienced first-hand. The majority of my diet consists of pure raw fruits and vegetables and I feel absolutely amazing for it. Raw food is made up of pure, whole, living, plant-based foods that are eaten in their natural state, without being cooked or processed. Raw foods include fresh leafy greens, vegetables, fruit, nuts and seeds. Cooking food, such as fruit and vegetables, can turn it from being highly alkalising, energetic food to pretty much dead food. This is because when heat is applied, especially at high temperatures, it drastically decreases the nutrients, destroys the enzymes, and changes both the chemistry and the electromagnetic energy of the food and even the way it is metabolised in the body. Remember, no other animal on this planet cooks their food before they eat it. If you are striving to improve your health, your focus should be to include an abundance of raw fruits and vegetables into your lifestyle. To begin with, this could be as simple as enjoying a salad or a smoothie, or choosing the lettuce wrap over the burger bun.

I often find that when people begin to include more raw, live foods into their diet, they begin to crave more and it gradually becomes a part of their everyday life.

8. Eat more fruit

Fruit, glorious, vibrant fruit is the true essence of a superfood, and in my opinion, Nature's most powerful food. Fruits are excellent brain and nerve foods, are high in antioxidants and astringents, and work as incredible cleansers in the body, making them vital for our natural detoxification process. Fruits are the perfect carbohydrate, providing pure energy as well as containing the easiest fibre for our digestive tract to break down, while keeping our intestinal walls clean. Many people are concerned about the sugar content in fruit. In my opinion, there is a misconception about the different types of sugar, including the effects they have on our health, and this discourages people from consuming too much fruit. While an excessive intake of refined sugar (such as the type found in processed foods) can be extremely harmful, whole fruits contain simple sugars that require minimal digestive effort and very efficiently energise and nourish our cells. They also aid alkalisation which hugely contributes to a healthy body. Often, fruit is associated with bloating. This can sometimes simply be because the fruit is eaten unripe and in terrible combinations with other food. For optimum digestion and to maximise the nutrients, aim to eat fruit alone and at least 30–60 minutes before consuming any other food.

9. Choose organic when possible
In our family, we prioritise our health and choose to spend our money on healthful foods. This includes organic where possible. Eating organic produce has many health benefits, especially when it comes to promoting positive ecosystems within our environment, avoiding synthetic pesticides and fertilisers, and maximising plants' nutrients. However, it's not always entirely possible, nor affordable, to source organically grown food. Planting a vege garden could provide the solution. This is not only a fantastic way to grow your own nutrient-dense plants, and in good-quality soil, but it is also an inexpensive way to eat organically, and an awesome way to include the whole family. I find when my children plant, nurture and gather their own greens from the garden, or pick fresh fruit from a tree, they are much more inclined to eat it. Do the best you can, wherever your budget allows, but at the end of the day you are far better off obtaining the nutrients from washed, non-organic fruit and veges than avoiding fruit and veges altogether. I often use a home-made fruit and vegetable wash on non-organic produce. Simply mix 2 cups of cold, filtered water, ¼ cup of white vinegar and the juice of 1 lemon together and pour into a spray bottle. Squirt it onto your produce three times, let it sit for a few minutes, then rinse under cold, filtered water before consuming.

10. Drink plenty of good-quality water
It's extremely important to ensure the water you are drinking is good quality. I believe it is essential to assess where your water is coming from. Many chemicals, such as chlorine, are added to the majority of town water supplies around the world. If you rely on drinking this water, I recommend getting a good-quality water filter that removes these harsh chemicals before they enter your body. Rainwater is ideal but, even then, contaminants from the catchment can leach into the water, so I would still recommend some form of filtration. Do your own research on this and find out the best solution for you. A common guideline as to how much water to drink is to aim for at least 8 glasses of water per day, but this will differ depending on your level of activity as well as how much you sweat. Use common sense and adjust to your day. Listen to your body. I always carry my drink bottle with me wherever I go and aim to drink at least 2–3 litres (70–100 fl oz) of

water each day. When I am consuming high quantities of fresh fruit, I find my hydration levels are much often higher.

11. Reduce toxic chemicals

What you breathe into your lungs and choose to put on your skin are two ways to bring the inharmonious outside world into your body. Our skin is the largest organ in our body. It has the potential to absorb every single substance applied to it, directly into the bloodstream. This is something I was incredibly ignorant about for many years when purchasing cosmetics, skincare and household cleaners. Unfortunately, we are exposed to many carcinogens in our environment that we have no control over, but we do have control over the products we use in our household and what we choose to use on our skin. There are now many natural alternatives to skincare and household cleaners available, but of course the more minimalistic we learn to become, the better.

12. Exercise, sleep, breathing, sunshine and happiness

I strongly believe that adequate sleep, rest, relaxation, exercise, breathing, fun, laughter and happiness are also extremely important in sustaining a healthy lifestyle, and I try to implement these factors into my life when possible. I religiously practised all of the above when I was detoxing and it absolutely shone through. The importance of a solid night of sleep is something I've come to greatly respect, as it plays a vital role in robust health. Sleep allows our body the crucial time it needs to repair and rejuvenate. Good sleep, or lack of it, also totally determines the outcome of our day: it affects our moods, reflexes, focus, drive, energy, appearance, eating habits and so much more. Exercise is also an extremely important factor. Keeping regularly active has been shown to have many positive health benefits, both physically and mentally, including the movement of one of the most vital systems in our body—the lymphatic system. Unlike blood, lymph fluid does not have a pump (heart) to keep it moving, so one of the methods it relies on is the contraction of our muscles, which are activated through movement and exercise. Also, when we stimulate the lymph system and allow our body to sweat, we encourage the elimination of toxins through our skin, as previously mentioned, the largest eliminative organ in the body. Take a walk in the sunshine, sweat, breathe, relax, smile, think positive thoughts, be grateful, rest, relax—and at the end of the day, ensure you prioritise a good night of sleep.

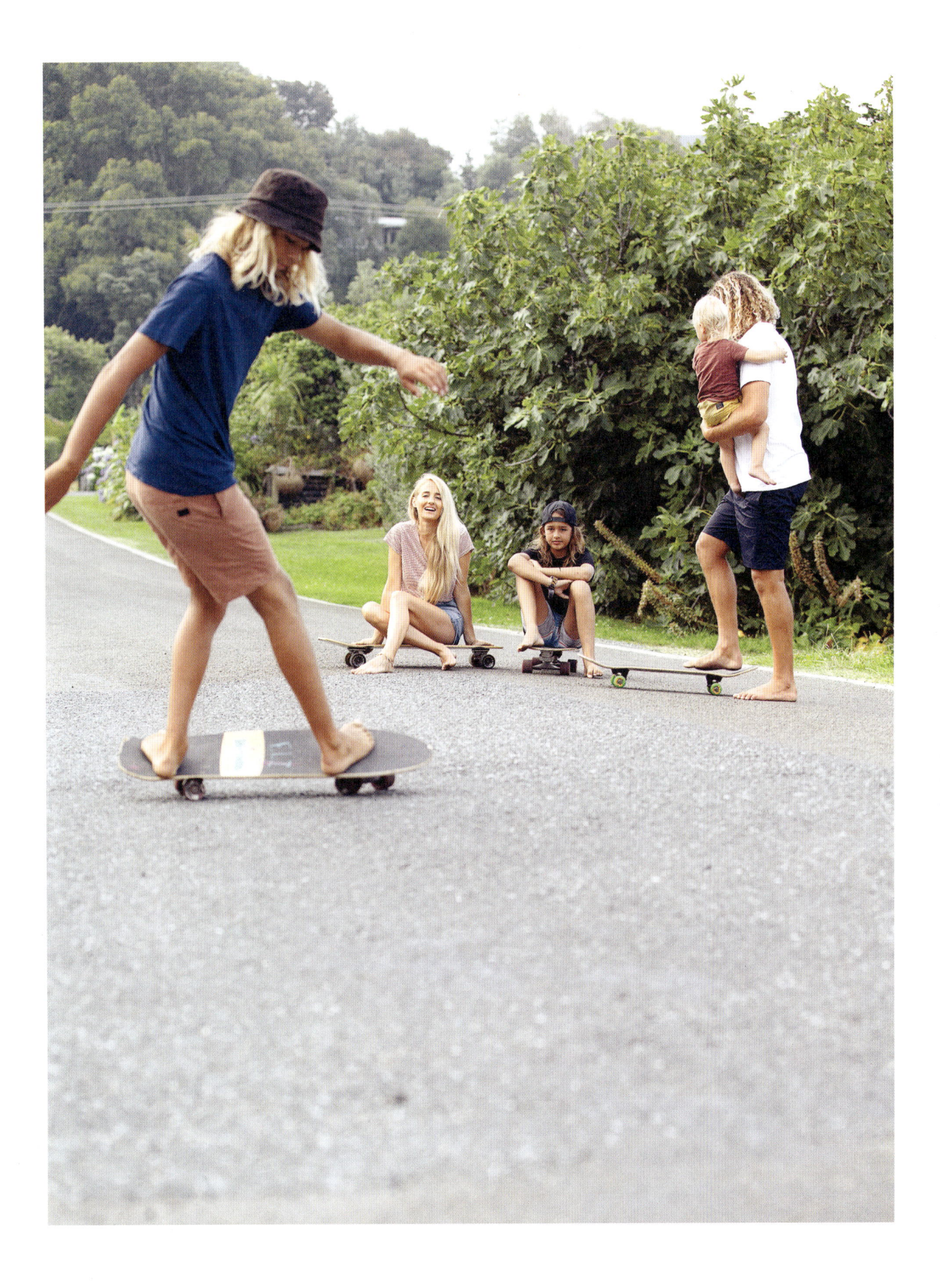

ENCOURAGING CHILDREN TO EAT MORE PLANTS

This is a really popular topic and if I'm honest, there really is no perfect answer. By no means do my three boys eat perfectly all of the time, but from personal experience, I found educating them was an absolute game-changer. This helped them to understand why we were making this enormous change in our family and how important it is to sustain a healthy diet, despite what they may see around them. Watching documentaries about health, wellness, the environment and plant-based amazingness together as a family is a fantastic way to achieve this—something we do all the time in our home. It really helps remind us all exactly why we are living this lifestyle.

Recreating the kids' favourite dishes, finding wholesome, plant-based recipes that they enjoy and involving them in the preparation is a fantastic way to encourage them to eat more plants. Another key factor is to eliminate processed packet foods from your home. This may seem difficult at first, but you'll be surprised at how quickly children will adapt. It is also important to ensure you then refill your pantry with plenty of healthy and readily available snacks, such as fresh fruit, dried fruit, nuts, bliss balls, home-made nut bars and smoothie essentials (smoothies are an amazing way to sneak in an abundance of nutrients into their bodies). Also, be consistent in creating healthful meals, and as time goes on, they will hopefully begin to enjoy them. My children are much more inclined to eat their fresh greens or salads when I provide a beautiful home-made dressing to drizzle over—and this book has plenty of quick and easy recipes for them.

In addition to this, being a good role model has definitely had a positive impact on my children, especially in encouraging their relationship with healthy food. I strongly believe that living a healthy lifestyle is one of the best things we as a society can do for our future generation, and is also one of the best ways to encourage them to do the same.

ESSENTIAL NUTRIENTS

While plant-based foods are jam-packed with essential nutrients, you will need to ensure you are getting adequate amounts to sustain a healthy, functioning body. Here are some of the best plant-based sources for protein, calcium, iron and vitamin B_{12}—the four nutrients in particular of common concern when it comes to following a plant-based diet.

Protein
Protein is important for building, growth and repair, and of the 21 amino acids in protein, there are nine that are labelled essential. Essential amino acids are the ones that cannot be synthesised by the body, so must be provided by the food we eat. Hempseeds and quinoa are plant-based foods that are known as a complete protein source—a food source containing all of the nine essential amino acids. Nuts and seeds, dark leafy greens (spinach, kale, collards), raw green beans, sunflower seeds, pea sprouts, pumpkin seeds, sesame seeds, brown rice, beans, legumes and tofu are also great sources of plant-protein.

Calcium
Calcium is an essential mineral our body requires for bone, cartilage, tendon and connective tissue strength and growth, as well as for many other important functions

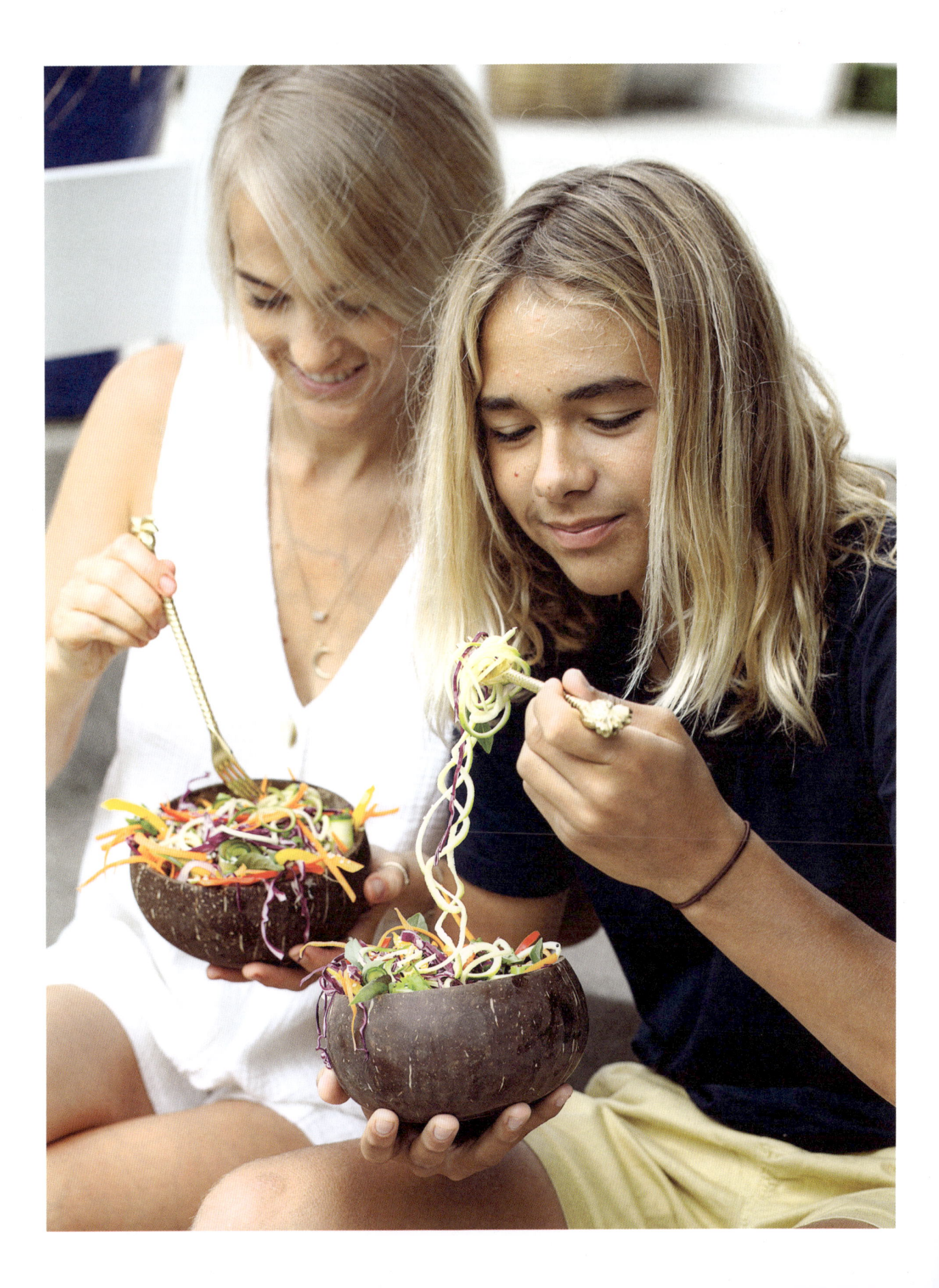

in our body. Calcium-rich plant-based foods include dark leafy greens, broccoli, kelp, carrots, oranges, papaya, walnuts, cashews, Brazil nuts, sunflower seeds, sesame seeds, brown rice and tofu, along with many other fruits and vegetables.

Iron

Iron is a trace mineral essential for the formation of red blood cells, and is primarily involved in the transfer of oxygen from the lungs throughout the body. Iron plays a vital role in maintaining energy levels, and also helps to strengthen the immune system, increasing resistance to colds and infections. A well-functioning digestive system can help with the absorption of iron, as well as eating iron-rich foods and vitamin C-rich foods together—vitamin C assists iron absorption. An abundance of iron can be found in dark leafy green vegetables, kelp, parsley, cucumbers, spinach, root vegetables, broccoli, green peas, Brussel sprouts, avocados, asparagus, carrots, oranges, grapes, bananas, prunes, raisins, figs, sesame seeds, pumpkin seeds, nuts such as almonds, cashews and hazelnuts, lima beans, wholegrains and many other fruits and vegetables.

Vitamin B_{12}

Vitamin B_{12} (cobalamin) can be a controversial topic because it's the only nutrient that is not reliably sourced from either plant-based foods or sun exposure. Made by microorganisms, bacteria, algae and fungi, Vitamin B_{12} is an important vitamin essential for the growth, production and regeneration of red blood cells. Plants cannot synthesise B_{12}, but some plants contain traces through contaminated soils. Because of vigorous washing and food safety practices, especially in developed countries, plants are not a reliable source of adequate B_{12} levels. The most common, readily available sources include animal foods—such as meat, eggs and cheese—and foods that have been fortified with B_{12}, the most popular being cereals, nut milks and nutritional yeast. If your diet is predominately plant-based, it is extremely important to keep a close eye on your vitamin B_{12} levels. At some point, you will likely need to supplement.

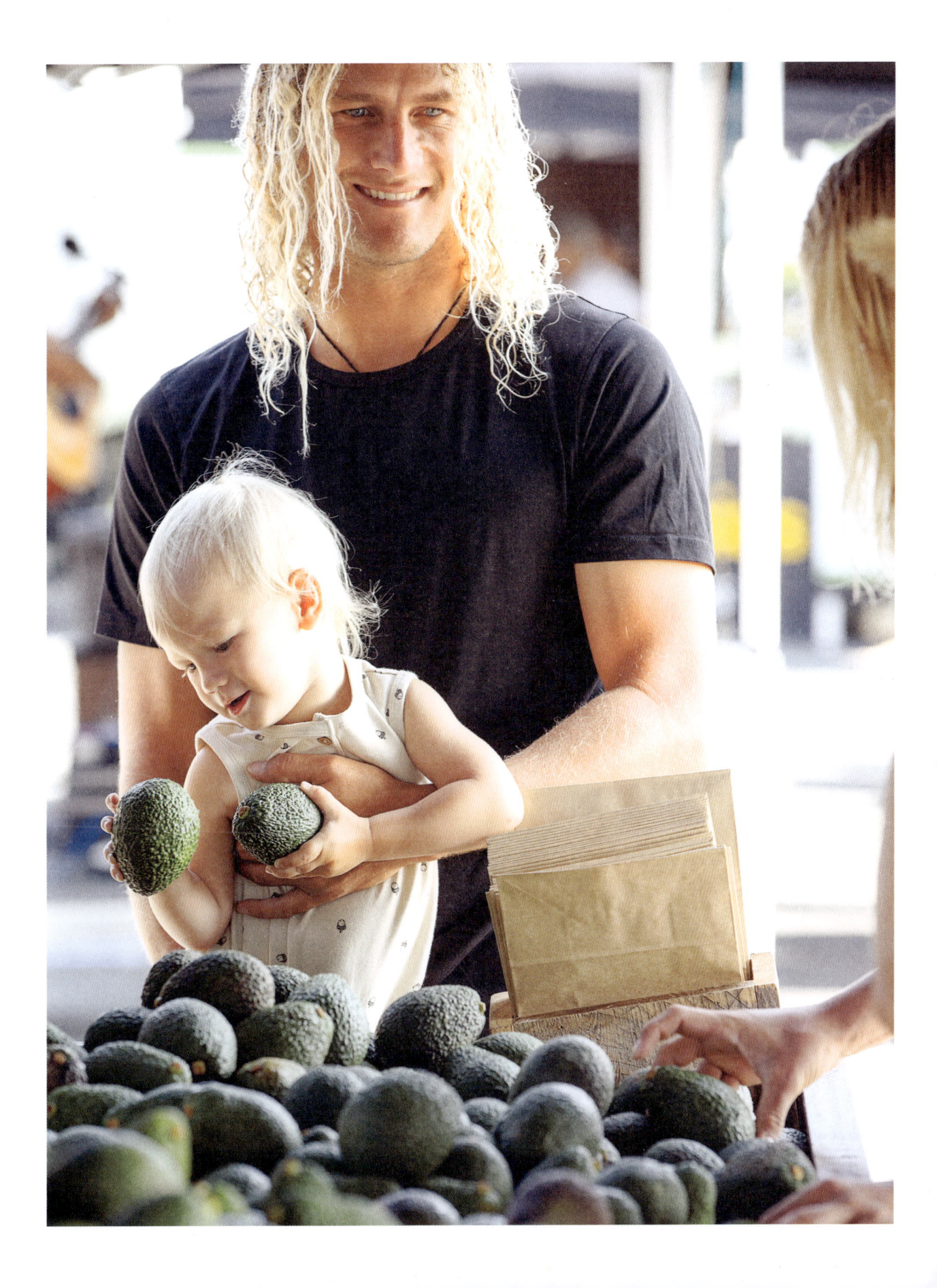

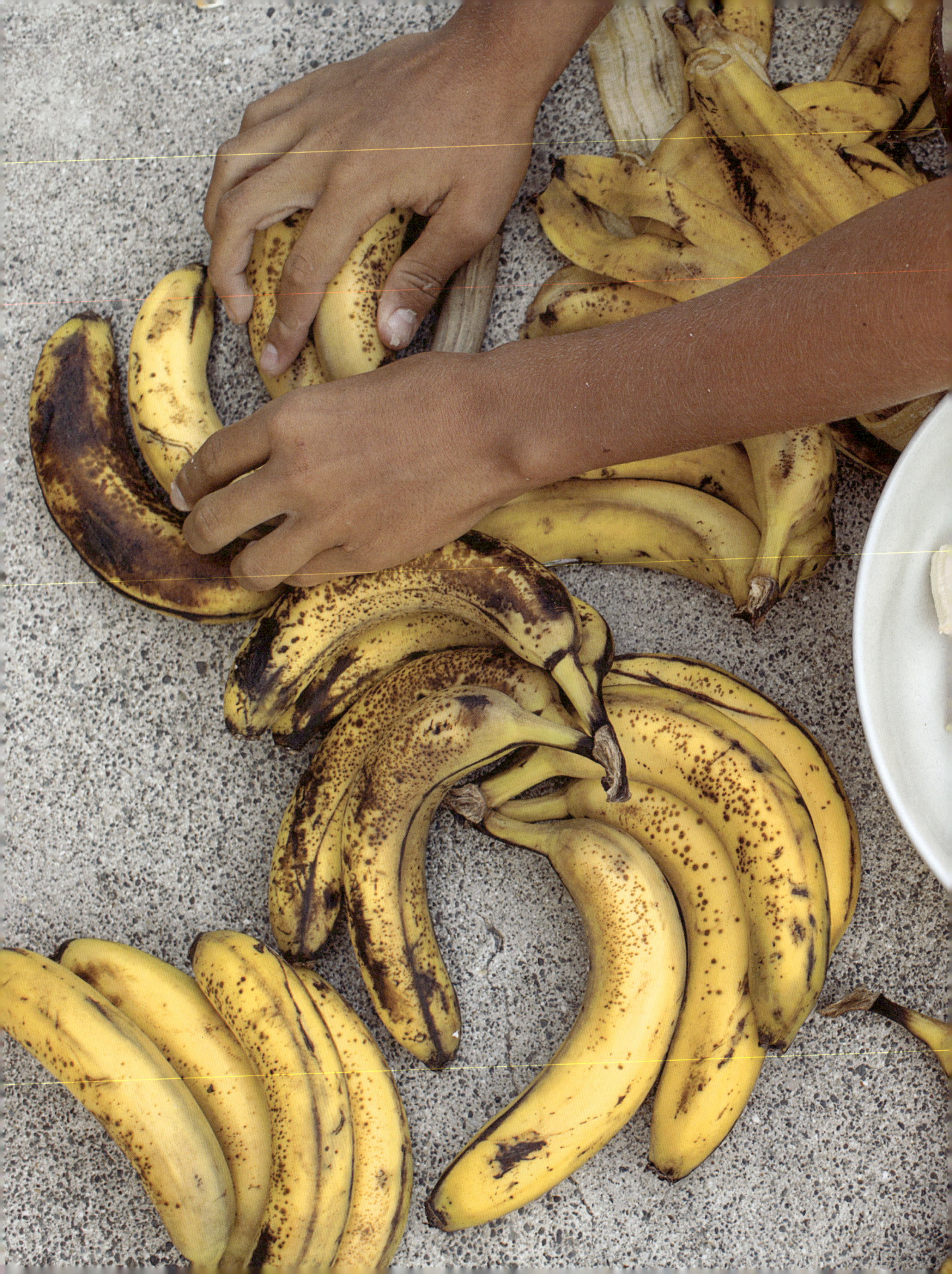

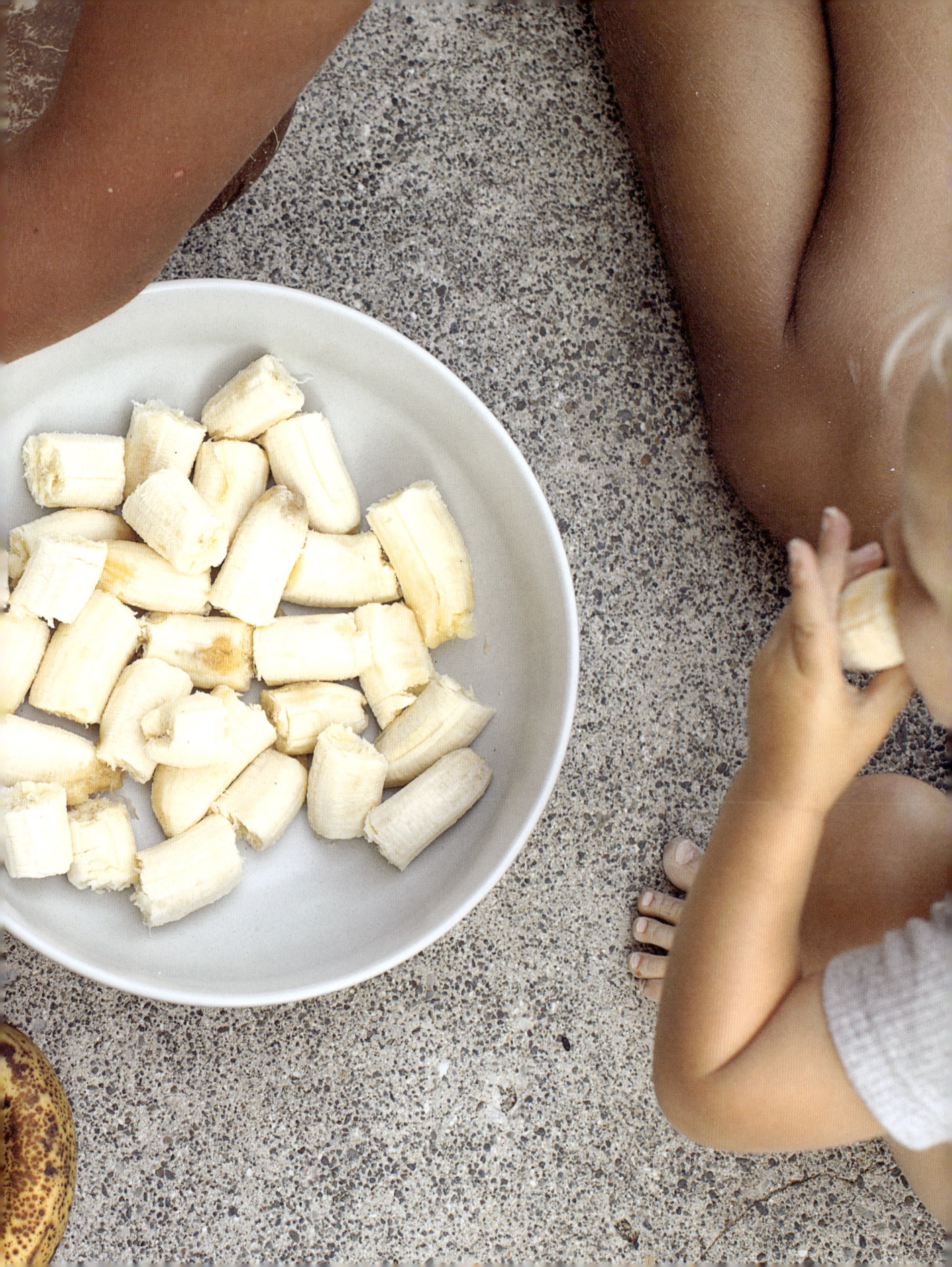

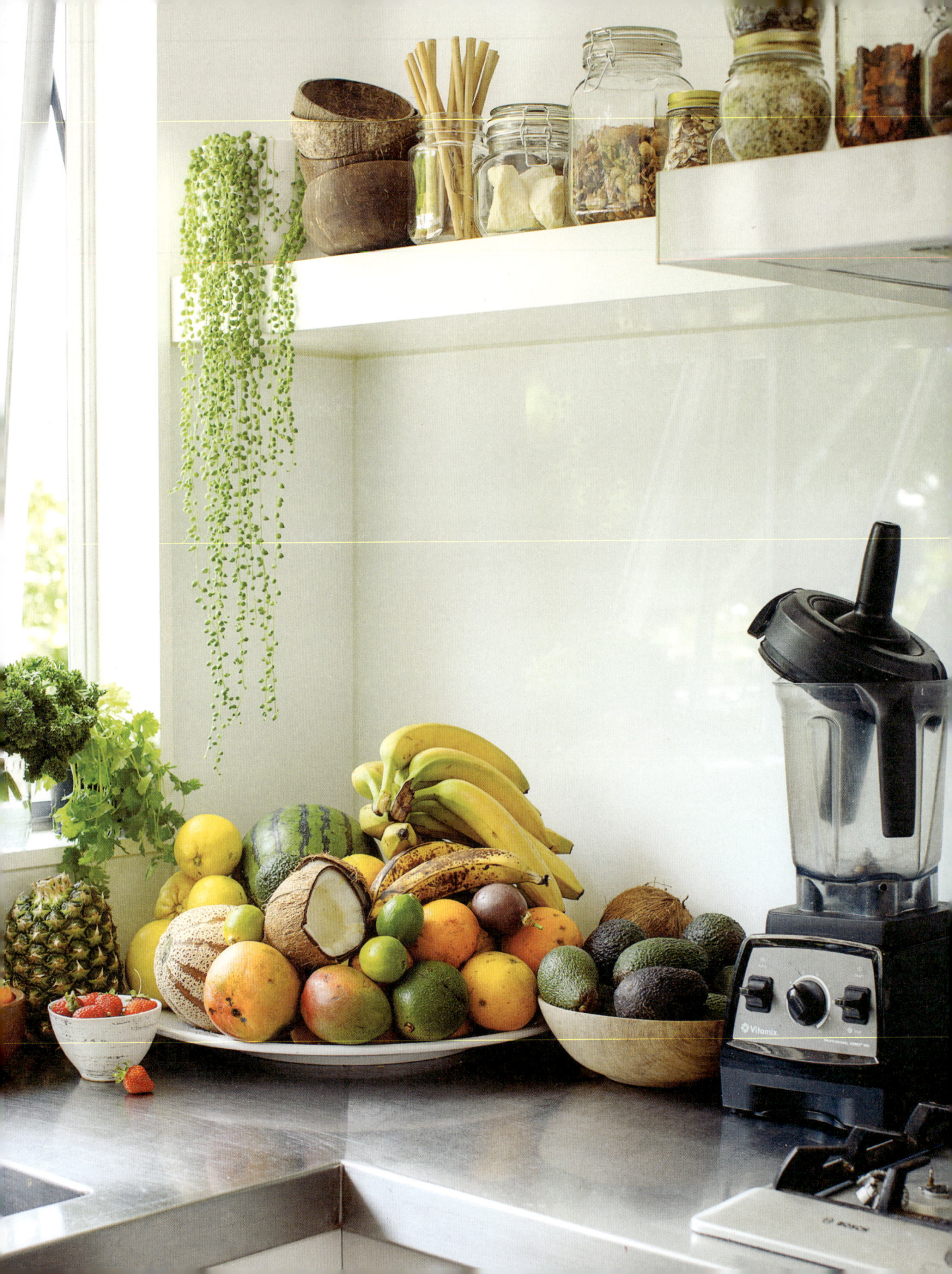

Kitchen + Pantry Basics

MY FAVOURITE KITCHEN EQUIPMENT

The following are my favourite kitchen tools, some of which are almost essential to this way of eating. Other than the basic kitchen utensils, a blender and a food processor are the two main items you will need to create the majority of the recipes in this book; you'll need a juicer and a spiraliser for a few of them, too. Other useful items are a good sharp knife (this might sound silly, but trust me, it makes a world of difference), a steamer, an ice-block mould and a nut-milk bag.

Blender

A blender is something I simply cannot live without. One glass of smoothie can so easily provide an abundance of beneficial nutrients, and my family and I enjoy a smoothie every single morning and quite often as a snack throughout the day. The blender we use, and the one I would highly recommend, is a Vitamix. They are powerful, efficient, high-speed blenders that will allow you to easily create a variety of liquid-based foods, including smoothies, nice creams, soups, dips and dressings. Before purchasing a Vitamix, I blew three different blenders up in one year! I've since owned my Vitamix for more than four years and it's still going strong, so for me personally it was definitely worth the investment. I would suggest you do your research and purchase the most powerful blender that fits within your budget.

Food processor

A good, high-quality food processor is another one of my absolute kitchen favourites. Yes, they are quite expensive, but I can assure you they truly do make a world of difference in the kitchen, so in my opinion they are definitely worth the investment. You can also get away with a cheaper one if need be—I used a cheapy for many years before taking the leap and although it didn't work to the same extent, it still did the trick. The beauty of these machines is that they make it so easy to make such a variety of food, including bliss balls, raw slices, dressings, dips, hummus and pesto. They are also fantastic for efficiently grating and cutting your produce, which can save you a lot of time in the kitchen. People often ask me what the difference is between a blender and a food processor, and if they should invest in both of these items. This is a really good question. Blenders require liquid to run, they have short blades and a very powerful motor as they work mostly with liquids—this is why they are also called liquidisers. In contrast, food processors mostly work with solid food items and will break down whatever you put into them, hence have different, longer blades and attachments. I personally use my blender more often than my food processor, but I would highly recommend both items, as they serve two very different purposes and are both incredibly useful and practical kitchen equipment for a plant-based lifestyle.

Juicer

A juicer is another highly beneficial kitchen asset. Juicing has so many amazing health benefits as it's a powerful way to get loads of nutrients in. I try to juice regularly using lots of in-season fruit and vegetables. My children enjoy juicing, too. I have a slow, cold-pressed juicer and I absolutely love it. It's also really easy to clean, which is something I would recommend considering when investing in one, as the clean-up can be a mission.

Water filter

In my opinion, a water filter is more of a necessity than a kitchen tool. Unless you are lucky enough to have your own rainwater supply, drinking tap water will expose you to chemicals such as chlorine, which are unfortunately put into our main water supply, as well as biological and heavy-metal contaminants. I believe a water filter is both essential and beneficial in any home, and you will absolutely taste and feel the difference from drinking good-quality, pure water.

Spiraliser

I wouldn't say a spiraliser is essential, but it's definitely a great kitchen tool, especially when it comes to preparing raw food. A spiraliser is amazing for creating a healthier and lighter alternative to noodles, such as zucchini or cucumber. It also makes for a fun way to dress up any meal, such as salads or Buddha bowls.

COMMONLY USED INGREDIENTS

All of my recipes are plant-based, dairy-free, refined-sugar-free and gluten-free, and here are some of the most common ingredients that I use in them, explained in a little more detail. This will give you a better understanding of how best to use them, and how to include them in your recipes.

Apple cider vinegar

Apple cider vinegar is a key ingredient I use for making dressings or for adding a sweet, tangy element to salads. It's also a great addition in baking, as it will help to make the batter light and fluffy. I always like to have a large glass bottle on hand.

Cashews

Raw cashews are my number one ingredient for making dips, dressings, sauces and raw treats as they have a mild flavour and a creamy, silky texture when blended. They will often need to be soaked prior to using (see Recipe Notes page 47), so keep this in mind. Cashews are also high in magnesium, making them a great snack or salad addition.

Chia seeds

Chia seeds are a fantastic pantry staple, loaded with nutrients such as essential amino acids, omega-3 fatty acids and fibre. They also work wonders as an egg replacement. When chia seeds are combined with liquid they become gelatinous, making them the perfect ingredient to use for binding in many recipes. Ground flaxseeds (linseed) will also do the same thing—another great binder or egg replacer.

Coconut

From coconut yoghurt and coconut milk to coconut oil and shredded coconut, go nuts for coconut as it has multiple purposes, especially for adding a thick and creamy consistency to hot pots, smoothies, salad dressings and raw treats. Always read the ingredient label when purchasing coconut products to ensure they do not contain any nasty additives.

Gluten-free flours

Gluten is the term used to describe the proteins that are found in wheat, barley, spelt and rye. As the name suggests, gluten acts as a 'glue' that holds food together. For me, maintaining a gluten-free diet is a personal choice. I simply choose to avoid gluten as I feel a lot more energised without it. The absence of gluten from my diet over the past four years has also immensely improved my digestive health. While gluten-free flours are wonderful alternatives, they don't always have quite the same flavour and texture as wheat-based flours, so can often take a little time to get used to. Buckwheat, an earthy-flavoured flour, is an ideal substitute to use in pizza bases, wraps, tacos and recipes that do not require the mixture to rise. Chickpea flour (besan or gram flour) is a heavier flour that is often used as an egg replacement in recipes such as vegan omelettes and frittatas. It also works well as a binder, but keep in mind that it has quite a strong, legume-like flavour that doesn't always appeal to all taste buds and can sometimes give a dry texture to a dish. Tapioca flour (starch), from the cassava plant, is commonly used as a thickener in sauces and pies; it also works well to attain a chewy texture in baking. I found it to be a great addition in my buckwheat pastry and chickpea tacos, as it helped to create a stretchy, 'break-free' recipe. Coconut flour and almond flour (or almond meal/ground almonds) are my favourite flours to use in raw treats. Both are light flours with a mild flavour, and work wonders in creating a 'biscuit' base in tarts and slices, along with cashews.

Gluten-free wholegrains

A wholegrain is a cereal grain that still contains the endosperm, germ and bran of the grain. The bran is the outer skin of the grain that is high in fibre. Unlike processed grains, such as white rice, wholegrains remain packed with many essential nutrients. Brown rice, millet, quinoa, buckwheat and sorghum are my favourite gluten-free wholegrains; similar in size and texture, they make a nutritious addition to salads, baking, and breakfast cereals, and are wonderful served as a nutritious side.

Hempseeds

Hempseeds, derived from the plant *Cannabis sativa*, are the true essence of a superfood. Although they are the same species as the cannabis plant, they are a different variety and only contain minute traces of the psychoactive constituent of cannabis, THC. Hempseeds are highly nutritious with an earthy, nutty flavour, and play an important role in a plant-based diet. The versatility and creaminess of these seeds mean you can add them to majority of your meals, from smoothies to salads, desserts to milks. Hempseeds are also a great source of complete protein as they contain all of the nine essential amino acids, as well as vitamin E, phosphorus, potassium, sodium, magnesium, sulphur, calcium, iron and zinc. Hempseeds are becoming increasingly easy to source and are now available in most big supermarkets.

Herbs and spices

Herbs and spices, both fresh and dried, are a key staple in any kitchen. They are a vital ingredient for bringing any dish to life, providing warmth, sweetness, spice and wonderful herby flavours. My favourite fresh herbs, and the ones I commonly use in my recipes, include fresh parsley, coriander, basil, mint and dill. Some of the dried herbs and spices I commonly use include cumin, sweet basil, ground turmeric, paprika (sweet, smoked and regular), curry powder, garlic powder, onion powder, ground coriander, fennel seeds, cayenne pepper, chilli flakes, ground ginger, mixed spice, allspice, oregano, thyme and rosemary, among others.

Jackfruit

Jackfruit is definitely my latest obsession. The jack tree is a tropical fruit tree that originates from south-west India. The fruit it bears are large and oval-shaped with edible fibrous flesh, seeds and pods. Jackfruit is becoming increasingly popular in plant-based cooking due to its pulled-pork-like texture when cooked. Jackfruit is high in fibre, rich in vitamins B and C and potassium, and works wonders as a flavoursome, marinated addition in tacos, nachos, burgers and curries.

Maple syrup

Naturally derived from the sap of maple trees, maple syrup is one of my favourite unrefined sweeteners. It provides a subtle sweetness to almost any dish, both sweet and savoury. I like to include it in my smoothies, salad dressings, hot pots and raw treats. When purchasing, always read the label to ensure the bottle contains 100 per cent pure maple syrup, without any additives, sweeteners or preservatives. Blackstrap molasses, sourced from the sugar cane plant, is another fabulous natural sweetener, as well as being a natural source of many essential minerals and trace elements. Other commonly used unrefined sweeteners include coconut sugar, agave nectar, brown rice syrup and date syrup.

Medjool dates

Medjool dates are naturally super-sweet, highly alkalising and nutritious, with a caramel-like flavour. People can often be confused about the difference between medjool dates and regular dates. Medjool dates are a soft, plump and chewy fresh fruit, whereas regular dates (commonly called Deglet Noor) are the dried version, usually smaller with a firmer flesh. Medjool dates are fantastic to use in vegan baking as they're big and sticky, which really helps with binding, especially in raw slices. Dates in general

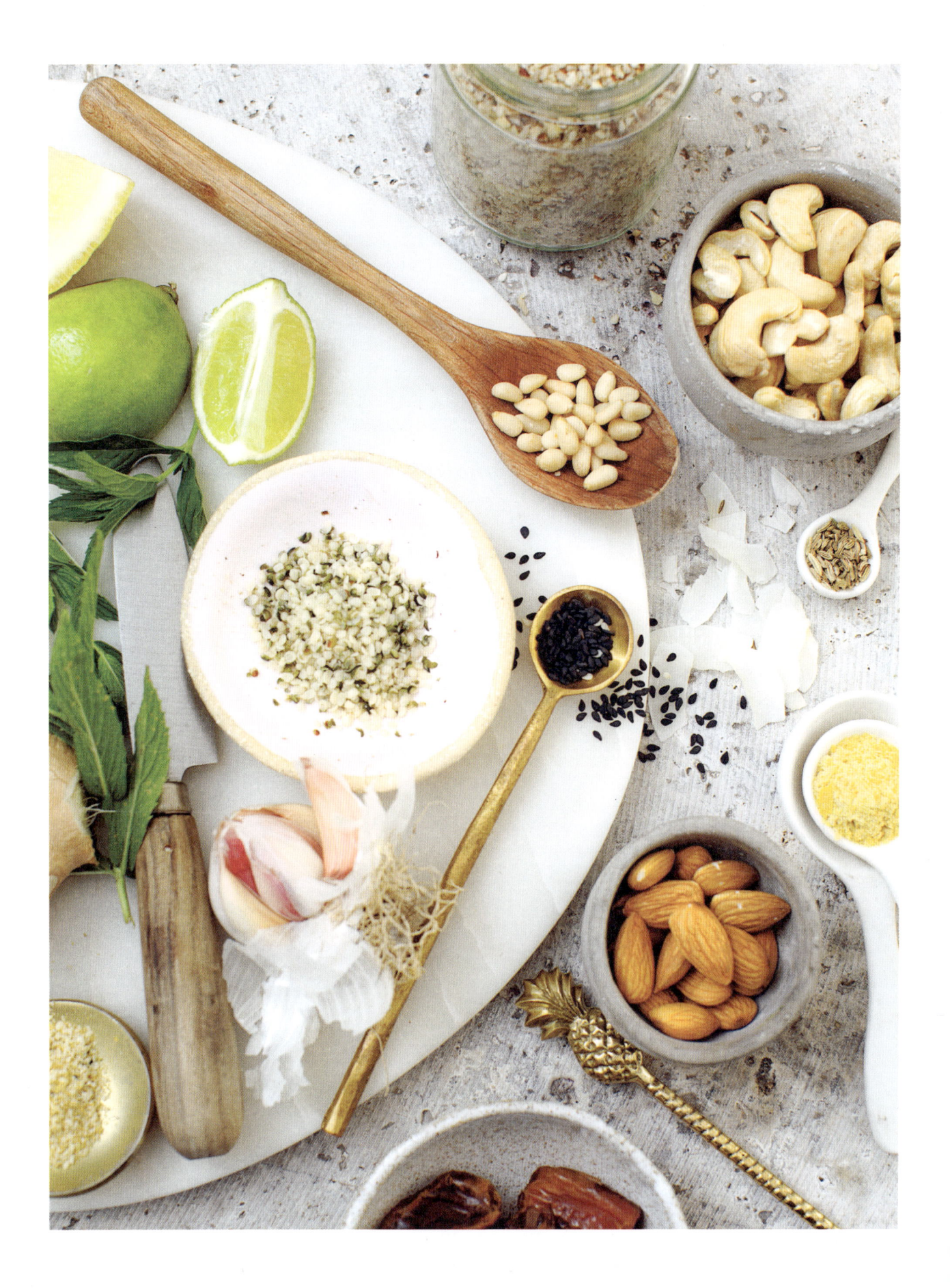

are one of my absolute favourite go-to wholesome snacks, and are also the perfect addition to sweeten smoothies, dressings and raw treats, as well as being blended into date syrup, a natural liquid-form sweetener.

Miso paste

Like tamari, miso paste is made from fermented soybeans; it has a similar flavour but is much thicker. You can also get brown rice miso paste, which is made from soybeans fermented with brown rice. Miso paste is a fabulous, slightly salty and rich addition to many dishes, especially to enhance the flavours of your favourite hot pots, soups, pastas and pies.

Nutritional yeast flakes

Nutritional yeast is an absolute game-changer in the kitchen, especially when it comes to adding a savoury, cheesy flavour to almost any dish. My mum bought us up on nutritional yeast toast, so it's a flavour I'm well accustomed to. I commonly use these super-fine flakes blended into sauces, dressings or sprinkled over savoury dishes, such as pastas, soups, pizzas and patties. Nutritional yeast, which is often fortified with vitamin B_{12}, is a deactivated yeast, so it will not rise or bubble in the same way as brewer's yeast or baker's yeast.

Nuts and seeds

Aside from hempseeds, chia seeds and cashews, some of the other nuts and seeds I commonly use include walnuts, macadamias, almonds, pumpkin seeds, sunflower seeds and sesame seeds, which are all highly nutritious, crunchy additions to include in your salads, main meals, raw treats or as a wholesome snack. Sunflower seeds can be used as an alternative to cashews in dips and dressings, as they have a similar, creamy texture when presoaked and blended (see Recipe Notes page 47).

Plant-based milks

Plant milks are another fantastic staple for adding a creamy consistency and texture to smoothies, dips and dressings, and they are really easy to make. Hemp milk is my favourite plant milk; as well as being a beautifully creamy, earthy and highly nutritious milk, it only takes about 30 seconds to make. If purchasing nut milks, make sure to read the ingredient list and look out for any nasty additives, such as carrageenan, commonly used as a thickener or stabiliser in many plant-based milks.

Quinoa

Quinoa is one of my favourite gluten-free wholegrains; it's high in fibre and contains all of the nine essential amino acids, making it a fabulous source of complete protein. It's also incredibly versatile and cooks really fast, so is a great staple to have on hand for a quick, easy and nutritious meal.

Raw cacao powder

My pantry is never short of this rich, chocolatey goodness; it's one of my favourite pantry staples. Raw cacao is pretty much the unprocessed version of cocoa, it's the ground-down cacao bean so is still packed with antioxidants, vitamins and minerals. You'll find cacao is used in many of my raw treat recipes to create the most divine chocolatey treats.

Tahini

Tahini is made from toasted, ground white or black sesame seeds. It comes in either a hulled or an unhulled form. Hulled tahini comes from sesame seeds with the outer shell removed and has a creamier taste. Unhulled tahini is made from whole sesame seeds and has a darker, slightly bitter flavour. Black tahini is made with black sesame seeds and works well for adding a depth of colour. In general, tahini is a fantastic staple ingredient, commonly used in many dips and dressing recipes.

Tamari/coconut aminos
Tamari, a wheat-free, fermented soy sauce, works wonders in adding a rich, savoury and salty flavour to many dishes. For a soy-free alternative, I also use coconut aminos. Coconut aminos is made from the fermented sap of the coconut palm. It has a similar, salty flavour to tamari. You can also buy it seasoned with chilli, garlic and onion, which makes for a flavoursome addition to salads and vegetables.

RECIPE NOTES

Here are a few notes on my recipes before you get started.

Coconut cream
When a recipe requires the use of coconut cream, try to ensure you scoop out the thick cream, often settled on the top half of the can. To easily access the thick coconut cream, place the can in the fridge overnight. By doing this, the cream will naturally settle towards the top of the can.

Oil
Generally, I cook with very little oil and use water to stir-fry my vegetables. When frying or baking vegetables, feel free to use more or less to suit your individual preferences, or, if you prefer to cook without oil, simply replace it with a splash of water.

Oven settings
I generally use fan bake for most of my cooking, on a fairly low-medium heat (180°C / 350°F), however if it's not specified in the recipe just use conventional bake. I have found that different ovens cook at slightly different rates, so please keep this in mind and adjust the cooking time if needed.

Packaged items
If a recipe calls for a packaged item, such as a can of coconut milk or a plant-based milk, ensure you purchase one without any nasty additives or preservatives—always read the ingredients list.

Salt
I use sea salt or Himalayan salt in my recipes. Feel free to substitute with whatever good-quality salt you prefer and adjust to suit your desired taste. Generally, I try to add very little salt in my cooking.

Soaking nuts and seeds
For some of the dressing recipes, cashews or sunflower seeds will need to be presoaked. Soaking your nuts will soften them, making them easier to blend, and will also decrease the anti-nutrients (such as phytate) that block our body's ability to absorb nutrients.

To do this, simply place the nuts/seeds into a bowl, cover with (preferably filtered) water and leave them to soak overnight, or for at least 8 hours. Drain and rinse. For a faster preparation time, add them to a bowl of just-boiled water and soak for at least 1 hour prior to using.

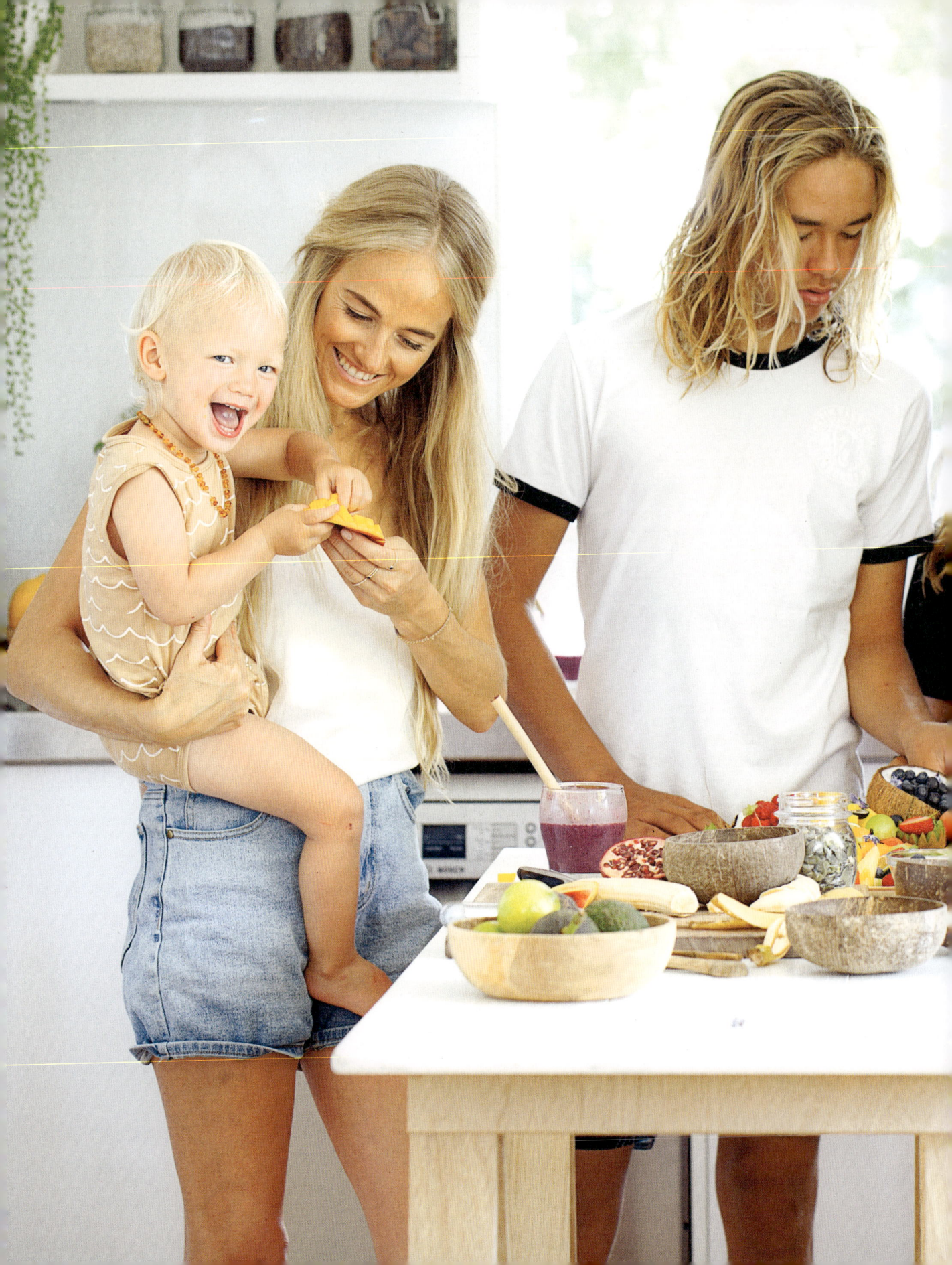

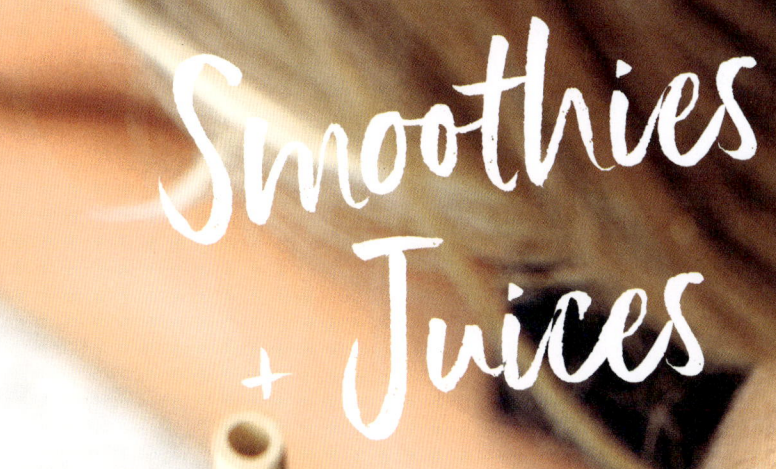

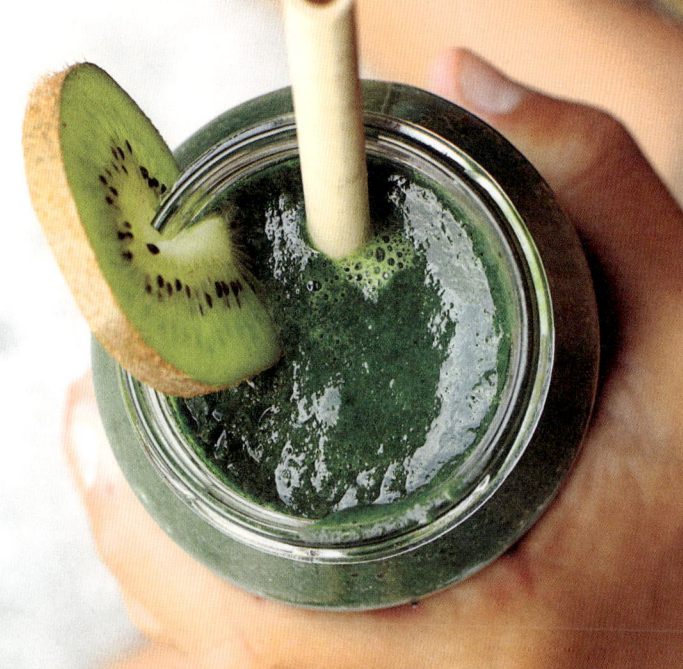

Smoothies + Juices

Smoothies + Juices

Smoothies are my world. Aside from fresh fruit, I believe smoothies are one of the simplest and most nutritious breakfasts or snacks you can create. My family and I religiously begin our day with a beautifully vibrant and healthful fruit concoction. So it was essential for me to begin this book with some of my favourite fruity recipes.

I think my Raw and Free family probably see me as one big smoothie bowl, and it's easy to see why. Along with mono meals of fresh seasonal fruit (see page 74), smoothies truly do make up many of my daily meals. I love how quick and easy they are to make, the endless combinations that can be created and, most importantly, how pure and energised they make me feel. Long gone are the days of offering a cup of tea for anyone who stops by; our home is always stocked with fruit to whip up a glass (or bowl) of goodness.

Juicing is another beneficial nutrient-booster to add to your daily routine. When you juice fresh fruit and vegetables, most of the fibre is removed, allowing your digestive tract to rest and making it simpler for your body to absorb a much larger, more concentrated dose of nutrients than you would normally consume in one sitting. Fruits are the body's cleansers and vegetables are the building blocks, containing high levels of minerals, chlorophyll and amino acids.

In this chapter you will find some of my favourite smoothies, smoothie bowls, nice creams (or as I like to call them, fruity whips) and juices—all incredibly wholesome additions to your diet.

SMOOTHIE AND SMOOTHIE BOWL TIPS

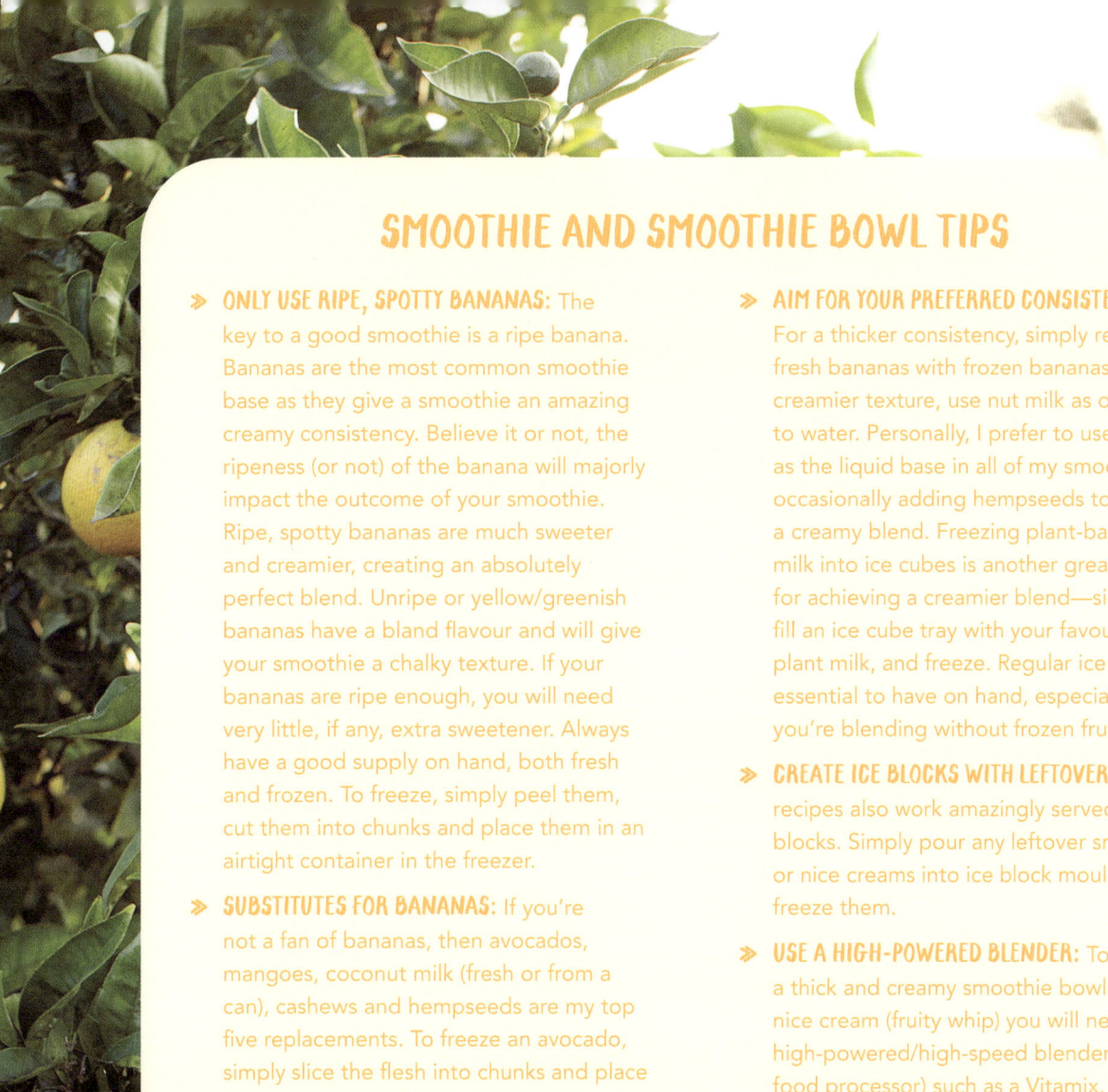

» **ONLY USE RIPE, SPOTTY BANANAS:** The key to a good smoothie is a ripe banana. Bananas are the most common smoothie base as they give a smoothie an amazing creamy consistency. Believe it or not, the ripeness (or not) of the banana will majorly impact the outcome of your smoothie. Ripe, spotty bananas are much sweeter and creamier, creating an absolutely perfect blend. Unripe or yellow/greenish bananas have a bland flavour and will give your smoothie a chalky texture. If your bananas are ripe enough, you will need very little, if any, extra sweetener. Always have a good supply on hand, both fresh and frozen. To freeze, simply peel them, cut them into chunks and place them in an airtight container in the freezer.

» **SUBSTITUTES FOR BANANAS:** If you're not a fan of bananas, then avocados, mangoes, coconut milk (fresh or from a can), cashews and hempseeds are my top five replacements. To freeze an avocado, simply slice the flesh into chunks and place in an airtight container in the freezer.

» **CHOOSE SPINACH:** The fibre content of spinach is much less dense than that of kale, collards or chard. This means that when spinach is blended with fruit it will be digested at a similar rate, and therefore you will receive the maximum nutrients from the smoothie. This makes spinach the best dark leafy green to use in fruit smoothies.

» **AIM FOR YOUR PREFERRED CONSISTENCY:** For a thicker consistency, simply replace fresh bananas with frozen bananas; for a creamier texture, use nut milk as opposed to water. Personally, I prefer to use water as the liquid base in all of my smoothies, occasionally adding hempseeds to create a creamy blend. Freezing plant-based milk into ice cubes is another great idea for achieving a creamier blend—simply fill an ice cube tray with your favourite plant milk, and freeze. Regular ice is also essential to have on hand, especially when you're blending without frozen fruit.

» **CREATE ICE BLOCKS WITH LEFTOVERS:** These recipes also work amazingly served as ice blocks. Simply pour any leftover smoothies or nice creams into ice block moulds and freeze them.

» **USE A HIGH-POWERED BLENDER:** To create a thick and creamy smoothie bowl or nice cream (fruity whip) you will need a high-powered/high-speed blender (or food processor) such as a Vitamix. Without a good blender you can still create an amazing flavour, but it will be tricky to achieve a thick, creamy, ice-cream-like consistency. A blending stick is another helpful tool; these often come as an accessory with a blender.

» **LET FRUIT DEFROST SLIGHTLY BEFORE BLENDING:** Allow the frozen fruits to defrost for about 5 minutes. This will allow you to use the least amount of liquid as possible, which will make it much easier to achieve a thick and creamy consistency.

BERRY BLISS

SERVES 1

This glass of berry bliss is one of my go-to breakfast smoothies. I absolutely love berry smoothies; berries are packed with antioxidants, and when blended with nutrient-rich hempseeds you have a wholesome, creamy smoothie that will keep you going.

1 large ripe banana, fresh or frozen
1 cup frozen mixed berries (blueberries, strawberries, raspberries, blackberries)
2–3 tablespoons hempseeds
1 cup filtered water or coconut water
1 large medjool date, pitted

GREEN GLOW

SERVES 1

Eat your greens and glow from the inside out. This smoothie is a great way to add more spinach into your daily diet; it tastes just like tropical mango, but has lots of green power.

1 large ripe banana, fresh or frozen
1 cup frozen mango pieces
1 cup fresh spinach leaves
1 cup filtered water or coconut water
1 large medjool date, pitted
1 tablespoon chia seeds (optional)

TO MAKE THE SMOOTHIES

Place all the ingredients in a blender and blend on high speed until smooth. Pour into a large glass or jar and enjoy.

ALKALISING REFRESHER

SERVES 1

This one's an old favourite of mine; it's an incredibly refreshing smoothie and great for those who don't like to use bananas as a base. It's an alkalising glass of greens, packed with sweet apples and refreshing mint and the hydrating power of fresh cucumber and celery.

1 cup fresh spinach
handful fresh mint
1 small stalk celery
½ cup chopped cucumber
1 large medjool date, pitted
1 cup filtered water or coconut water
1 green apple, cored
1 cup ice

SPIRULINA ENERGISER

SERVES 1

I grew up on earthy green spirulina; from a young age my mum would pack the energy-boosting powder into a smoothie for my siblings and me. Spirulina, a nutrient-rich blue-green algae, is high in protein and contains a number of important nutrients, such as calcium and magnesium. Spirulina powder also works wonders as a natural food colour; use it to tint your food in wonderful shades of green.

1 large ripe banana, fresh or frozen
1 cup fresh spinach leaves
2 kiwifruit, peeled
1 orange, peeled
1 teaspoon green spirulina powder
1 large medjool date, pitted
1 cup ice
1 cup filtered water

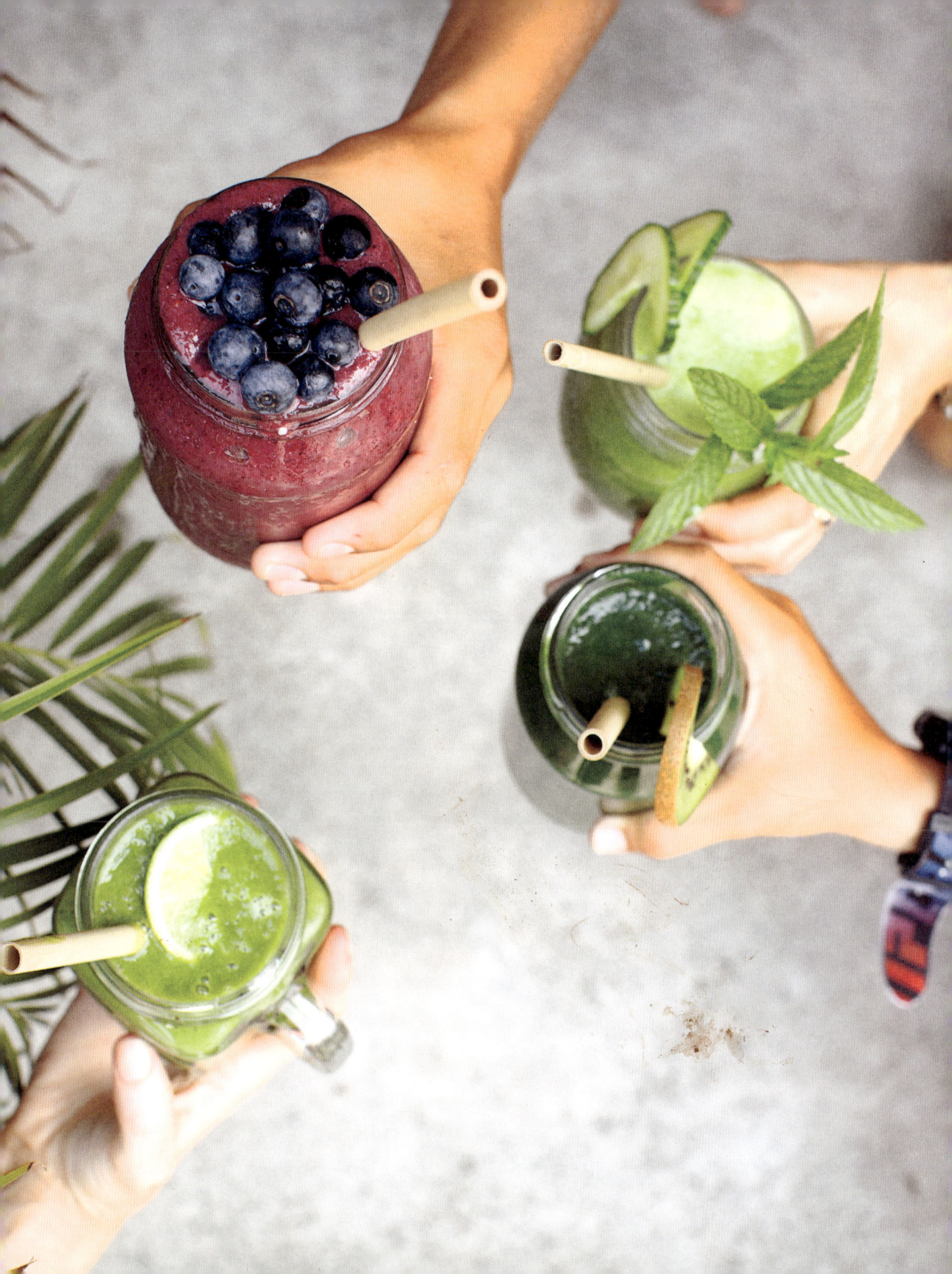

PINEAPPLE PARADISE

SERVES 1

I highly recommend this creamy pineapple blend—it truly is pure paradise in a glass. The sweet pineapple, creamy coconut and fresh ginger are such a dreamy combo —one I'm a little obsessed with.

1 cup fresh pineapple pieces
1 large ripe banana, fresh or frozen
½ cup coconut milk
½ cup filtered water
1 cm (½ in) piece fresh ginger, peeled
1 large medjool date, pitted
1 cup ice

ZESTY STRAWBERRY

SERVES 1

I go through phases with smoothies and end up having the same flavour over and over again— this one's my latest obsession. I absolutely love the zesty kick of lime with the dreamy combination of creamy strawberries, mango and banana.

1 large ripe banana, fresh or frozen
½ cup frozen strawberries
½ cup frozen mango
juice of ½ lime
1 large medjool date, pitted
2 tablespoons hempseeds
1 cup coconut water

TO MAKE THE SMOOTHIES
Place all the ingredients in a blender and blend on high speed until smooth. Pour into a large glass or jar and enjoy.

TROPICAL LOVE

SERVES 1

When we lived on the Gold Coast a few years ago, this smoothie was one of our absolute staples—especially for the boys after a long morning in the surf. With the combination of beautiful tropical flavours it makes the most refreshing glass of fruity goodness. Don't omit the ice, it's not quite the same without it.

1 large ripe banana, fresh or frozen
1 orange, peeled
1 cup fresh pineapple pieces
½ cup frozen mango pieces
1 large medjool date, pitted
1 cup coconut water
pulp of 1 passion fruit
1 cup ice

HEAVENLY HAZELNUT

SERVES 1

You will become obsessed with this smoothie. It's perfectly sweet, silky, creamy, nutty and chocolatey—a Nutella-lover's dream. Pure organic cacao powder is rich in antioxidants, iron and magnesium. Be sure to also try my absolute favourite Hemp Chocolate Shakes (see page 268) for another heavenly chocolate drink.

1 cup frozen ripe banana
2 tablespoons hempseeds
2 large medjool dates, pitted
handful hazelnuts
2 teaspoons cacao powder
¾ cup coconut water
¼ cup coconut milk
½ cup ice

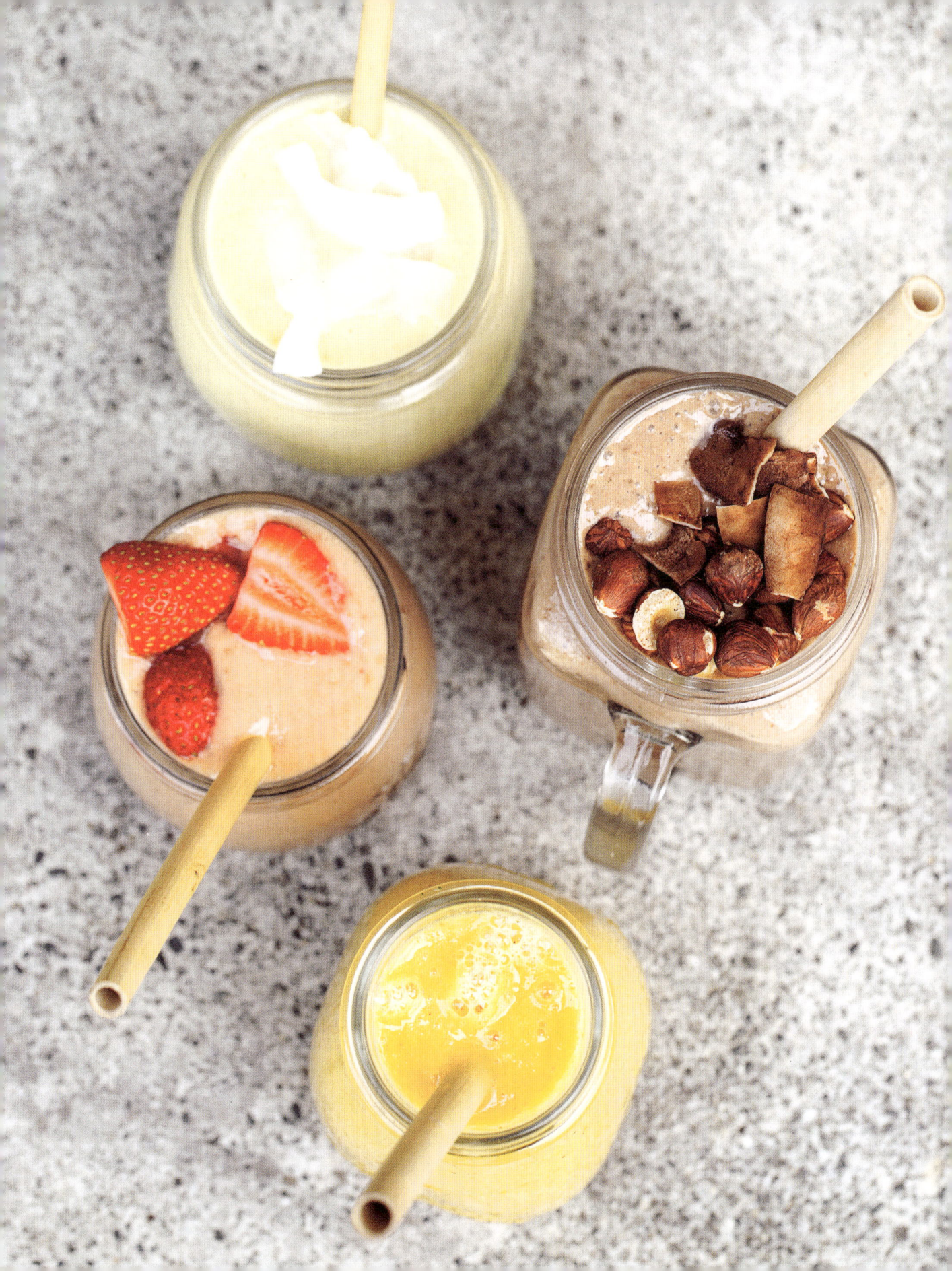

SUNRISE AÇAÍ BOWL
with GRANOLA, CACAO NIBS and FRESH FRUIT

SERVES 2

3 frozen ripe bananas
½ cup frozen blueberries
200 g (7 oz) frozen açaí
½–1 cup coconut water (depending on desired consistency)

Toppings per bowl
½ cup Chewy 'n' Nutty Vanilla Maple Granola (see page 82) or store-bought granola
1 cup fresh fruit (such as kiwifruit, banana, berries, mango)
1 tablespoon coconut flakes
1 teaspoon cacao nibs

Açaí bowls are the perfect way to refresh and refuel and are a long-time family favourite; wherever we travel as a family, we are almost guaranteed to find a nourishing açaí to cool our taste buds. Açaí is a powerful reddish-purple berry, incredibly rich in antioxidants. It's cultivated from the açaí palm tree, which is native to Central and South America, and usually comes in a frozen purée or powder form. It can be found in some supermarkets, most health food stores, or, alternatively, ordered online.

Place all the ingredients in a high-powered blender and let sit for at least 5 minutes, to allow the fruit to slightly defrost. This is an important step as it will make it easier for you to obtain a thick and creamy blend, using little liquid.

Start by blending on a low speed, using a blending stick to help assist with moving the fruit, then slowly increase to a high speed as the fruit begins to easily blend. You will probably need to stop the blender, mix and blend again, until you get a thick, creamy swirl.

Transfer into 2 serving bowls and arrange the toppings on top. Serve immediately.

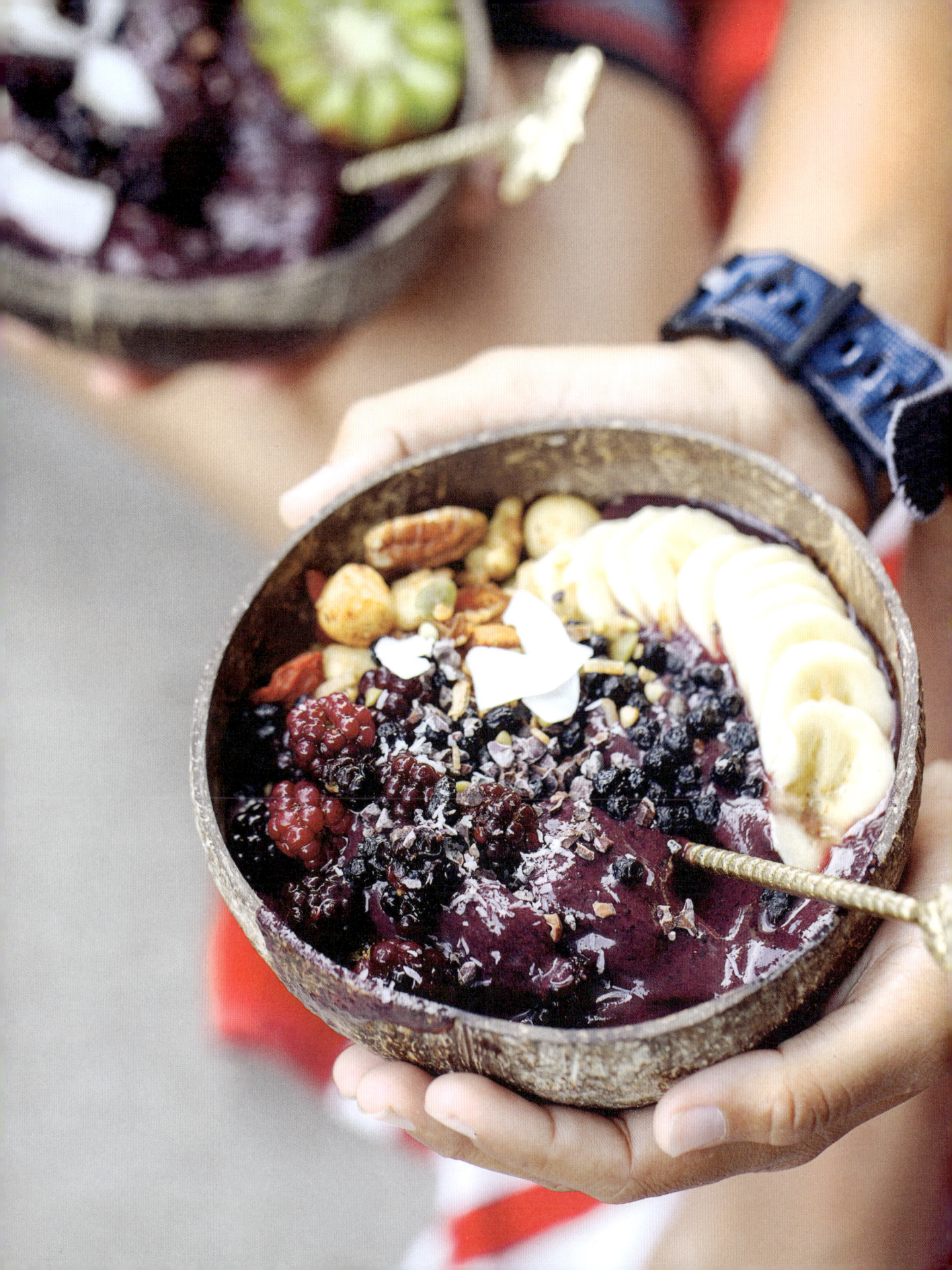

MANGO MADNESS BOWL
with GRANOLA, COCONUT and FRESH FRUIT

SERVES 2

3 frozen ripe bananas
3 cups frozen mango
juice of 1 large lime
1 tablespoon pure maple syrup (optional)
½–1 cup coconut water (depending on desired consistency)
pinch of ground turmeric (optional for colour)

Toppings per bowl
½ cup Chewy 'n' Nutty Vanilla Maple Granola (see page 82) or store-bought granola
1 cup fresh fruit (mango, banana coins)
1 tablespoon shredded coconut
lime wedges

Kick-start your day in a nourishing way with this refreshingly creamy mango smoothie bowl. The squeeze of lime takes this bowl to a whole new level, while a touch of turmeric will really help to pop that naturally vibrant colour. This magical fruity bowl is both highly nutritious and delicious; perfect for any time of the day, served with all of your favourite toppings.

Place all the ingredients in a high-powered blender and let sit for at least 5 minutes, to allow the fruit to slightly defrost. This is an important step as it will make it easier for you to obtain a thick and creamy blend, using little liquid.

Start by blending on a low speed, using a blending stick to help assist with moving the fruit, then slowly increase to a high speed as the fruit begins to easily blend. You will probably need to stop the blender, mix and blend again, until you get a thick, creamy swirl.

Transfer into 2 serving bowls and arrange the toppings on top. Serve immediately.

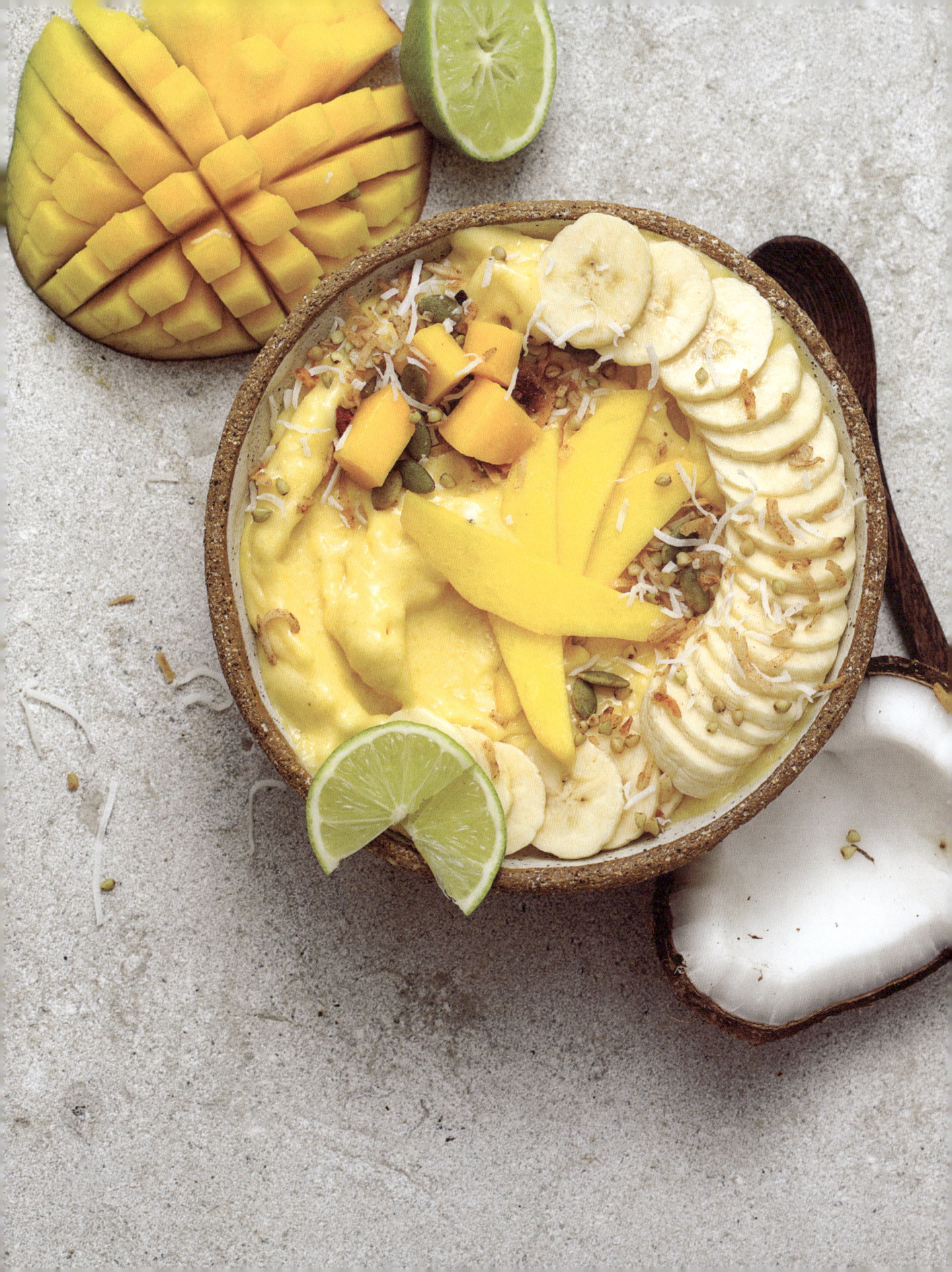

SWEET STRAWBERRY FIELDS
with FRESH STRAWBERRIES and COCONUT

SERVES 2

3 frozen ripe bananas
3 cups frozen strawberries
¼ cup coconut yoghurt
¼ cup hempseeds
½–1 cup coconut water (depending on desired consistency)
1 tablespoon pure maple syrup (optional)

Toppings per bowl
¾ cup fresh strawberries, sliced
½ teaspoon desiccated coconut

This creamy smoothie bowl is a sweet strawberry sensation. It's absolutely dreamy with the perfect balance of yoghurt flavour and texture, from both the blended hempseeds and the coconut yoghurt.

Place all the ingredients in a high-powered blender and let sit for at least 5 minutes, to allow the fruit to slightly defrost. This is an important step as it will make it easier for you to obtain a thick and creamy blend, using little liquid.

Start by blending on a low speed, using a blending stick to help assist with moving the fruit, then slowly increase to a high speed as the fruit begins to easily blend. You will probably need to stop the blender, mix and blend again, until you get a thick, creamy swirl.

Transfer into 2 serving bowls and arrange the toppings on top. Serve immediately.

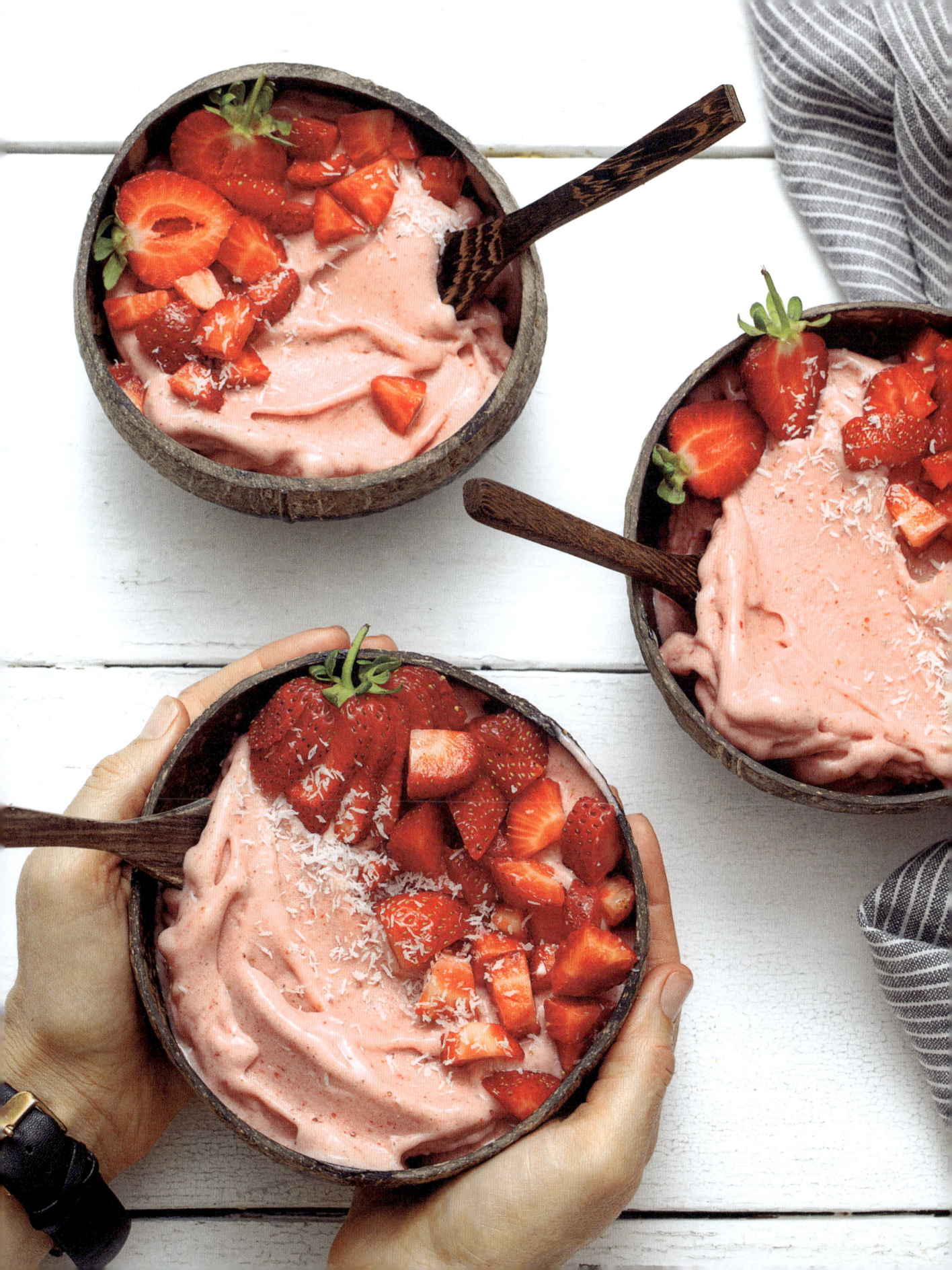

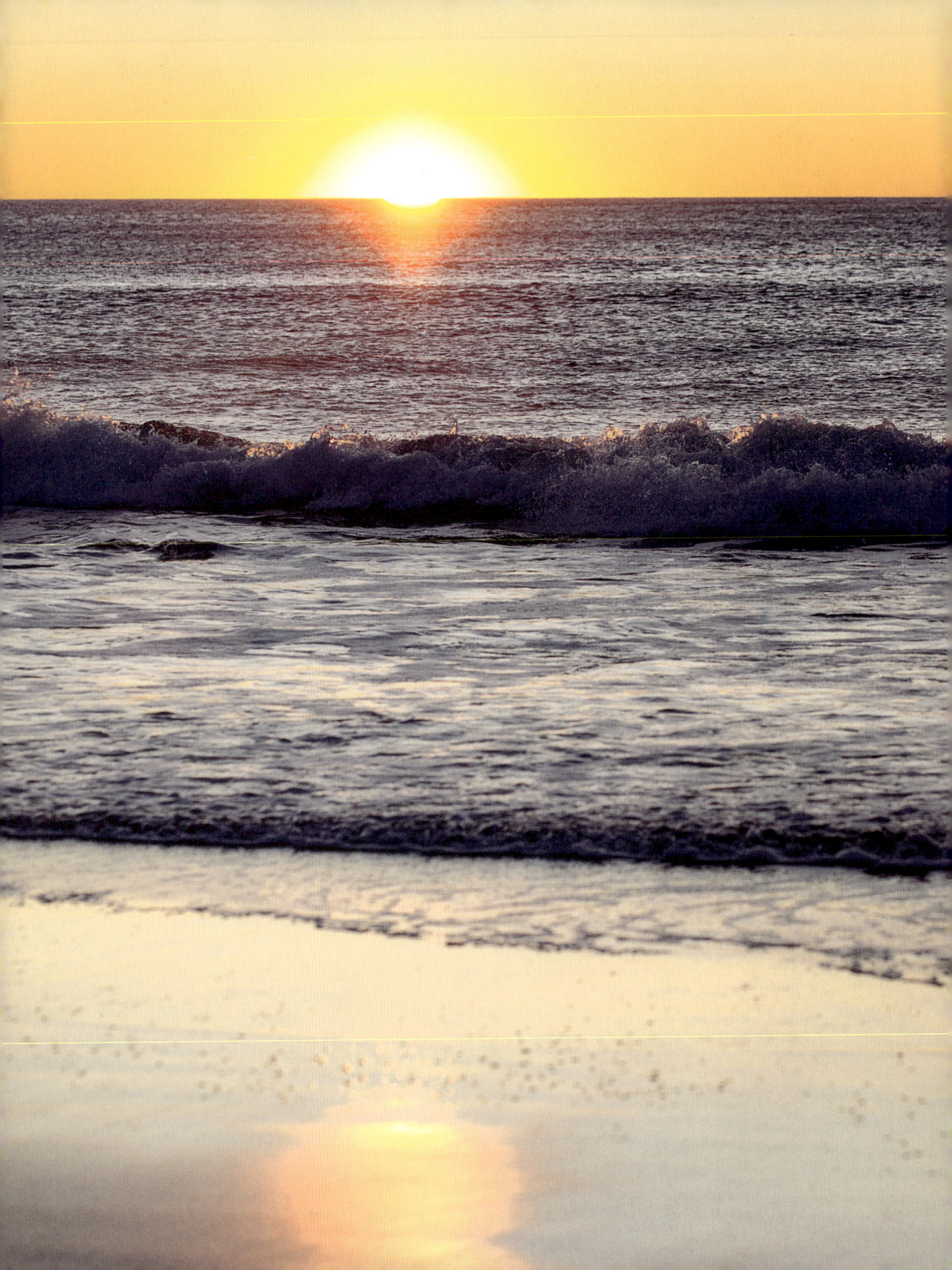

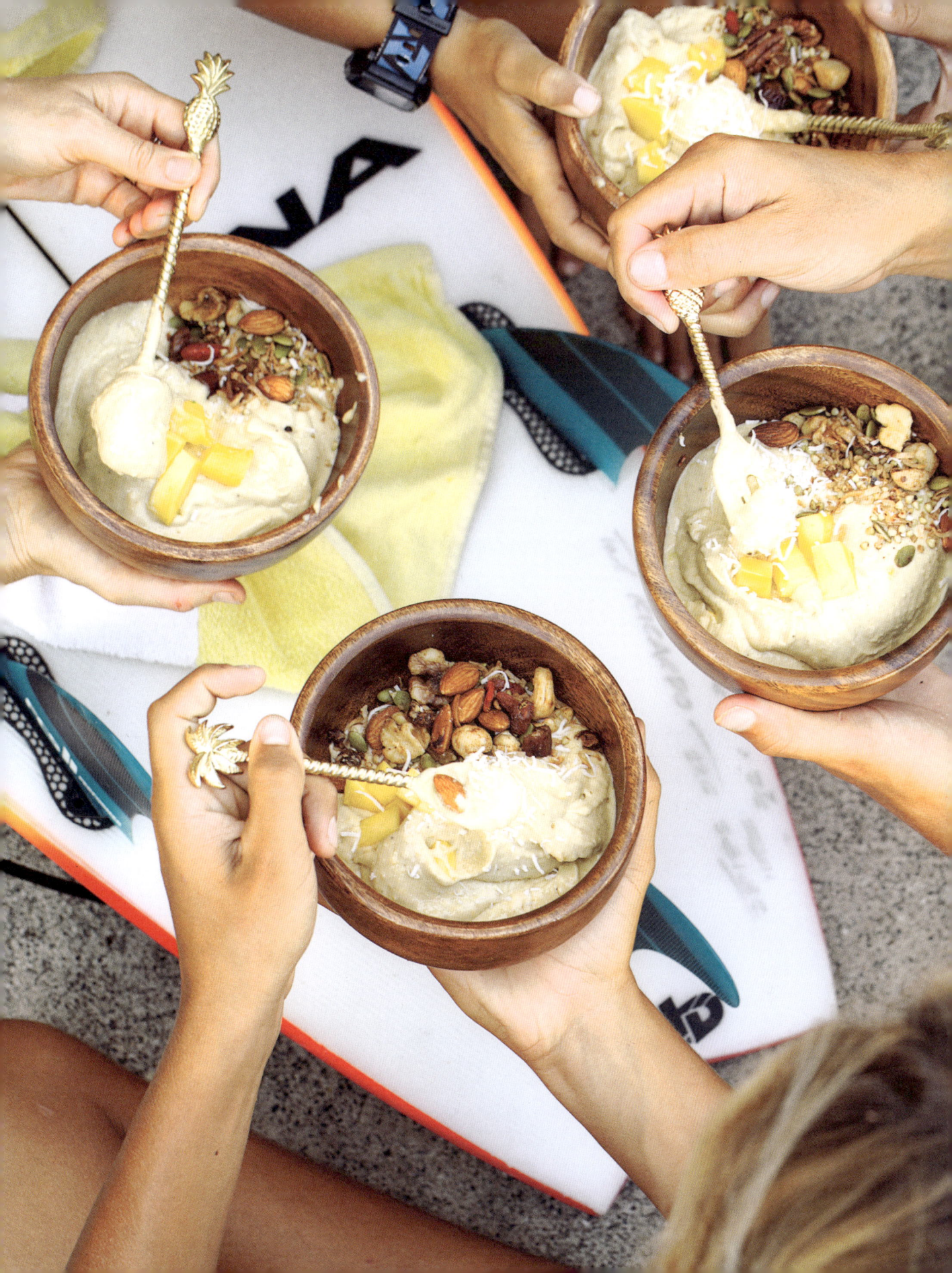

RASPBERRY and MANGO FRUITY WHIP

SERVES 2–3

2 frozen ripe bananas
1 cup frozen mango
1 cup frozen raspberries (or strawberries)
¼–½ cup coconut water
1 tablespoon pure maple syrup (optional)

Toppings (optional)
frozen raspberries
hempseeds

When I was detoxing, I enjoyed this beautiful combination almost every single morning for breakfast. I loved the sweet flavours and the thick consistency. For a zesty kick, add in a squeeze of lemon or lime juice. It's amazing with hempseeds and a little more coconut water to create a creamy, smoothie-like consistency, and you could also replace the raspberries with strawberries for another beautiful blend.

Start by blending on a low speed, using a blending stick to help assist with moving the fruit, then slowly increase to a high speed as the fruit begins to easily blend. You will probably need to stop the blender, mix and blend again, until you get a thick, creamy swirl.

Transfer into serving bowls or glasses, and sprinkle with optional toppings. Serve immediately.

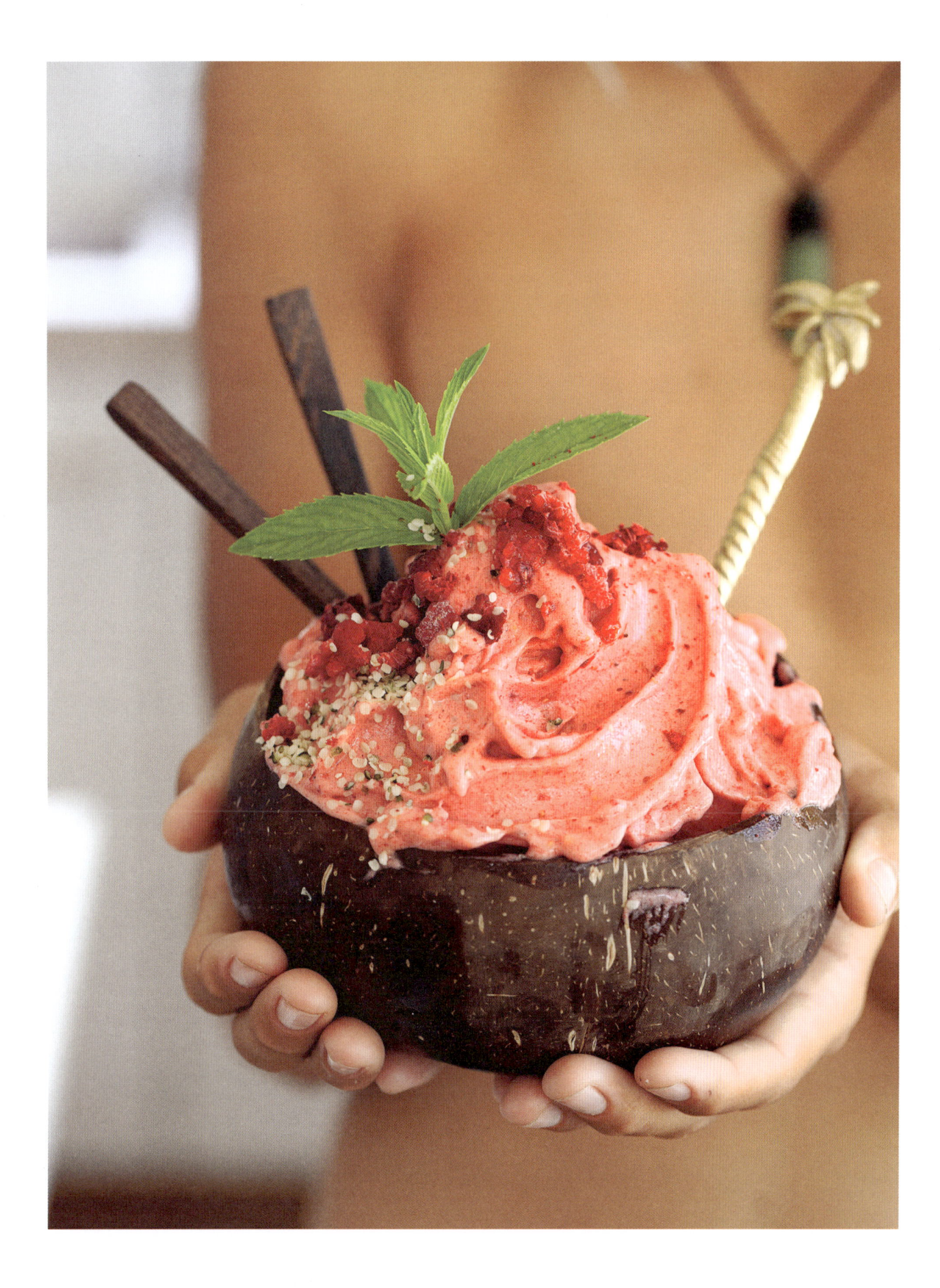

AVOCADO, LEMON and PISTACHIO FRUITY WHIP

SERVES 2–3

2 frozen ripe bananas
2 frozen ripe avocados
2 tablespoons lemon juice
1 tablespoon pure maple syrup (optional)
¼–½ cup coconut milk

Toppings (optional)
pistachios
sprig of fresh mint

Avocados are amazing for creating a really creamy smoothie or fruity whip, and they taste divine too. This flavour combo is a must-try and even better finished with a few crunchy pistachios.

Place all the ingredients in a high-powered blender (or a food processor) and let sit for about 5 minutes, to allow the fruit to slightly defrost. This is an important step as it will make it easier for you to obtain a thick and creamy blend, using little to no liquid.

Start by blending on a low speed, using a blending stick to help assist with moving the fruit, then slowly increase to a high speed as the fruit begins to easily blend. You will probably need to stop the blender, mix and blend again, until you get a thick, creamy swirl.

Transfer into serving bowls or glasses, and sprinkle with optional toppings. Serve immediately.

TROPICAL PASSION FRUIT FRUITY WHIP

SERVES 2–3

2 frozen bananas
2 cups frozen mango
⅓ cup passion fruit pulp
¼–½ cup coconut water

Toppings (optional)
passion fruit pulp
coconut flakes

Cool your taste buds while recreating those tropical vibes with this sweet passion fruit whip. I'm the biggest fan of passion fruit and absolutely love a mono meal of about twenty in a row. This beautiful creamy whip makes a perfect breakfast or snack idea, one your body will love you for.

Start by blending on a low speed, using a blending stick to help assist with moving the fruit, then slowly increase to a high speed as the fruit begins to easily blend. You will probably need to stop the blender, mix and blend again, until you get a thick, creamy swirl.

Transfer into serving bowls or glasses, and sprinkle with optional toppings. Serve immediately.

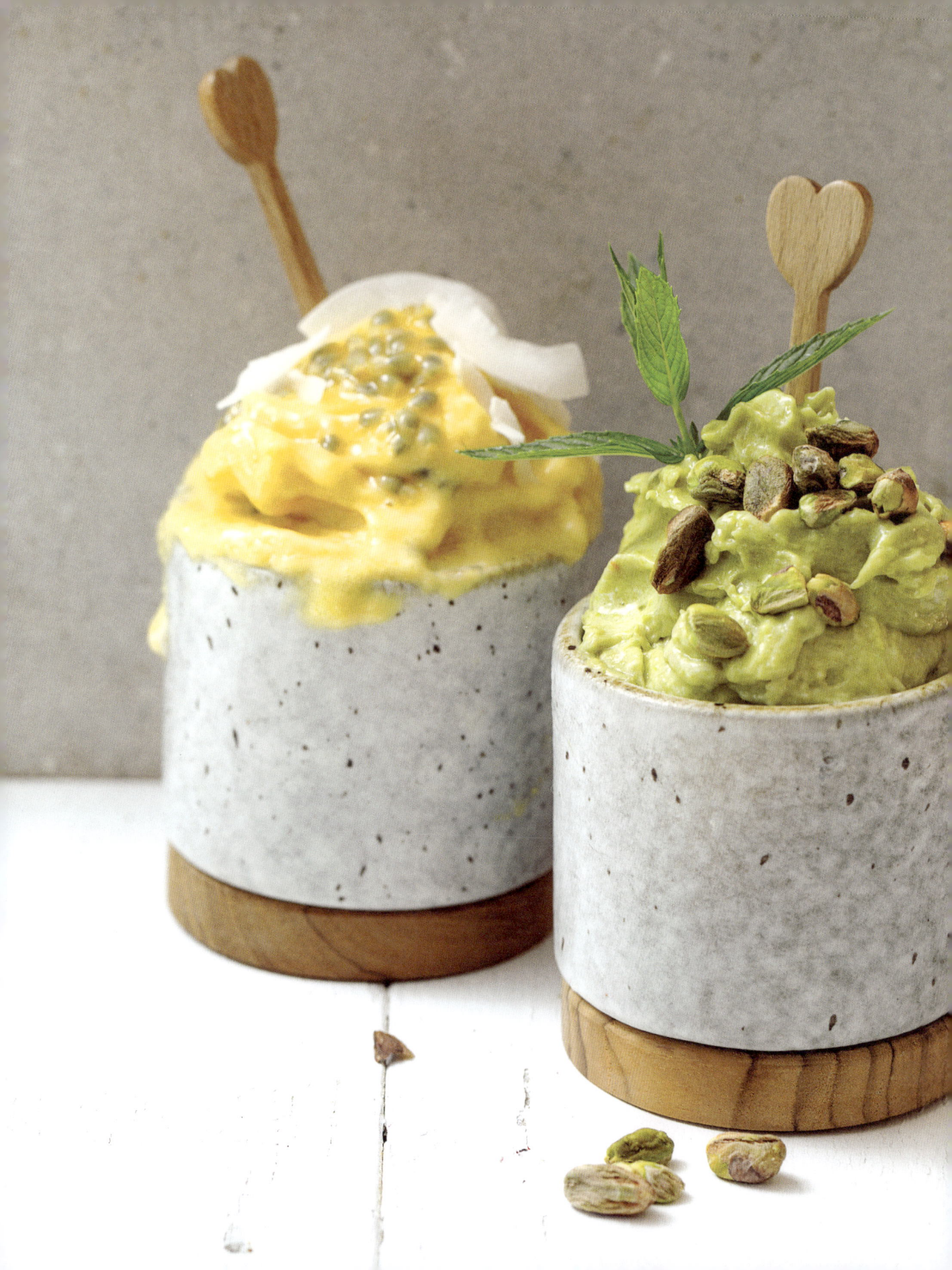

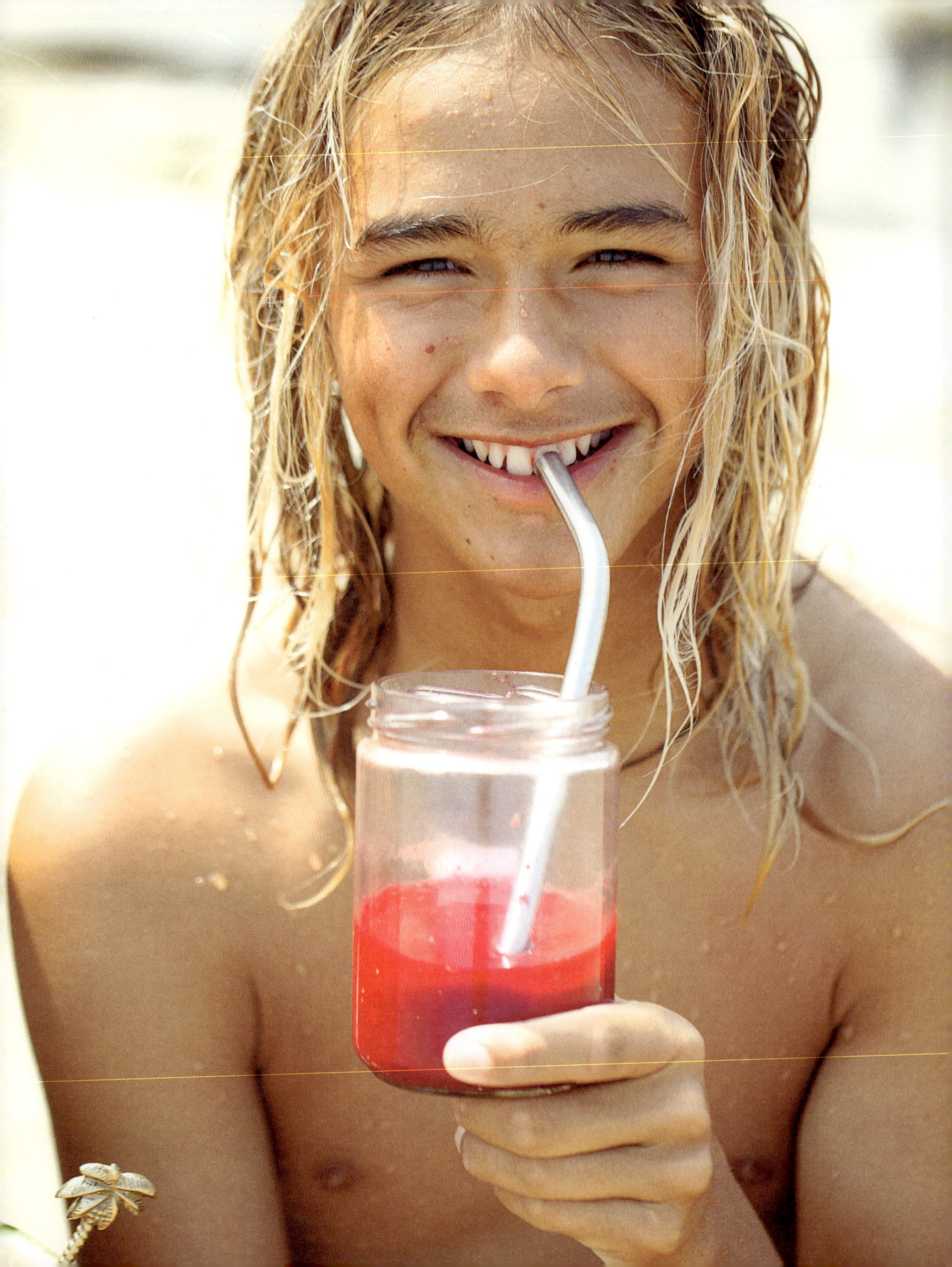

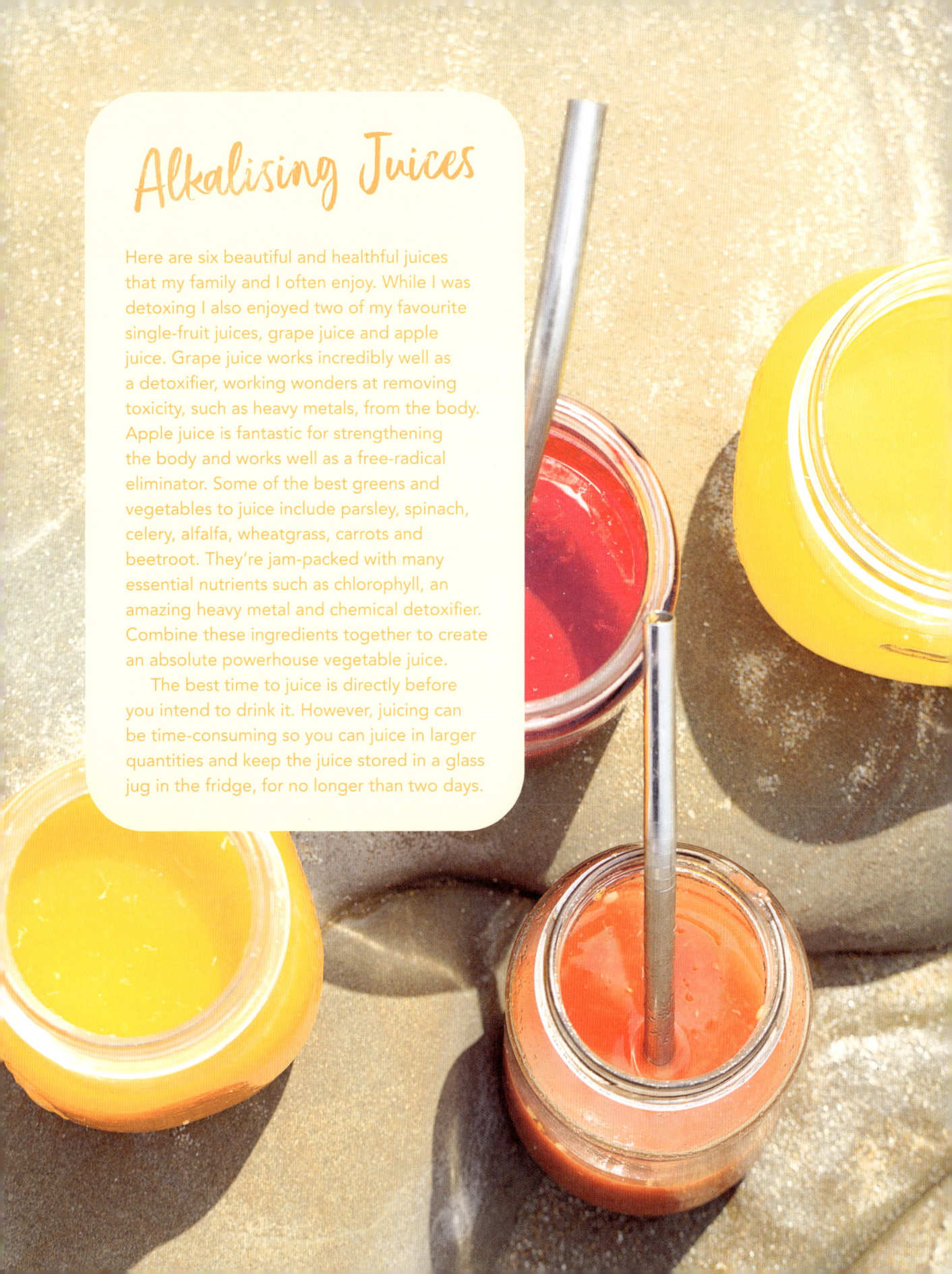

Alkalising Juices

Here are six beautiful and healthful juices that my family and I often enjoy. While I was detoxing I also enjoyed two of my favourite single-fruit juices, grape juice and apple juice. Grape juice works incredibly well as a detoxifier, working wonders at removing toxicity, such as heavy metals, from the body. Apple juice is fantastic for strengthening the body and works well as a free-radical eliminator. Some of the best greens and vegetables to juice include parsley, spinach, celery, alfalfa, wheatgrass, carrots and beetroot. They're jam-packed with many essential nutrients such as chlorophyll, an amazing heavy metal and chemical detoxifier. Combine these ingredients together to create an absolute powerhouse vegetable juice.

The best time to juice is directly before you intend to drink it. However, juicing can be time-consuming so you can juice in larger quantities and keep the juice stored in a glass jug in the fridge, for no longer than two days.

WATERMELON AND MINT

MAKES 1 LARGE GLASS

Watermelon juice is one of my favourite juices; it's unbelievably hydrating and incredibly alkalising, making this a glass of pure goodness—perfect on a hot day, served with a handful of ice.

500 g (1 lb 2 oz) watermelon flesh, cut into chunks to fit juicer
small handful mint

GREEN GOODNESS

MAKES 1 LARGE GLASS

Eat more greens! This powerhouse of a juice provides a perfectly subtle way to pack in more greens, without that overpowering, earthy taste. The pear and apple provide all the sweetness you need to balance out the flavours.

1 pear
1 apple
2 large stalks celery
½ large cucumber
2 large handfuls fresh spinach

VITAMIN C BLAST

MAKES 1 LARGE GLASS

If you're after a blast of vitamin C, this super-sweet juice will provide you with just that. Another one of my favourite combos. With an added handful of ice, this vibrant juice will cool your taste buds and sweeten your day.

½ fresh pineapple, skin removed (about 400 g / 14 oz)
2 oranges, peeled
½ lemon, peeled

CITRUS TURMERIC JUICE

MAKES 1 LARGE GLASS

This is a favourite combination of mine; I love the super-sweet carrots and oranges, with the tangy lemon and earthy turmeric to match. Turmeric works wonders as a natural anti-inflammatory but can also be left out for a sweeter juice.

4 oranges, peeled
4 carrots
1 small lemon, peeled
1 cm (½ in) piece fresh turmeric

REVITALISE JUICE

MAKES 1 LARGE GLASS

Vibrant in colour, this popular combination is a cleansing glass of goodness; one I often give to my boys if they're feeling run-down. It's naturally sweet, with a slight hint of spicy ginger.

1 large red apple
1 large orange, peeled
1 small–medium beetroot
2 large carrots
1 cm (½ in) piece fresh ginger

SWEET CELERY JUICE

MAKES 1 LARGE GLASS

Celery juice is having a massive movement in the health world. This juice has the added sweetness of apples and fresh ginger to liven it up.

2 large green apples
5 stalks celery
1 cm (½ in) piece fresh ginger

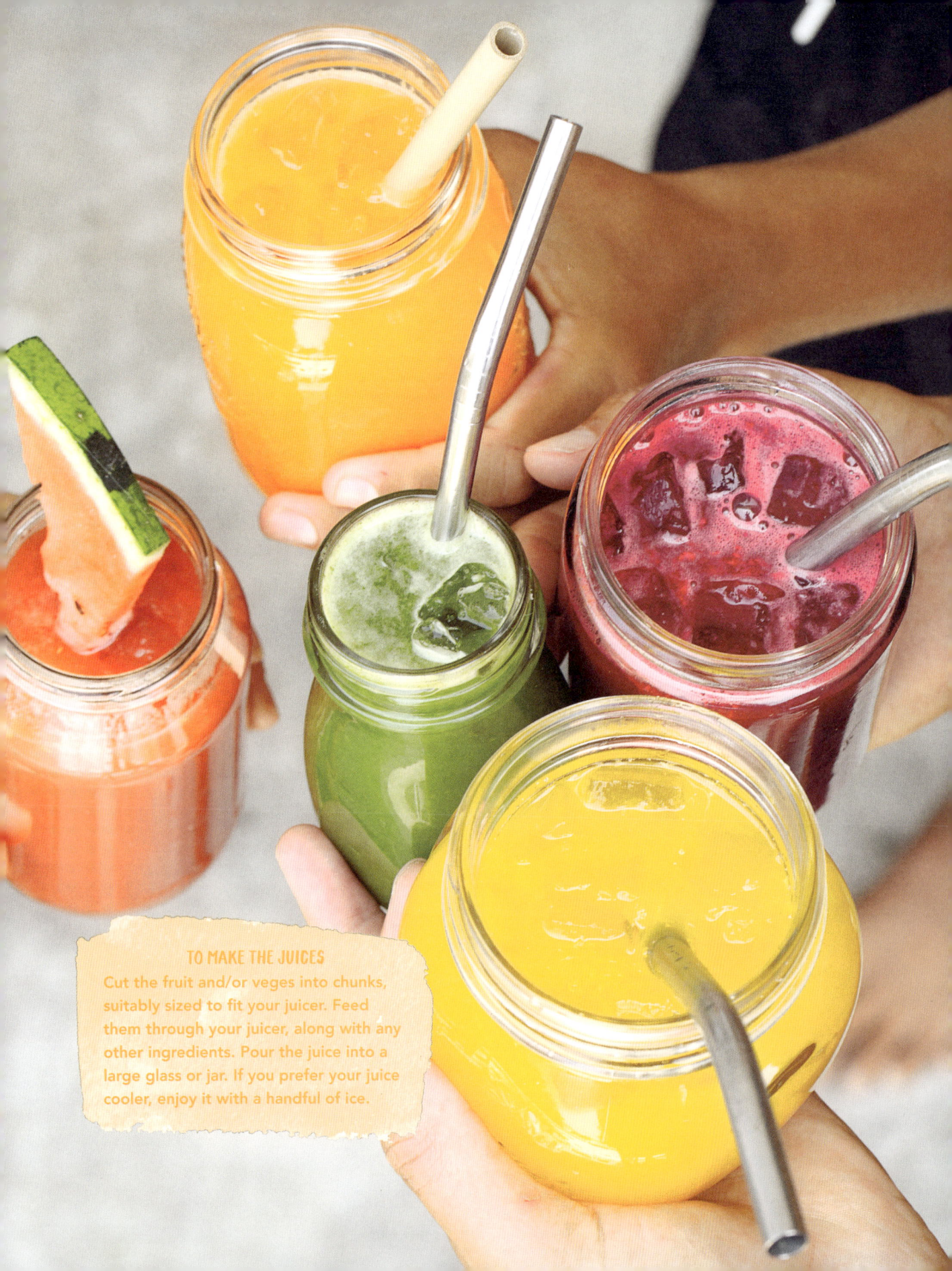

TO MAKE THE JUICES
Cut the fruit and/or veges into chunks, suitably sized to fit your juicer. Feed them through your juicer, along with any other ingredients. Pour the juice into a large glass or jar. If you prefer your juice cooler, enjoy it with a handful of ice.

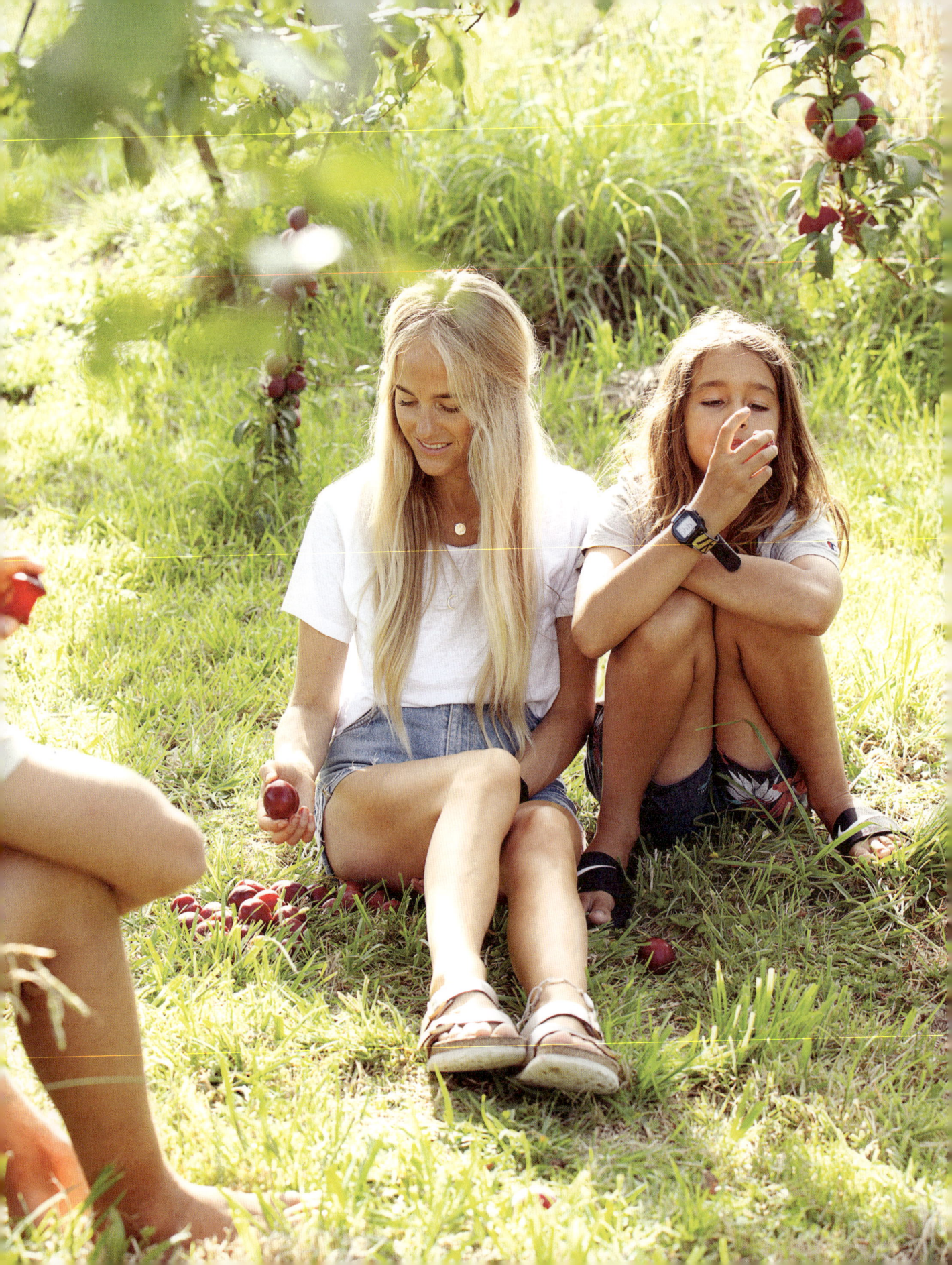

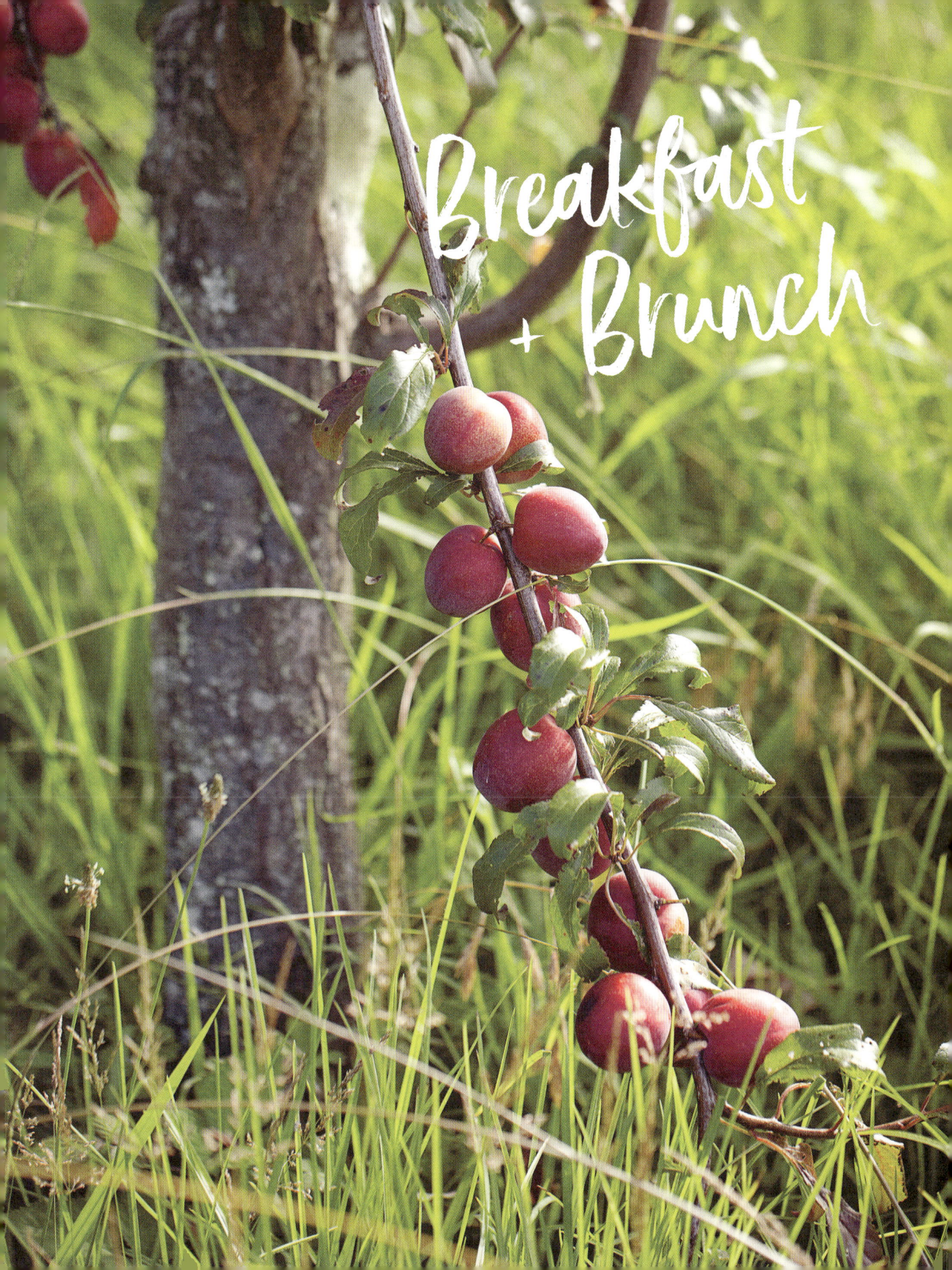

Breakfast + Brunch

Breakfast + Brunch

Breakfast is an important meal as it breaks your overnight fast, replenishes your glucose levels and helps to set you up for the day ahead. While I always begin my day with a large smoothie (see pages 52–66 for recipes) or an alkalising bowl of fresh seasonal fruit, this chapter provides you with recipes for other breakfast alternatives, which also make for great snacks throughout the day. It's time to ditch the unhealthy, highly processed foods, such as refined sugary breads and cereals, and begin your day with energy-boosting fresh fruit and healthful wholefoods. It will truly make a world of difference to the day ahead.

Another fantastic breakfast (or lunch or snack) is a mono meal of fresh seasonal fruit. A mono meal is a meal consisting of just one food, typically a raw fruit or vegetable, eaten in a sufficient quantity to provide fullness and satisfaction. A mono meal, such as a bowl of melons, mangoes or oranges, can result in better food digestion and nutrient absorption than eating a combination of different foods, because it allows the food to be efficiently digested by engaging in only those specific digestive processes needed for that one particular food. Proper food combining is a really interesting topic, one I recommend researching further, especially for anyone with a sluggish digestive system. Mono meals of fresh fruit are a big part of my daily meals. It may sound a little boring to consume one single fruit as a meal, but I love the simplicity of it, and I can absolutely feel the benefits. I take advantage of seasonal fruits; this way I can eat them in abundance—some of my favourites in New Zealand are feijoas, watermelons, navel oranges, grapes and berries. Can you imagine how excited I get when travelling to tropical countries? I could just about live on pink dragon fruit, mangoes and papaya.

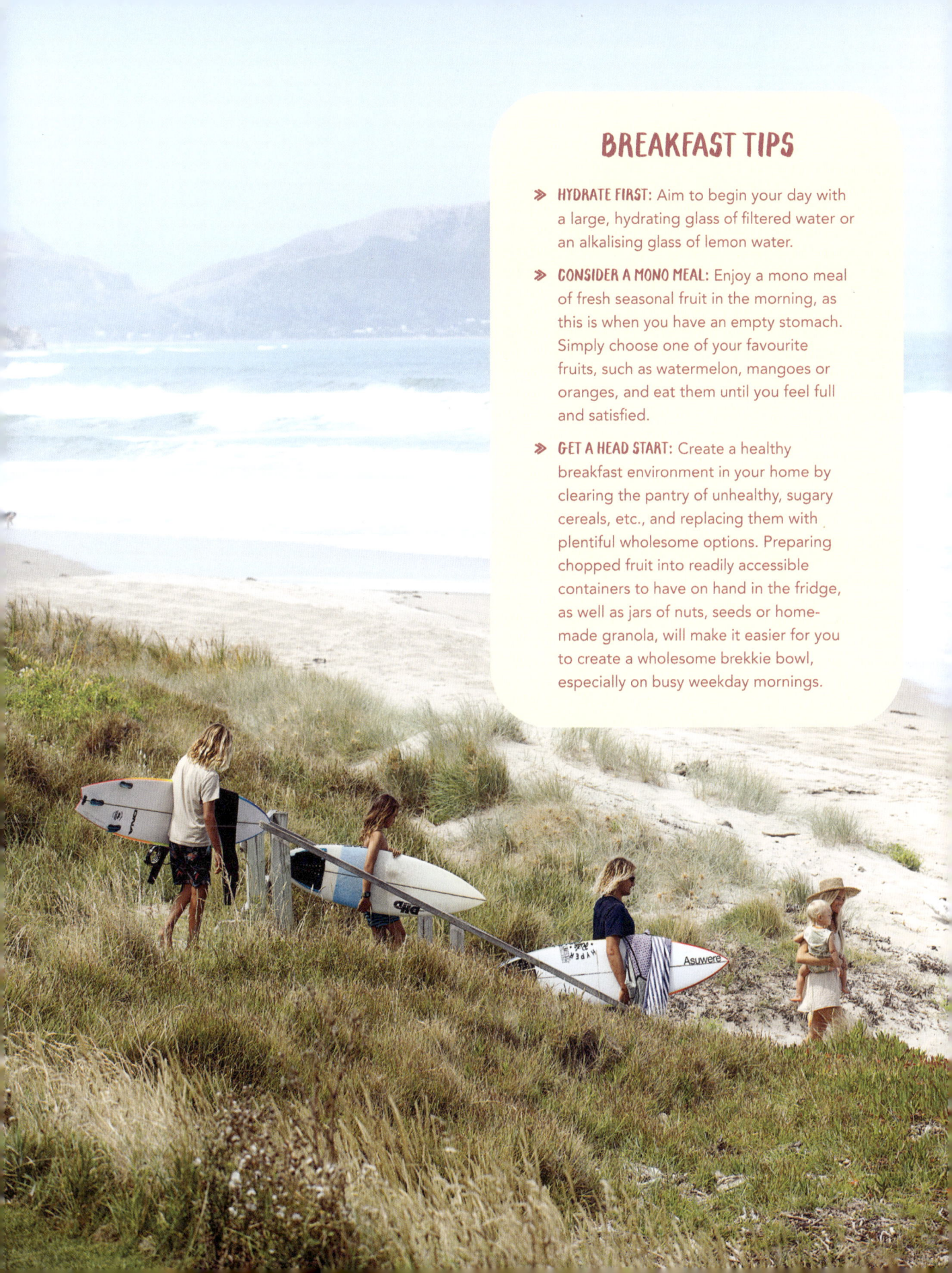

BREAKFAST TIPS

» **HYDRATE FIRST:** Aim to begin your day with a large, hydrating glass of filtered water or an alkalising glass of lemon water.

» **CONSIDER A MONO MEAL:** Enjoy a mono meal of fresh seasonal fruit in the morning, as this is when you have an empty stomach. Simply choose one of your favourite fruits, such as watermelon, mangoes or oranges, and eat them until you feel full and satisfied.

» **GET A HEAD START:** Create a healthy breakfast environment in your home by clearing the pantry of unhealthy, sugary cereals, etc., and replacing them with plentiful wholesome options. Preparing chopped fruit into readily accessible containers to have on hand in the fridge, as well as jars of nuts, seeds or home-made granola, will make it easier for you to create a wholesome brekkie bowl, especially on busy weekday mornings.

VERY BERRY ANTIOXIDANT CHIA PUDDING

MAKES 4 CUPS

1½ cups frozen mixed berries
1½ cups frozen raspberries
2 cups plant milk of your choice
2 tablespoons pure maple syrup
½ teaspoon pure vanilla extract or paste
½ cup chia seeds

To serve (optional)
fresh mixed berries
granola
coconut flakes

Chia seeds are a fantastic source of calcium, fibre, protein and omega-3 fatty acids, making them an awesome addition to a plant-based diet. This beautiful antioxidant pudding is a really simple recipe that can be made the night before eating; it makes a great up-and-go brekkie or wholesome snack idea, and is amazing served with fresh seasonal berries, granola and a dollop of almond butter.

Place all the ingredients in a large jar (or bowl). Secure the lid and shake well to combine. Leave for 5–10 minutes, then shake or stir again, ensuring the ingredients are well combined,

Place in the fridge to set overnight, or for at least 2 hours.

Serve alone or topped with berries, granola and coconut flakes.

Store in an airtight container in the fridge for up to 5 days.

NOTE: Place the mixture in ice block moulds and freeze for berry ice blocks.

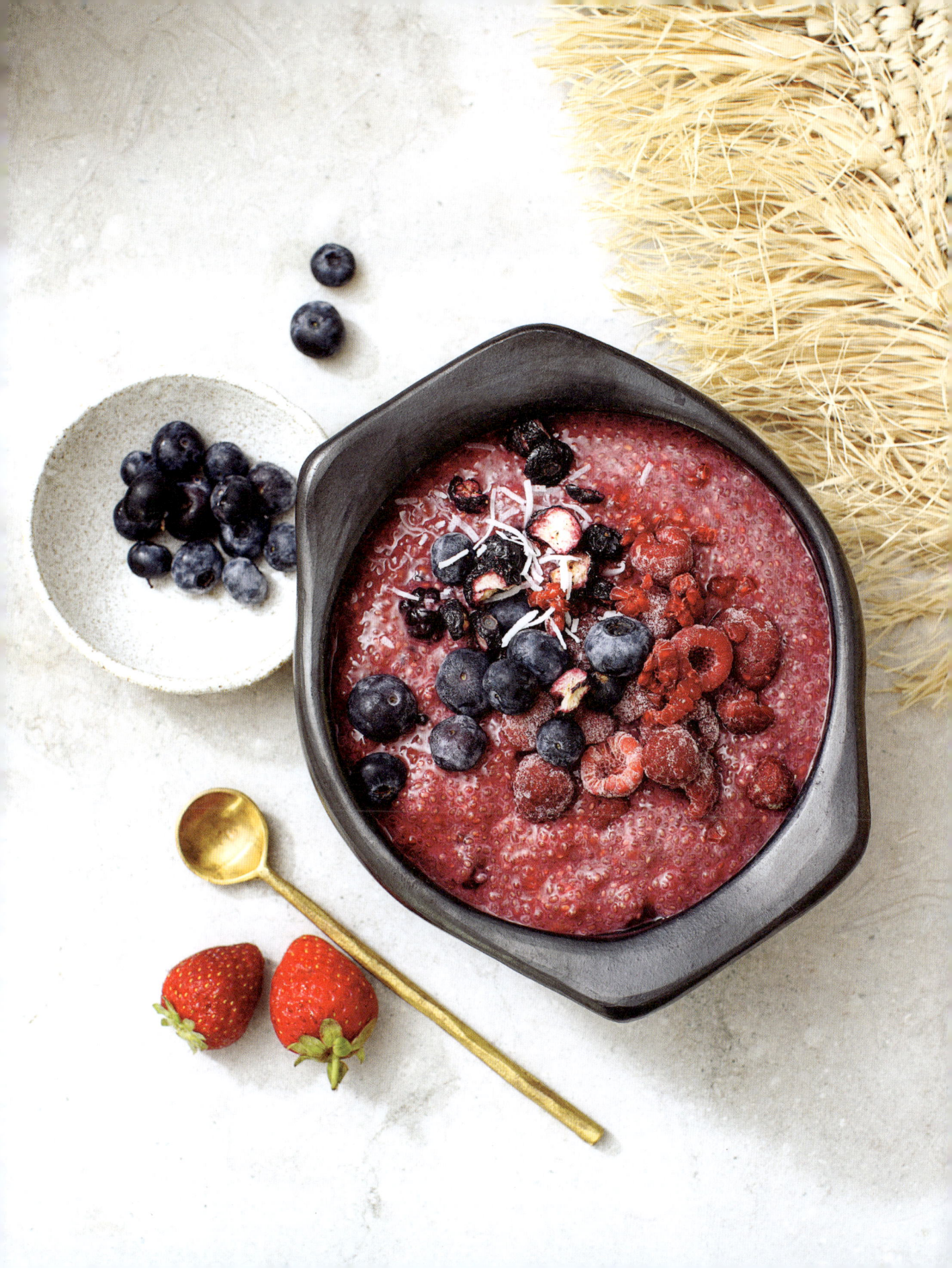

RAW ZESTY HEMP 'NOLA

MAKES 4 CUPS

1½ cups dried figs
1 cup medjool dates, pitted
¼ packed cup orange zest
1 cup gluten-free oats
1 cup desiccated coconut
¼ teaspoon ground ginger
⅓ cup hempseeds

This chunky raw granola is really quick to make, provides you with ample energy and is incredibly versatile. Simply throw it over some fresh seasonal fruit, use it as a smoothie bowl topper (see pages 56–66) or lunch-box filler, roll it into bliss balls (see page 236) or grab a handful on the go. The figs and citrus are a beautiful combination of sweet and zesty flavours with a slightly tropical feel. Figs are one of my favourite dried fruits to snack on; they're highly alkalising, super-sweet and really addictive.

Place all the ingredients in a food processor and blend and pulse for about 15 seconds, until all the ingredients are broken down into the desired consistency. Combine the mixture together with your hands if needed, to create larger and chunkier pieces.

Store in an airtight jar in the fridge for up to 2 weeks.

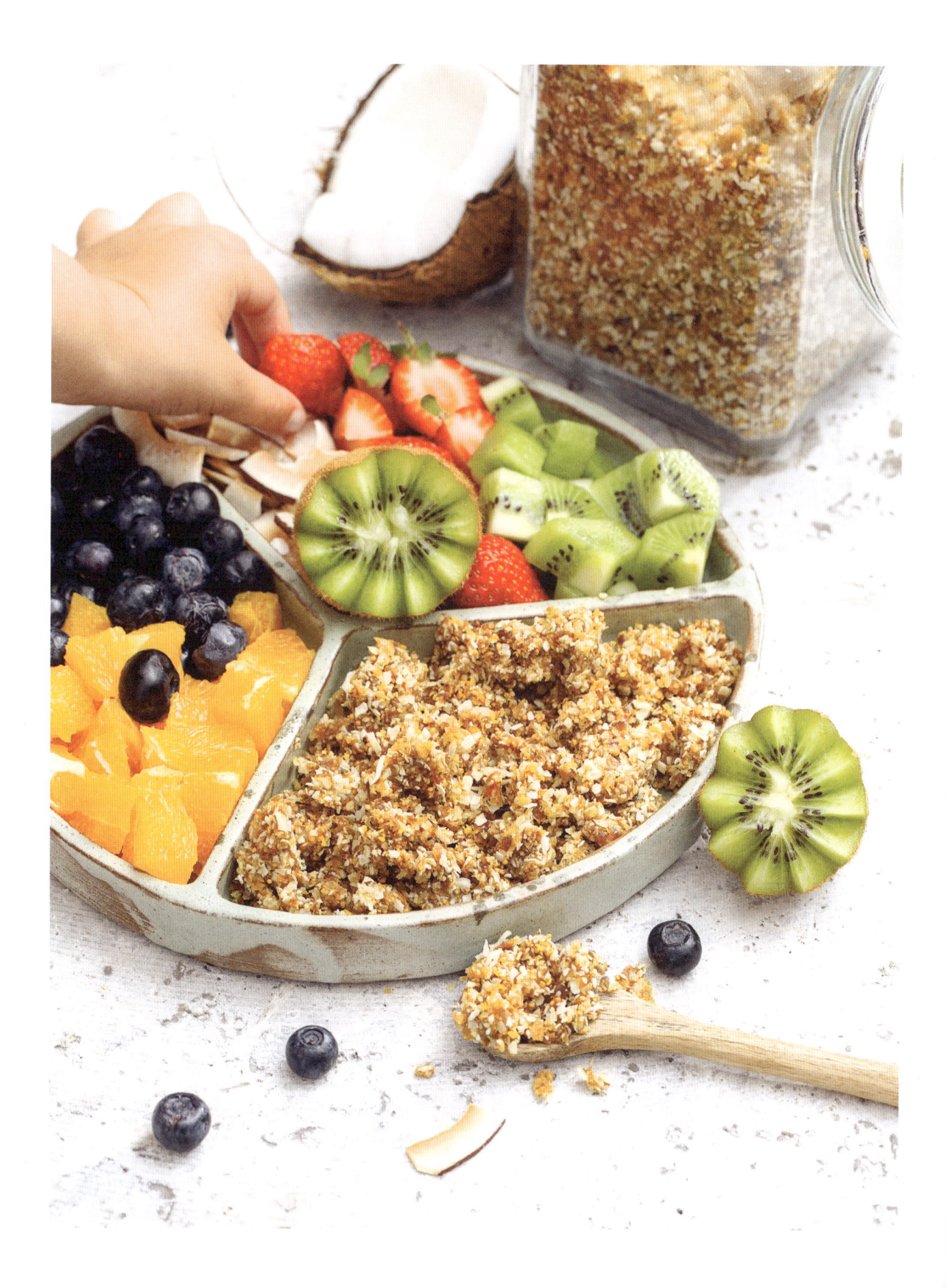

MANGO, HEMP and CHIA YOGHURT

MAKES 4 CUPS

3 cups frozen mango pieces
400 ml (14 fl oz) can coconut milk
¾ cup rice milk (or any other plant milk)
¼ cup hempseeds
2 tablespoons pure maple syrup
½ cup chia seeds

To serve (optional)
fresh fruit
coconut flakes

This creamy mango bowl of goodness makes for a beautiful on-the-go brekkie or snack idea. It's our family's version of mango yoghurt, a nutritious alternative to dairy; perfect eaten alone or topped with fresh fruit and coconut flakes. Hemp and chia seeds are two of my favourite everyday superfoods that provide a long list of nutrients including fibre, amino acids and essential fatty acids. I often make a batch on a Sunday evening, as it makes for a healthy addition to the boys' lunches for the week ahead.

Place the mango, coconut milk, rice milk, hempseeds and maple syrup in a blender and blend for about 30 seconds until smooth.

Transfer to a large bowl. Add the chia seeds and stir to combine. Leave for 5–10 minutes, then stir again.

Place in the fridge overnight to set, or for at least 2 hours.

Serve alone or as a parfait with fresh fruit and a sprinkle of shredded coconut.

Store in a sealed container in the fridge for up to 5 days.

NOTE: Place the mixture in ice block moulds and freeze for mango ice blocks.

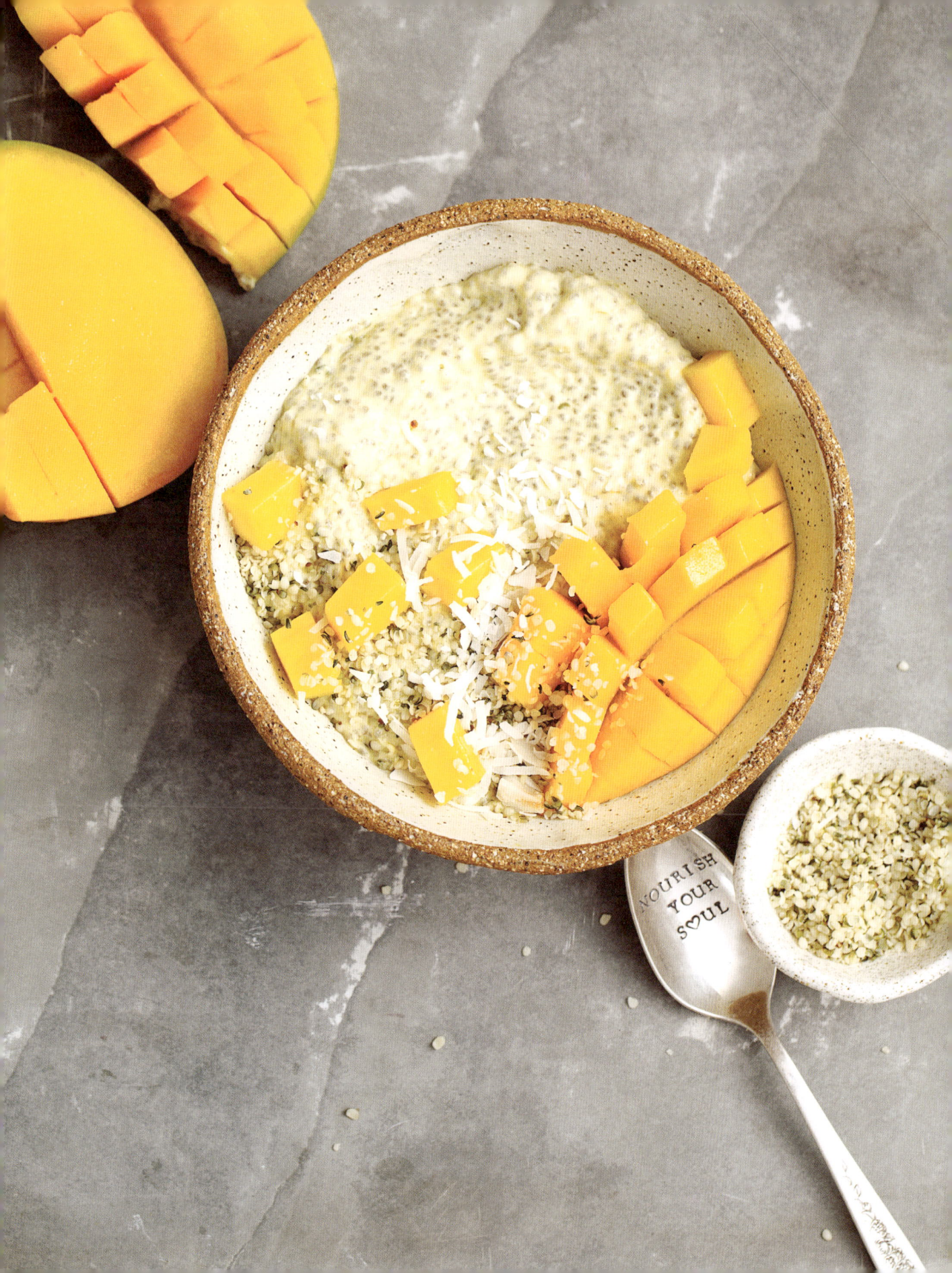

CHEWY 'N' NUTTY VANILLA MAPLE GRANOLA

MAKES 6 CUPS

- 10 medjool dates, pitted and finely chopped
- 3 cups mixed nuts (almonds, walnuts, pecans, hazelnuts)
- ½ cup pumpkin seeds
- ⅓ cup buckwheat grouts
- 1 cup shredded coconut
- 2 teaspoons pure vanilla extract
- 1 tablespoon lemon zest
- 1 teaspoon ground cinnamon
- ½ teaspoon mixed spice
- 1 tablespoon coconut oil
- 3–4 tablespoons pure maple syrup (depending on your desired sweetness)
- 1 cup goji berries (optional)

A nice granola is great to have on hand for a quick brekkie, snack or even dessert. A good way to make this recipe more economical is to visit your local bulk-bin store; this way you can purchase each ingredient in the smaller quantities you need. This is a beautiful granola with sweet chewiness from the dates and lots of crunch from the nuts. Enjoy served over fresh seasonal fruit, coconut yoghurt or as a topping on smoothie bowls.

Preheat the oven to 160°C (325°F) fan bake. Line a large baking tray with baking paper.

Place all the ingredients except the goji berries in a bowl and mix to combine. Tip onto the baking tray and spread out in a single layer. Bake for about 12–15 minutes, tossing once or twice, until golden and crunchy. Watch closely for the last few minutes as it will burn quickly.

Let cool before mixing through the goji berries, if desired, and transfer to a large jar.

Store in an airtight jar/container for up to 2 weeks.

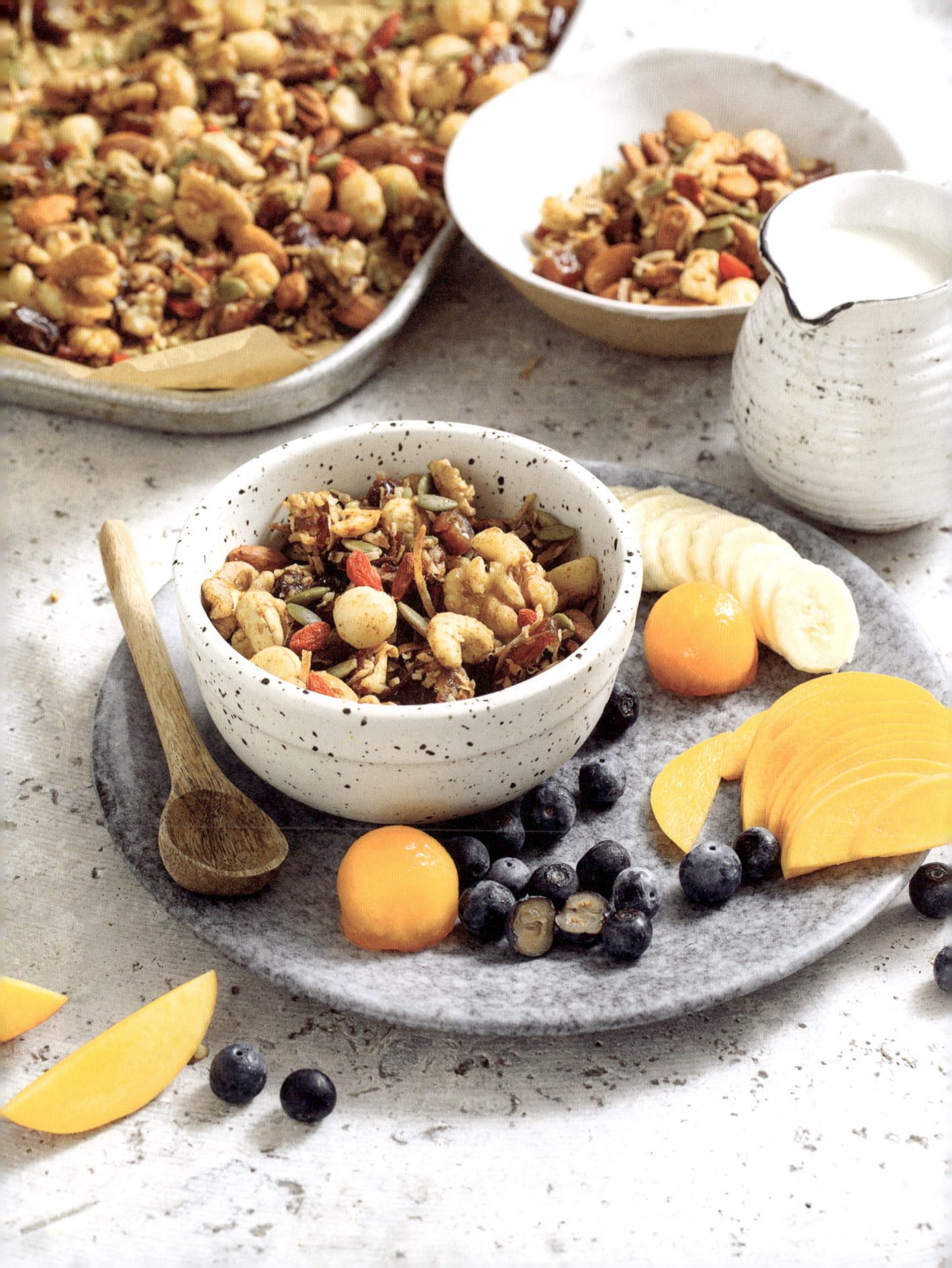

WHOLESOME CACAO POPS

MAKES 4 CUPS

6 cups puffed brown rice
¼ cup coconut cream (see Recipe Notes page 47)
⅔ cup coconut flakes
¼ cup pure maple syrup (or coconut nectar)
3 tablespoons cacao powder
2 tablespoons melted coconut oil
1½ teaspoons pure vanilla extract
⅓ cup shredded coconut

To serve
¾ cup Hemp Milk (see page 290) per serving

I created this recipe for Eli and Milo. Milo's my little sweet tooth boy; he often eyes up the sugary chocolate cereals that never quite make it into our trolley, so when he discovered a batch of this home-made coconutty cacao crunch in our pantry he was pretty stoked. It's amazing served with a creamy splash of highly nutritious Hemp Milk (see page 290) and works wonders as a chocolatey topping on smoothie bowls (see pages 56–66).

Preheat the oven to 180°C (350°F) fan bake. Line a large baking tray with baking paper.

Place all the ingredients except the shredded coconut in a large bowl and mix to combine. Tip onto the baking tray and spread out in a single layer. Bake for about 12 minutes. Watch carefully for the last few minutes as it will burn quickly.

Remove from the oven and let cool. Once cooled, mix through the shredded coconut and serve with creamy hemp milk and a little fresh fruit if desired.

Store in an airtight container for up to 7 days.

NOTE: You can also use a mix of different puffed gluten-free grains, such as brown rice, quinoa, amaranth and sorghum.

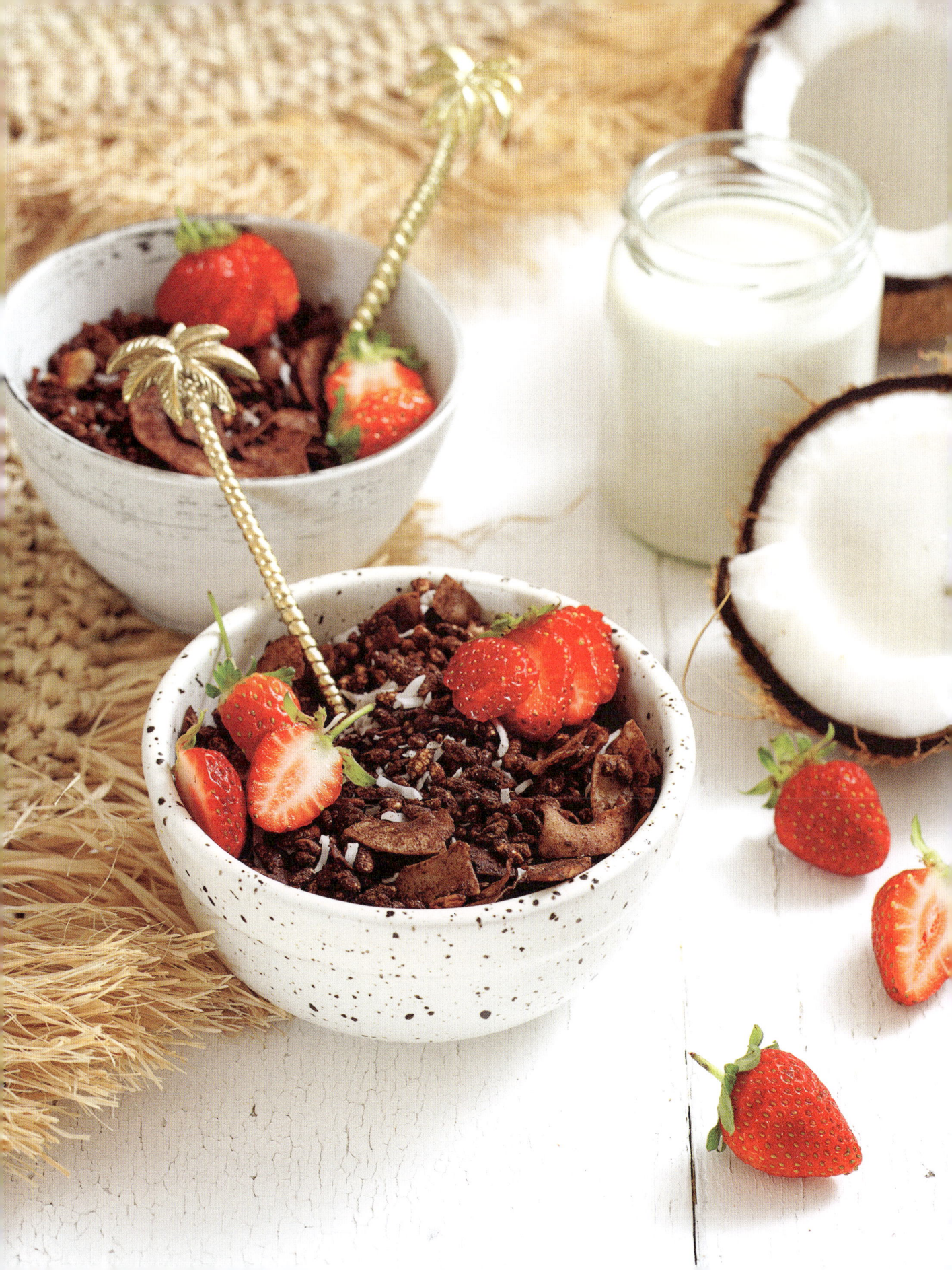

FRUITY NUT BOWL with POPPYSEED YOGHURT

SERVES 1

Poppyseed yoghurt
¼ cup coconut yoghurt
½ teaspoon poppyseeds
1 teaspoon pure maple syrup

Fruity nut bowl
1 small banana, sliced
1 cup prepared fresh fruit (green apple, blueberries, peaches, apricots, etc.)
1 cup mixed nuts (walnuts, almonds, cashews, etc.)

Toppings (optional)
chia seeds
hempseeds

This fruity nut mix is so easy to throw together, and creates an energising, healthful bowl for any time of the day. Mix it up with any fresh fruit, nuts or seeds you have on hand, and for those busier mornings simply take it on the road with you in a jar.

Place the coconut yoghurt, poppyseeds and maple syrup in a small bowl and mix to combine.

Place the fruit and nuts in a serving bowl and toss to combine. Top with the Poppyseed Yoghurt, and seeds if using.

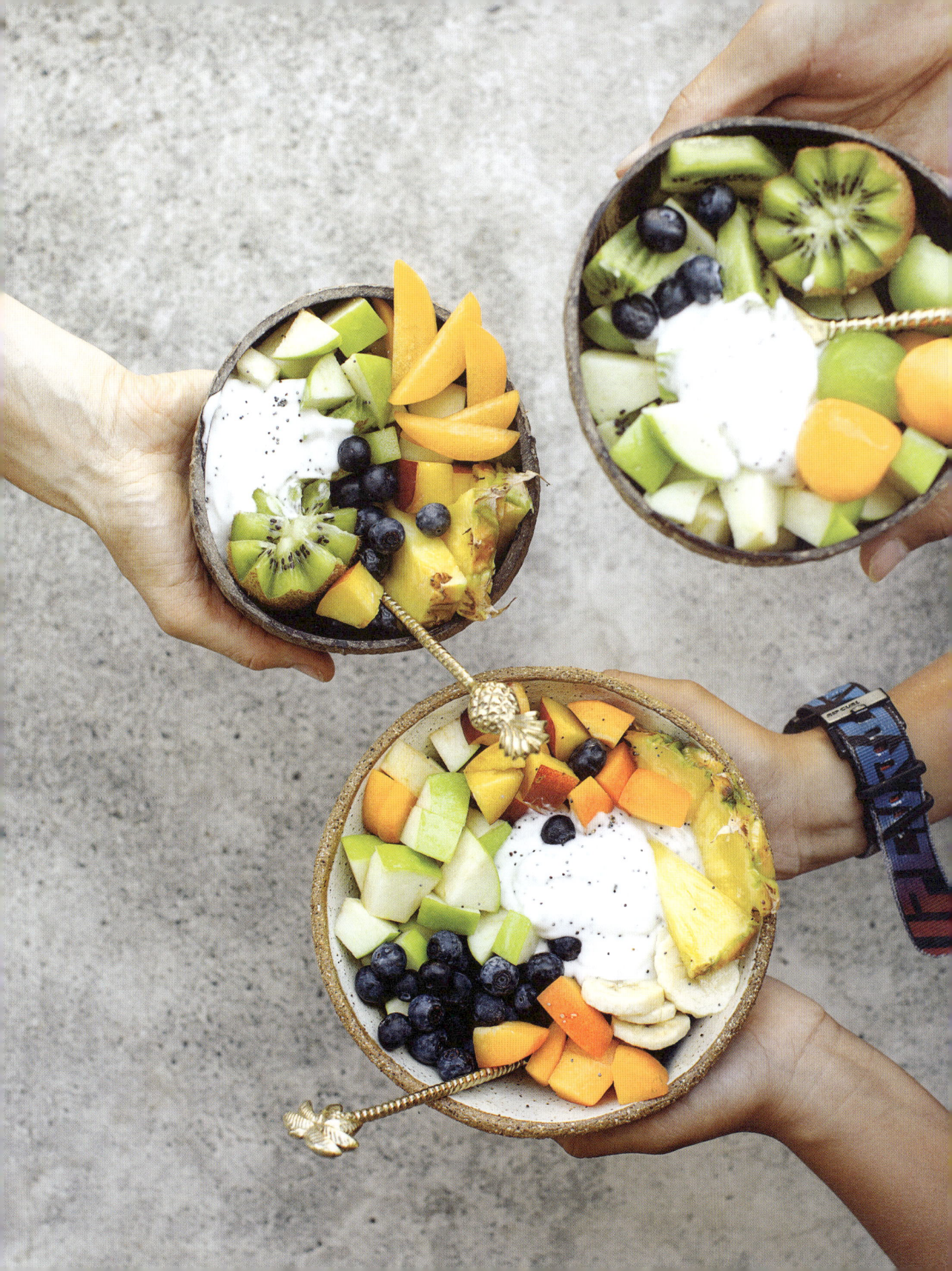

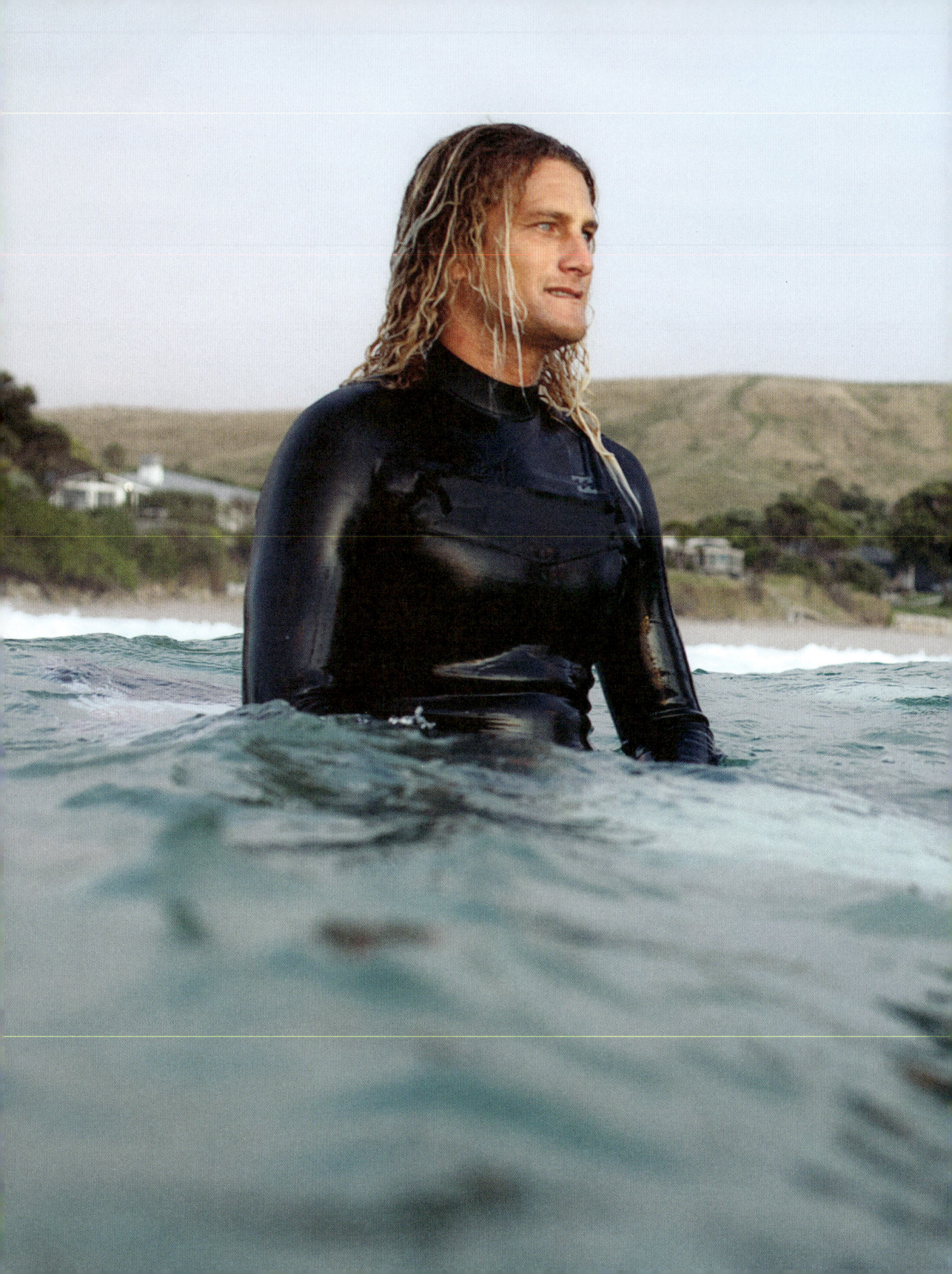

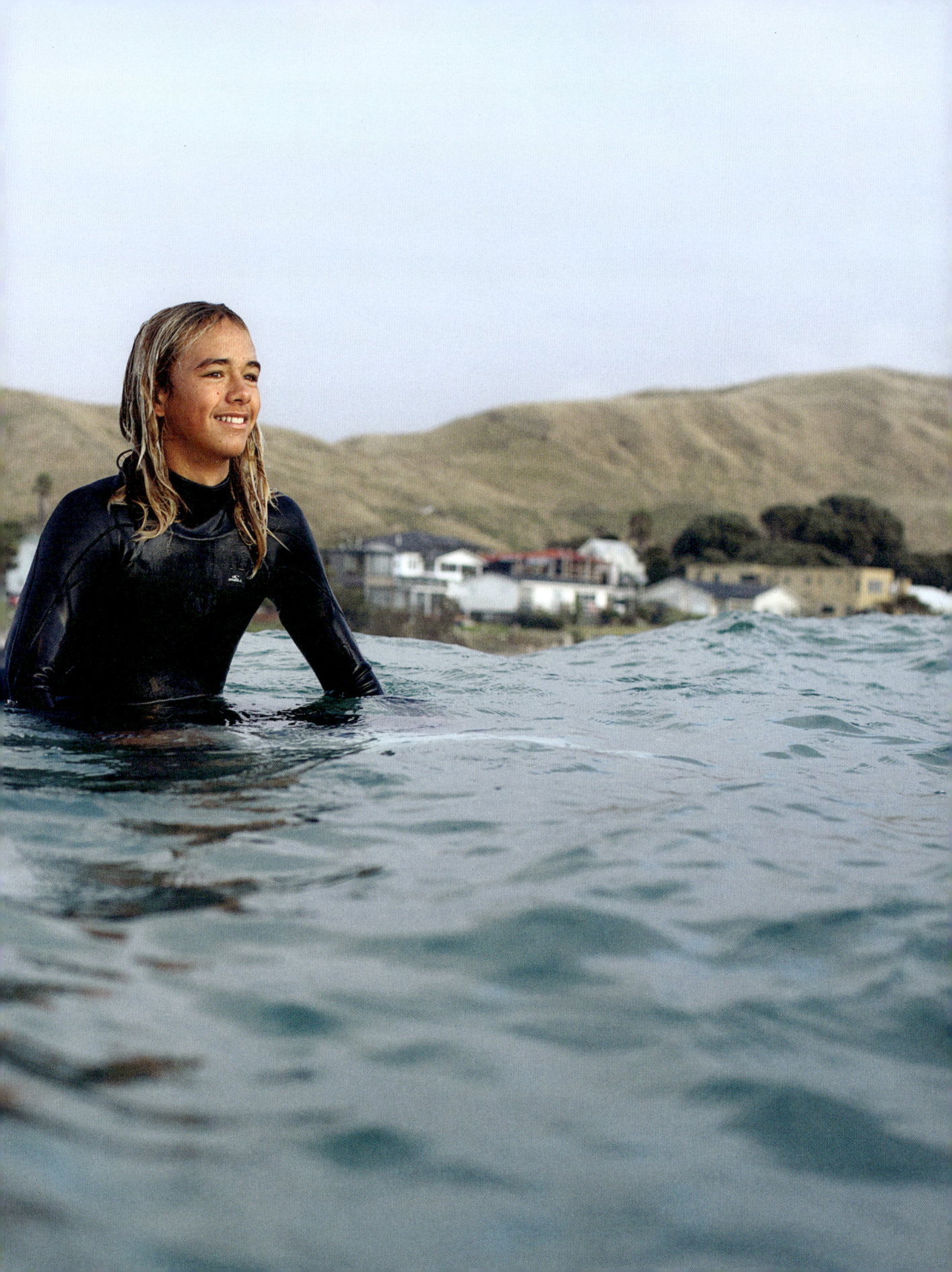

LINSEED and CACAO BIRCHER with RASPBERRY JAM

SERVES 1

Bircher
⅔ cup gluten-free oats
⅔ cup almond milk
1½ teaspoons cacao powder
2 teaspoons linseeds (flaxseeds)
½ teaspoon pure maple syrup

Toppings
⅓ cup Raw Raspberry Chia Jam (see page 287)
½ banana, sliced
1 tablespoon chopped almonds
1 tablespoon coconut flakes
dollop of nut butter (optional)

Bircher is super-quick to put together, and can be made in a jar for an easy, up-and-go brekkie—simply add your toppings of choice and go. The beauty of bircher is that you can make it in larger batches and have it readily available in the fridge. This recipe is one of my sister's favourites; raspberry chia jam is absolutely divine, and along with the cacao, linseeds and crunchy toppings it completes this jar perfectly for a nutritious breakfast.

For the bircher, place all the ingredients in a bowl (or jar) and mix to combine. Place in the fridge overnight.

To serve, remove from the fridge and add the toppings.

NOTE: Gluten-free oats can be found in health food stores; if not, order them online.

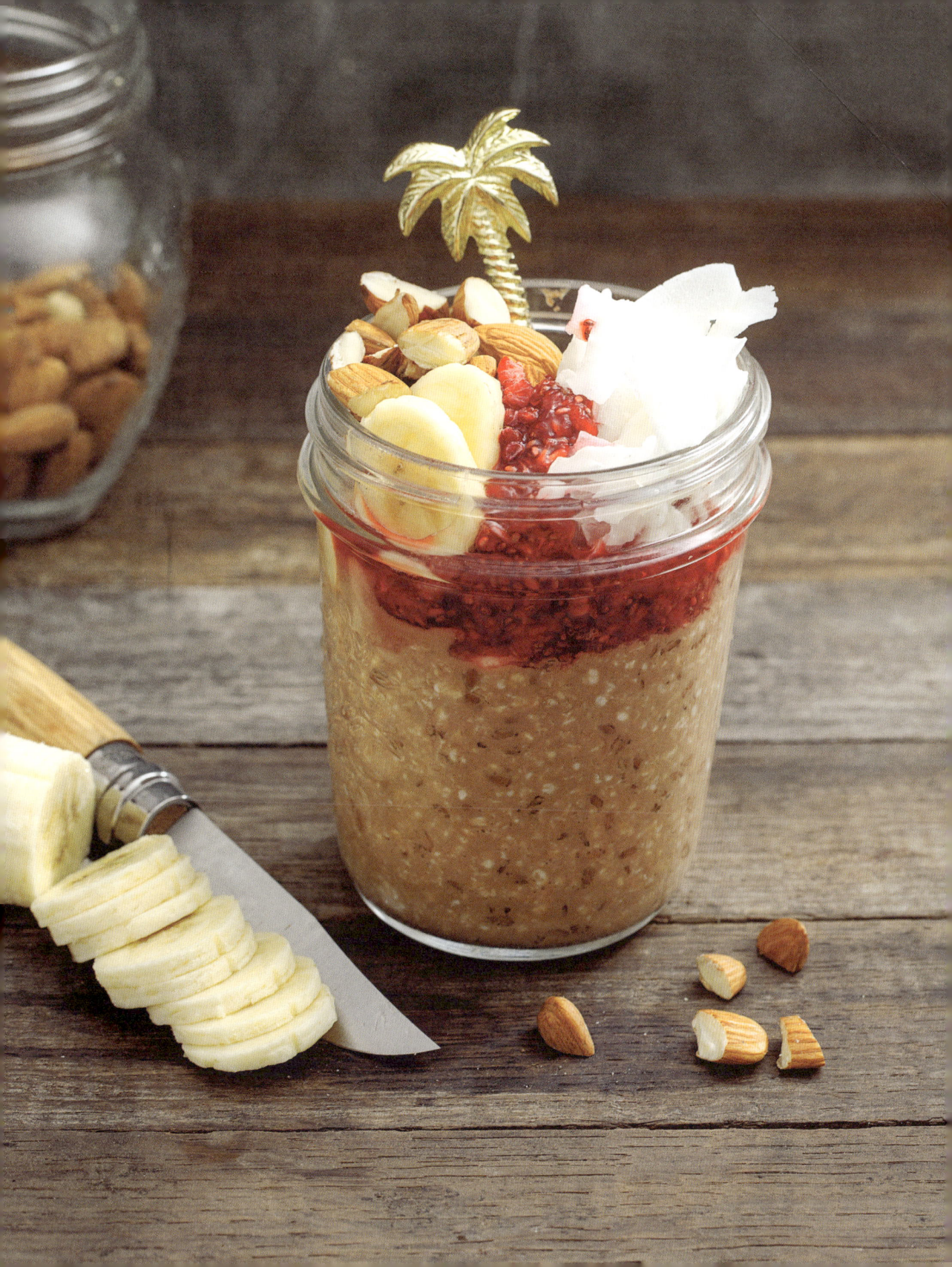

WALNUT, PEAR and FIG LOAF

MAKES 1 LOAF

1½ cups buckwheat flour
1 teaspoon baking powder
1 teaspoon baking soda
2 teaspoons ground cinnamon
½ teaspoon ground ginger
2 cups diced pear (dice into large chunks)
1 cup dried figs, sliced, plus extra to top
¾ cup sultanas (or raisins)
1½ cups walnuts, crushed, plus extra to top
1 cup nut milk
¼ cup pure maple syrup
¼ cup melted coconut oil (or olive oil)

As this lovely loaf bakes in the oven you'll smell the most beautiful, warming aromas wafting through the house. It's a lightly spiced and fruity loaf with sweet and chewy figs and crunchy walnuts to match. Buckwheat flour is used as the base, which is a great gluten-free flour alternative to use in baking. Enjoy a warm slice on its own, or try it with Raw Raspberry Chia Jam (see page 287) or your favourite wholesome condiment, such as almond or cashew butter.

Preheat the oven to 160°C (325°F). Line a loaf tin with baking paper.

Sift the buckwheat flour into a large bowl. Add the baking powder, baking soda, cinnamon and ginger. Mix to combine. Add the pear, figs, sultanas and walnuts and mix again.

In a separate bowl, combine the nut milk, maple syrup and coconut oil. Add to the dry ingredients and mix to combine.

Tip the mixture into the prepared loaf tin and spread out evenly. Arrange the extra sliced figs and crushed walnuts on top. Bake for 75–90 minutes, until golden. You will need to watch it closely for the last 15 minutes. To test, insert a sharp knife into the centre of the loaf. It should come out clean when the loaf is ready.

Remove from the tin and set aside to cool before slicing and serving.

Store in an airtight container for 3–5 days.

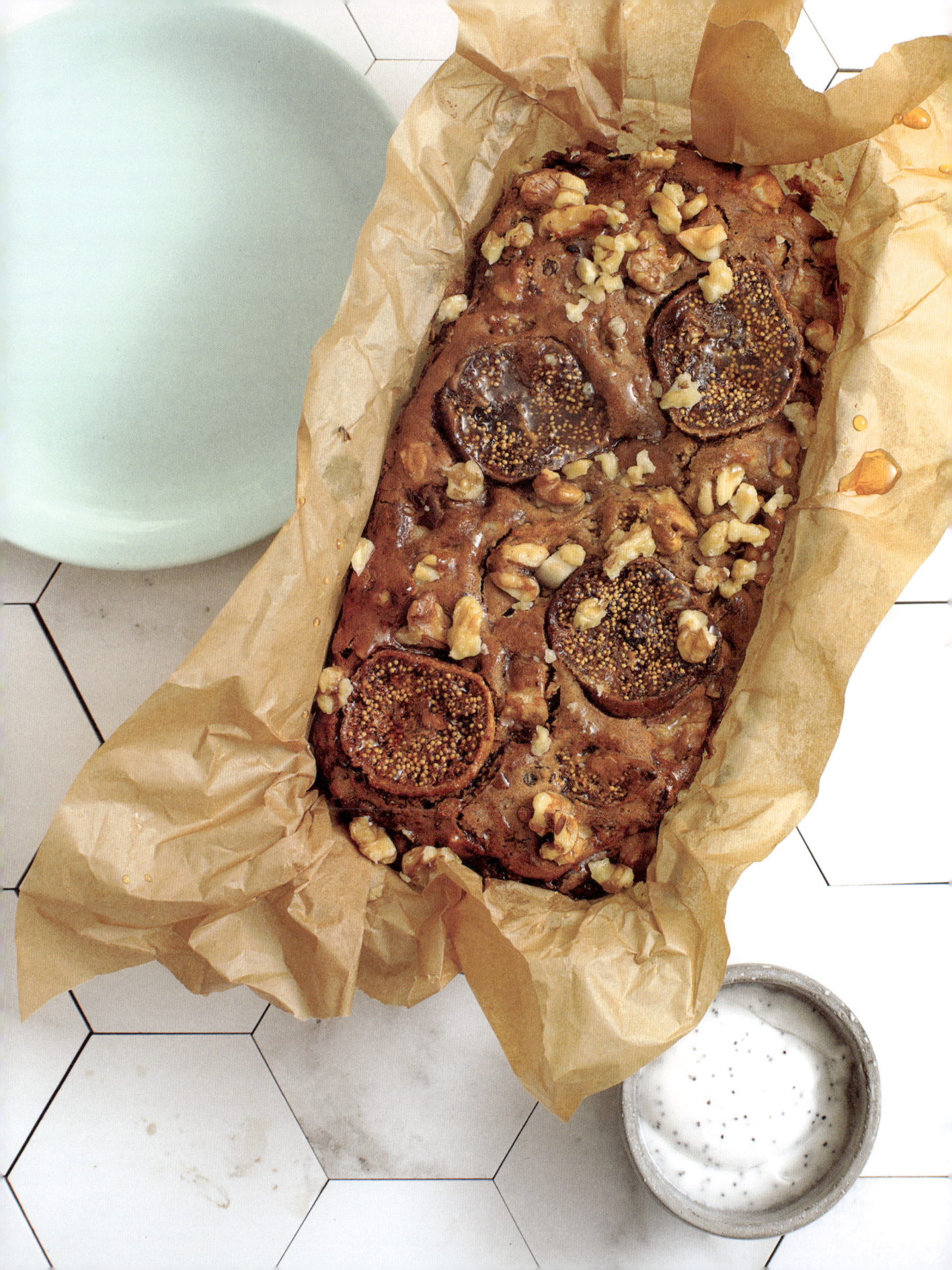

MINI HERB and FENNEL FRITTATAS

MAKES 12

1 teaspoon olive, avocado or coconut oil (optional), plus extra for greasing
1 white onion, sliced
3 cloves garlic, diced
¾ cup sliced mushrooms
1 red capsicum, diced into large chunks
2 cups spinach, sliced
1½ cups chickpea flour
1 teaspoon baking powder
1¾ cups water
handful fresh parsley, chopped
1 teaspoon fennel seeds
2 teaspoons dried oregano
¼ cup nutritional yeast
2 teaspoons tamari (optional)
cracked pepper, to taste
fresh chives

To serve (optional)
Raw Sweet Chilli Sauce (see page 280)
avocado slices

These vege frittatas make an ideal brunch, snack or lunch-box filler. Fennel seeds and oregano make for a delish aromatic combo, the mushrooms and capsicum add a little moisture and juiciness, and the nutritional yeast provides a cheesy flavour. Chickpea flour (besan) is an awesome gluten-free flour often used in vegan savoury recipes.

Preheat the oven to 180°C (350°F) fan bake. Lightly grease a 12-hole muffin tray with olive or coconut oil.

Heat the oil in a frying pan over medium-high heat. Once hot, add the onion, garlic and mushrooms and cook for 5–7 minutes, stirring frequently, until soft and fragrant.

Add the capsicum and spinach and cook for another 1–2 minutes, until the spinach is wilted.

Place the flour, baking powder and water in a bowl and mix until well blended. Add the cooked vegetables, parsley, fennel seeds, oregano, nutritional yeast and tamari, if using, and gently mix to combine all the ingredients.

Divide the mixture among the holes of the prepared muffin tray. Season with cracked pepper and sprinkle over fresh chives.

Bake for 30 minutes until golden. Remove from the oven and let stand for 15–20 minutes. This is an important step as it will allow the frittatas to set. Gently loosen the sides with a knife before removing.

Serve warm or cold with chilli sauce and avocado slices, if desired.

Once completely cooled, store in an airtight container for up to 5 days.

NOTE: The tamari is optional but recommended for a more flavourful frittata.

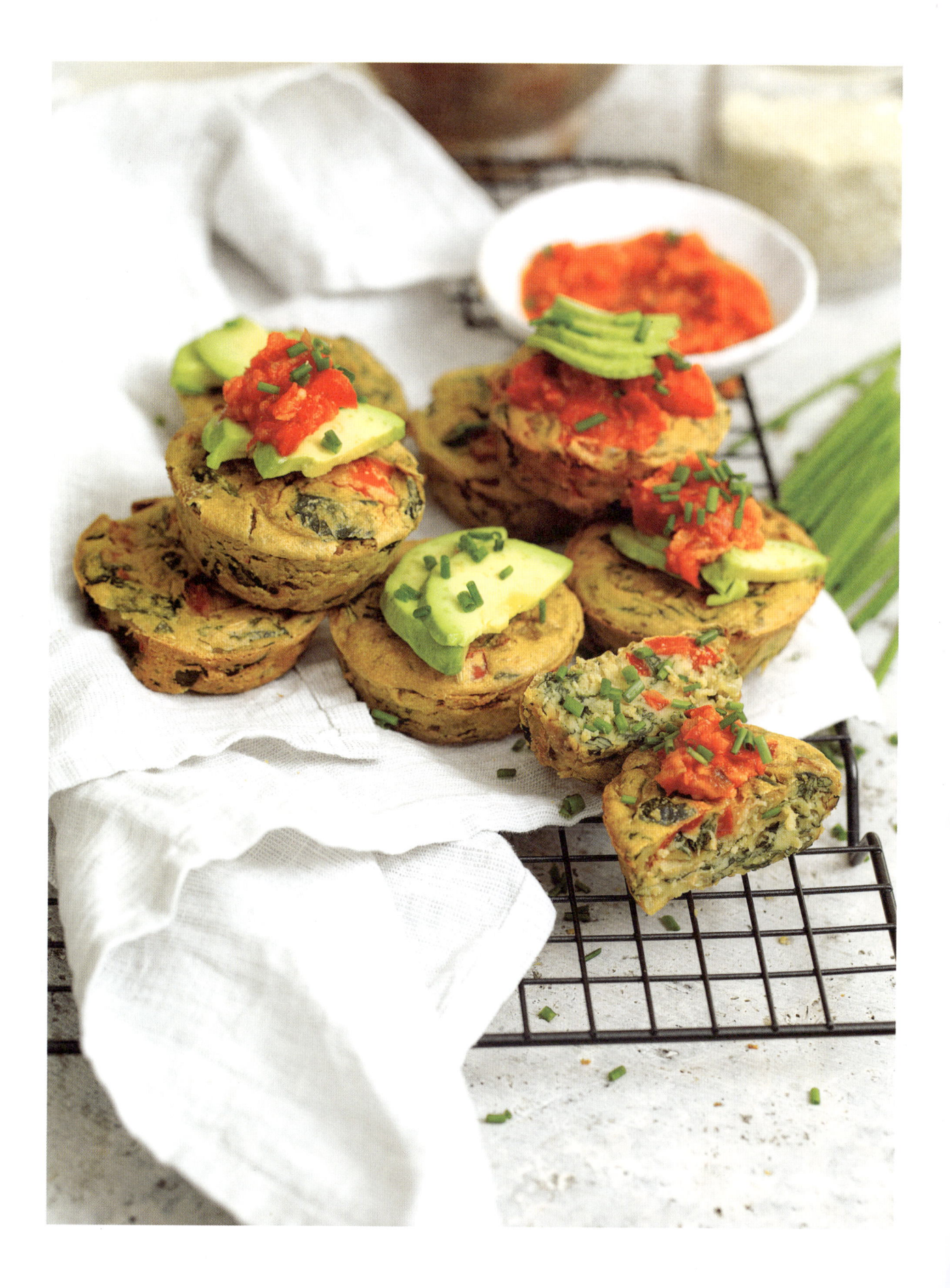

MILLET and QUINOA LOAF

MAKES 1 LOAF

Loaf
- ¾ cup millet
- ½ cup quinoa
- 1¼ cups filtered water
- 3 tablespoons psyllium husk powder
- 1¼ cups gluten-free rolled oats (or almond meal/ground almonds)
- 1 tablespoon baking powder
- ½ teaspoon baking soda
- 1 teaspoon sea salt
- 2 tablespoons olive oil
- 2 tablespoons pure maple syrup

Toppings
- 2 tablespoons seeds (pumpkin, sesame, chia, sunflower)
- 1 tablespoon gluten-free oats

I created this wholesome bread about four years ago after struggling to find a natural gluten-free loaf. After successfully nailing the recipe—using the two most alkalising grains, millet and quinoa—I shared it on my Raw and Free blog and it's been a hit ever since. For someone who hasn't eaten bread in nearly five years, it's become my favourite loaf to bake and my boys love it, too. You will need to presoak the grains, but other than that it's a really easy process. This nutrient-dense loaf is amazing served fresh or lightly toasted with all of your favourite toppings.

Place the millet and quinoa in a bowl of water, enough to cover the grains. Cover and set aside to soak overnight, or for at least 10 hours.

Preheat the oven to 165°C (330°F). Line a loaf tin with baking paper.

Combine the water and psyllium husk powder. Set aside to thicken for 5 minutes.

Pour the soaked quinoa and millet into a mesh strainer and rinse well. Drain thoroughly, then place in a food processor with ¾ cup of the oats, and the baking powder, baking soda, sea salt, oil and maple syrup. Add the psyllium mixture and blend until completely combined and the grains are mostly broken down.

Add the remaining ½ cup oats and blend again for 1 minute, or until the dough forms into a ball in the food processor.

Transfer the dough to the prepared loaf tin and spread out evenly. Sprinkle with oats and seeds of choice. Using a sharp knife, score the top of the loaf in several places.

Bake for 40 minutes. Remove and re-cut the places where you scored. This will allow the air out of the dough to ensure it can cook through. Bake for an additional 40 minutes.

Remove from the tin and set aside to cool. Slice and enjoy with your favourite toppings.

Store in an airtight container for 3–5 days.

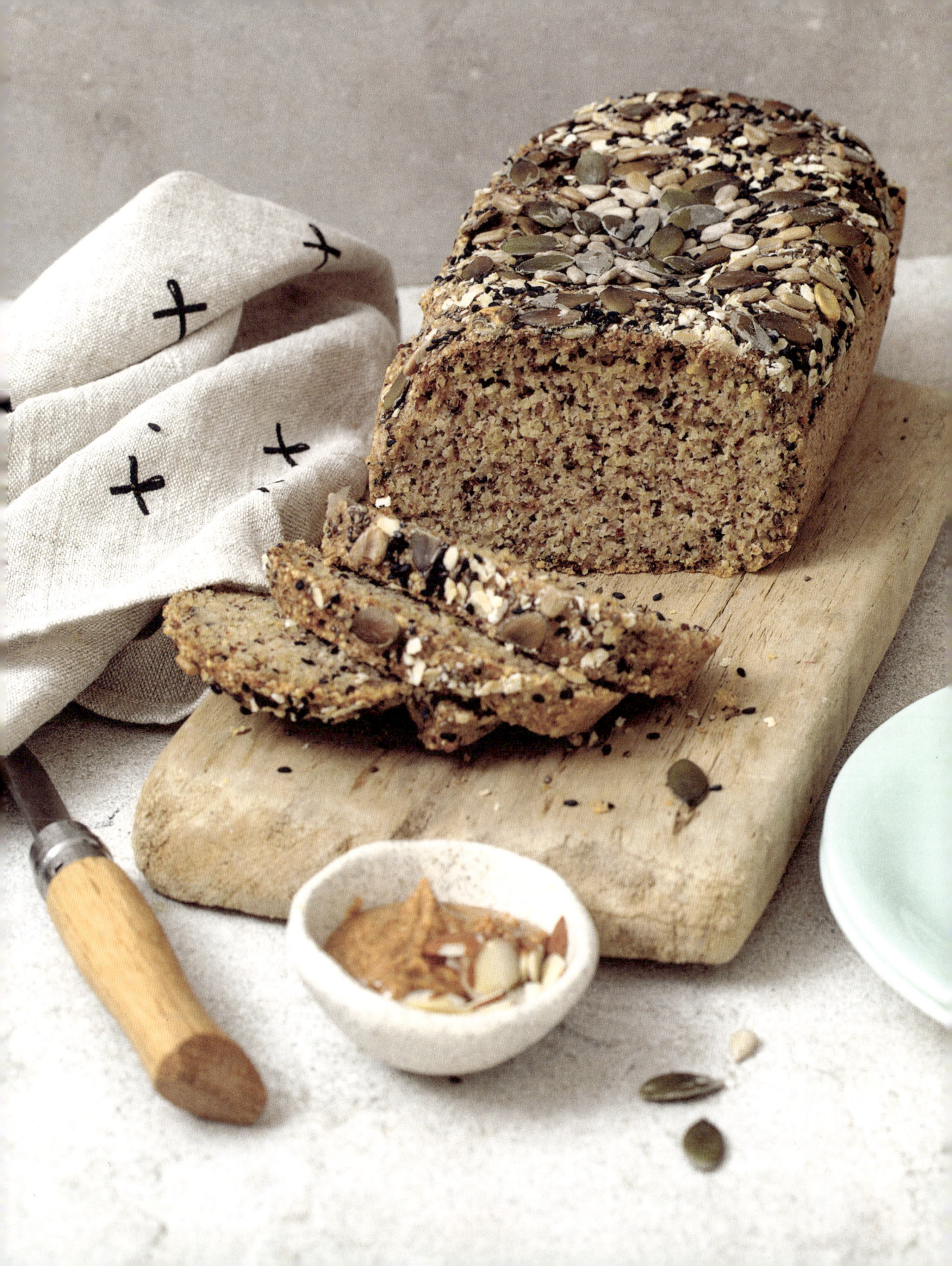

BUTTER BEAN, LIME and AVOCADO SMASH

SERVES 2–3

400 g (14 oz) can butter beans, drained and rinsed
flesh of 2 small avocados
2 large spring onions, sliced
juice of 1 lime
⅛ teaspoon white pepper
⅛ teaspoon Himalayan salt

To serve
4–6 slices of Millet and Quinoa Loaf (see page 96) or store-bought gluten-free bread, lightly toasted
¼ teaspoon white sesame seeds, per slice of toast
¼ teaspoon flaxseeds (linseed), per slice of toast

This scrumptious smash is perfectly balanced with tangy lime, spring onions and pepper. It will last in the fridge for a few days, and is great to have on hand for an easy protein-packed brunch or snack, as a toast topper or sandwich filler. It's particularly perfect served with my Millet and Quinoa Loaf (see page 96).

Place the beans and avocado in a bowl and mash with a fork until fairly smooth. Add the spring onions, lime juice, white pepper and Himalayan salt and mix to combine.

To serve, spread on a slice of toast and sprinkle with sesame seeds and flaxseeds.

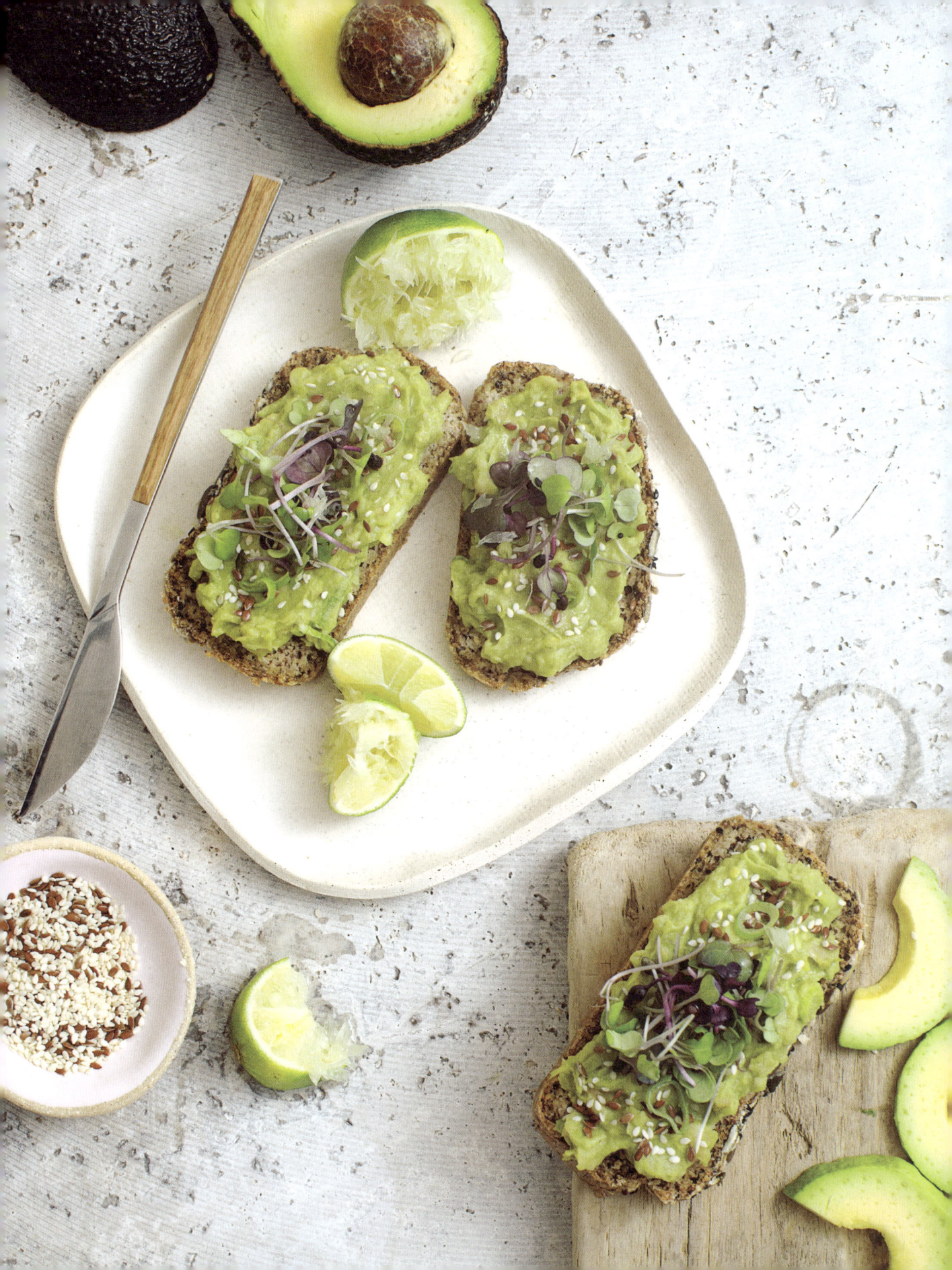

ALL-DAY BREKKIE BUDDHA BOWL with BALSAMIC YOGHURT MUSHROOMS

SERVES 2

- ⅓ cup black quinoa (or gluten-free grain of your choice)
- ⅔ cup water
- 2 cups baby spinach leaves
- 1 cup cherry tomatoes, halved
- ¼ small red onion, finely diced
- 1 large avocado, stoned and sliced
- ½ cup Hemp, Spinach and Basil Pesto (see page 222) or store-bought vegan pesto

Balsamic yoghurt mushrooms
- 1 teaspoon olive, avocado or coconut oil (optional)
- 200 g (7 oz) button mushrooms, sliced
- ½ teaspoon fresh or dried thyme
- 2 tablespoons balsamic vinegar
- 1½ tablespoons coconut yoghurt

If you're someone who loves a traditional savoury brunch, then you'll love this nourishing Buddha bowlful of goodness. It's an epic nutrient-packed bowl for any time of the day.

Place the quinoa and water in a saucepan, cover and bring to a boil. Once boiling, reduce the heat to low and cook for 12–15 minutes, until the water has been absorbed and the quinoa is soft and fluffy.

For the mushrooms, heat the oil in a large frying pan over medium-high heat. Add the mushrooms and cook for 5 minutes, stirring frequently, until soft. Add the thyme and balsamic vinegar, reduce the heat to low and cook for a further 5 minutes, stirring frequently. Remove from the heat and mix through the coconut yoghurt.

To serve, divide the quinoa, mushrooms and remaining ingredients between 2 shallow round bowls, finishing each with a dollop of pesto.

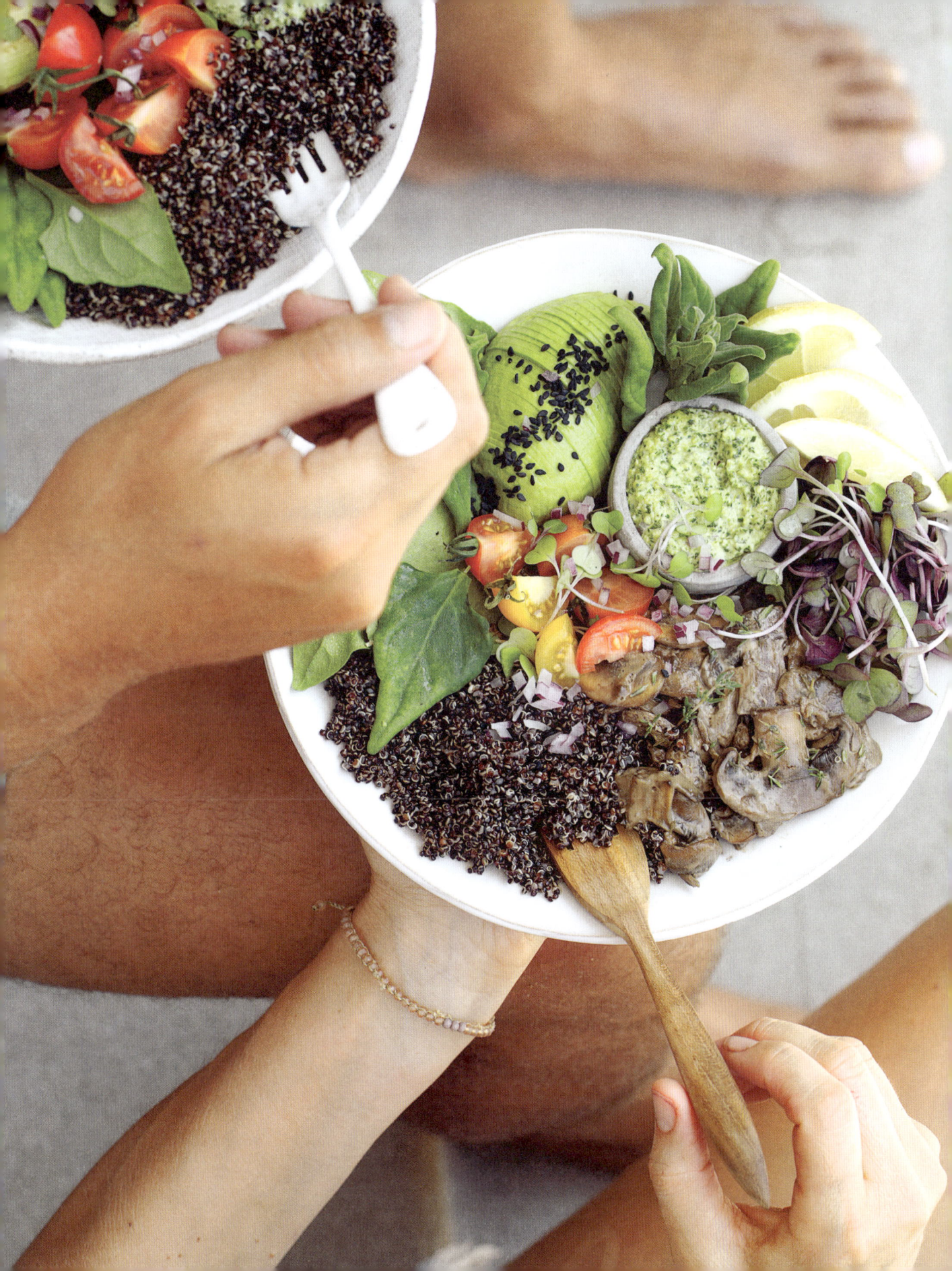

QUICK 'N' EASY CARROT FRITTERS

MAKES 8

Fritters
1¼ cups chickpea flour
1 cup water
3 large carrots, peeled and grated (approx. 2½ packed cups)
handful fresh parsley, finely chopped
2 teaspoons cumin seeds
½ teaspoon baking powder
½ teaspoon sea salt
⅛ teaspoon white pepper
oil for cooking

To serve
fresh greens
Raw Relish (see page 283) or Lime, Dill and Yoghurt Dressing (see page 202) or Raw Sweet Chilli Sauce (see page 280)
sprouts, chives or parsley
cumin seeds

These simple fritters make for a perfect weekend brunch with their sweet, earthy and aromatic flavours. They also work well served alongside a variety of different salads and are awesome served as a patty in a burger. They go beautifully with a variety of different dressings: try them with a dollop of my favourite Lime, Dill and Yoghurt Dressing (see page 202), Raw Sweet Chilli Sauce (see page 280) or Raw Relish (see page 283).

Preheat the oven to 80°C (175°F) fan bake.

In a large bowl, whisk together the chickpea flour and water until all clumps are smoothed away. Add the carrot, parsley, cumin seeds, baking powder, salt and pepper and mix to combine.

Heat the oil in a non-stick frying pan over medium heat. Place ¼ cup of the batter into the pan (I do about 3 at a time) and cook for 3–4 minutes until bubbles form on the surface. Flip and cook for an additional 3–4 minutes, until both sides are golden and crispy. Be careful not to have the heat up too high as the fritters will burn quickly.

Place on a plate in the oven to keep warm and repeat with the remaining batter.

Serve warm on a bed of greens topped with a dollop of the dressing of your choice and garnished with sprouts or fresh herbs and cumin seeds.

NOTE: It is important to use a good non-stick frying pan to cook these fritters.

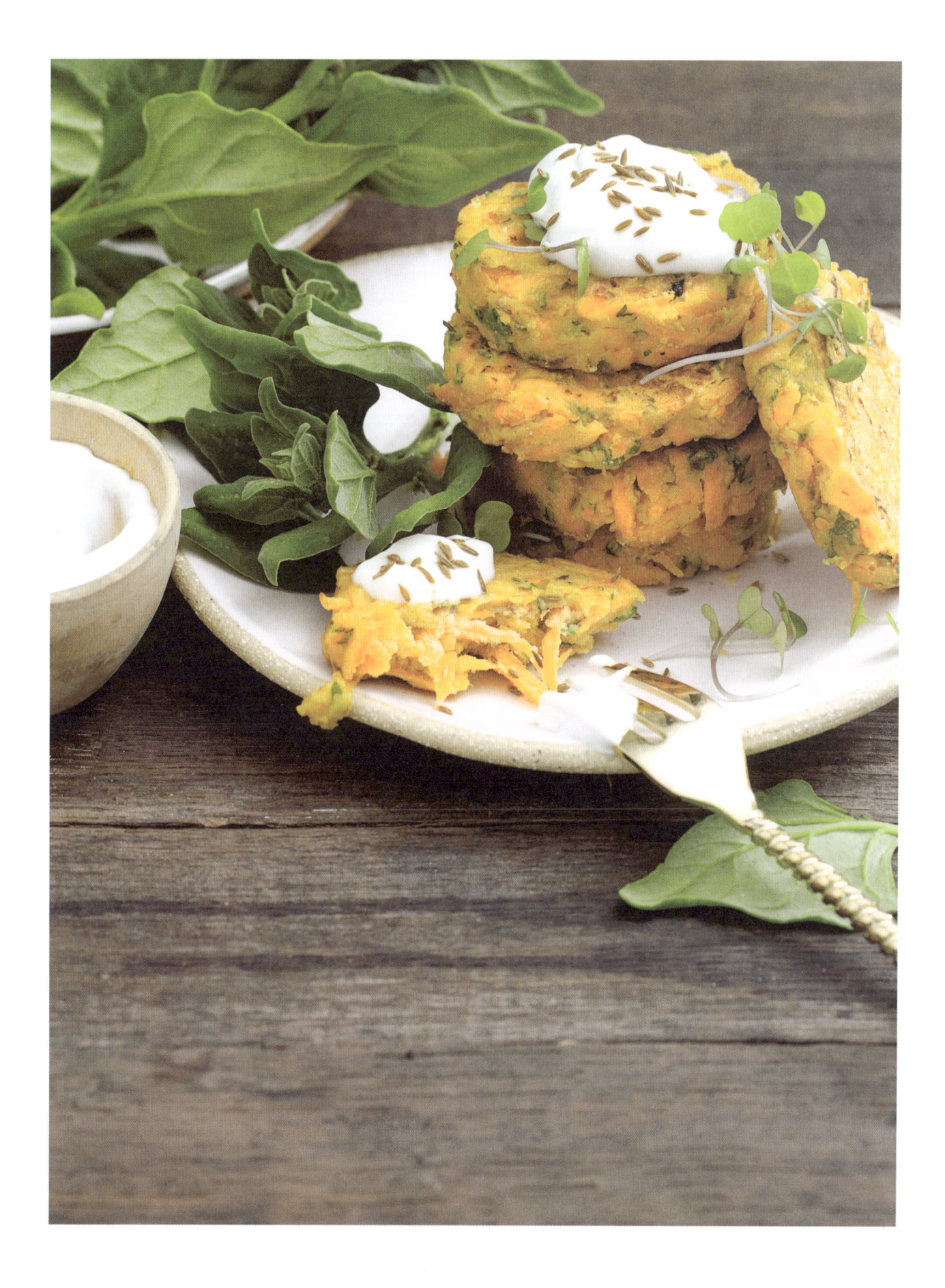

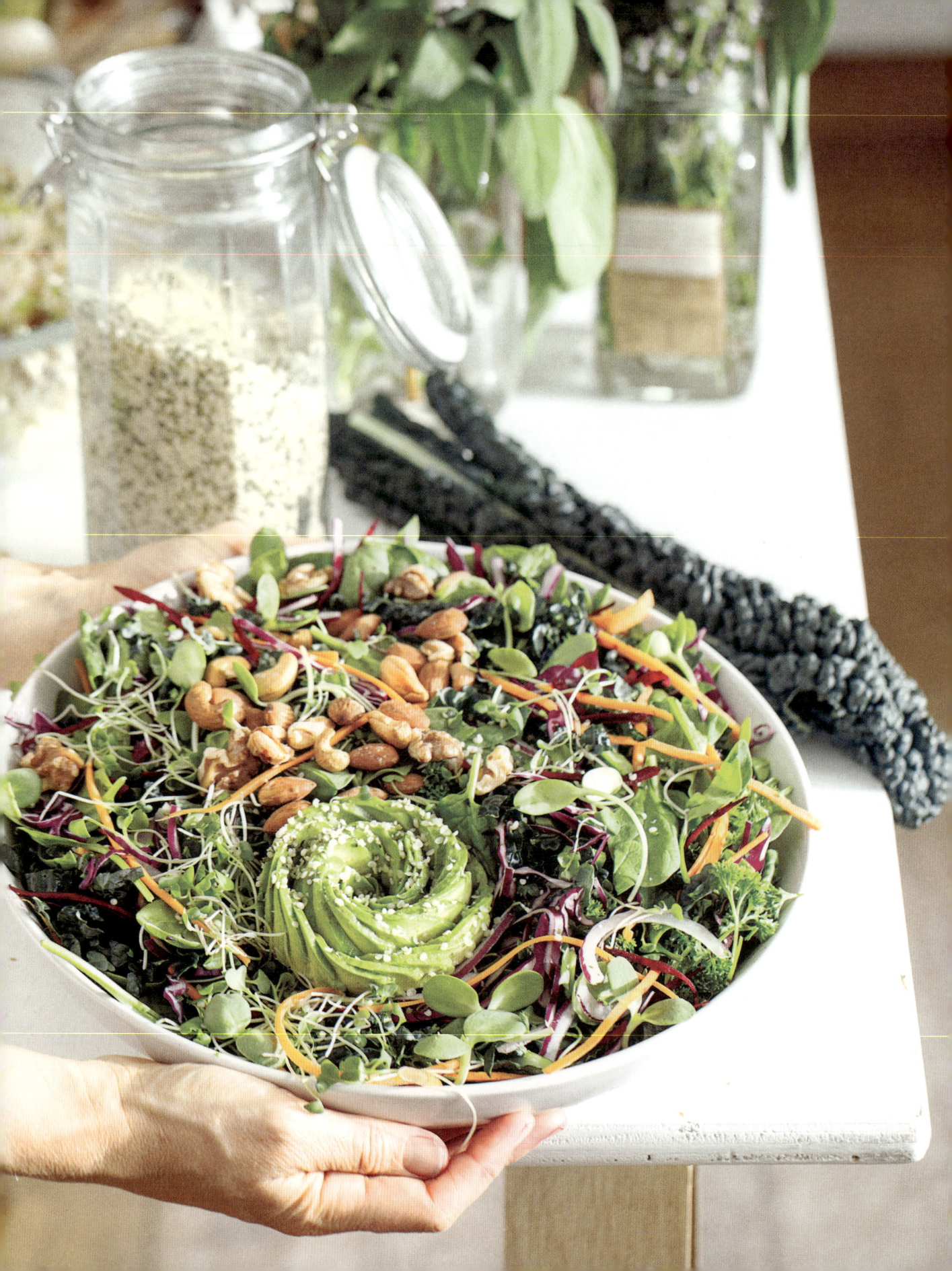

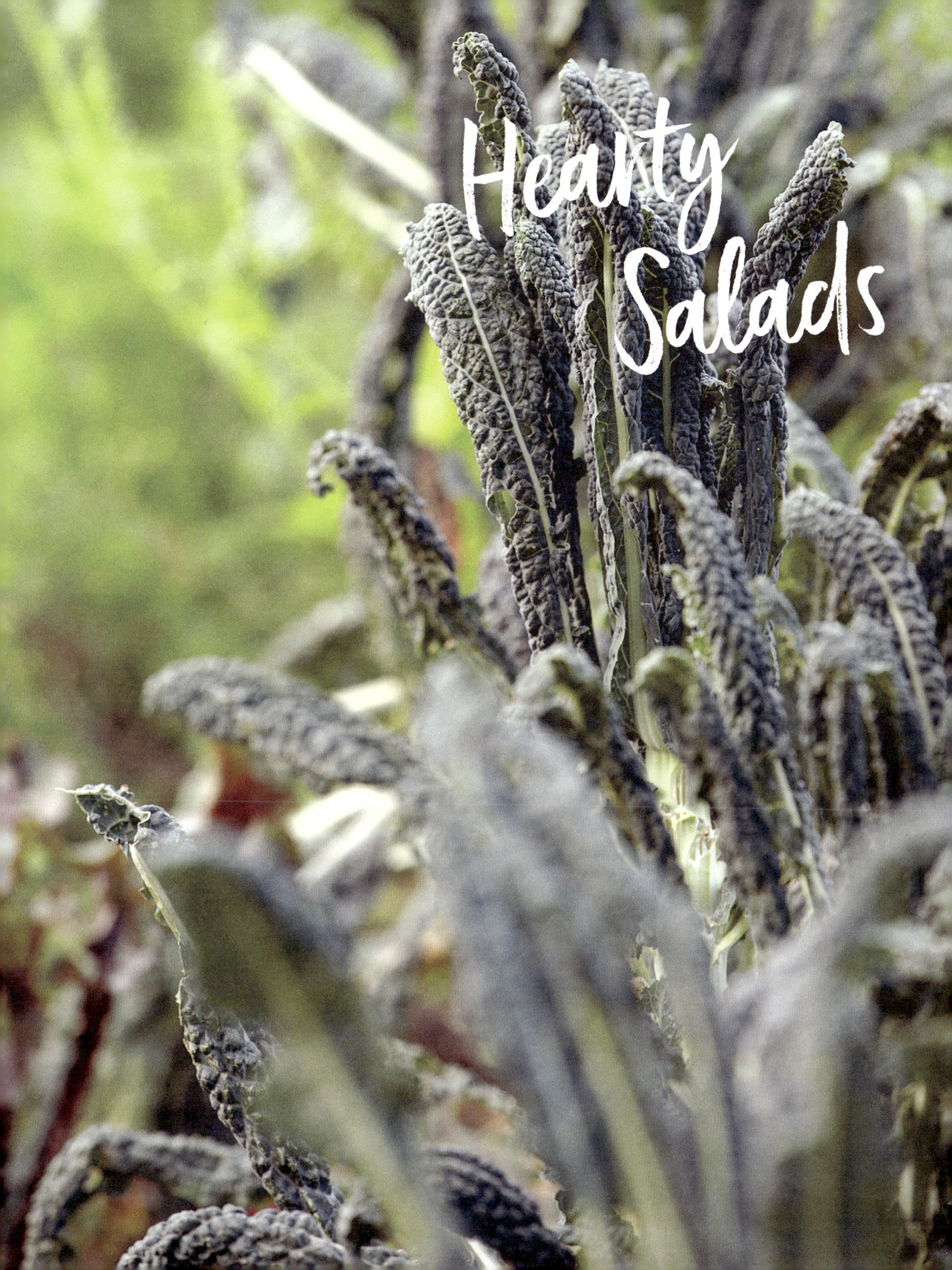

Hearty Salads

Hearty Salads

Salads are such a big part of my diet; a plant-based staple that, along with fresh fruit, makes up the basis of my daily meals. When you eat a good salad you're enjoying a wide variety of flavours, textures, colours and food groups while also benefitting from an abundance of raw nutrition.

These salads are so much more than just a plate of lettuce. My goal for this chapter was to create easy, family-favourite recipes that will encourage you to eat more plants, while emphasising how delicious they can be. These flavoursome and highly nutritious salads are either voluminous and hearty or light and refreshing, leaving you feeling satisfied, energised and amazing from the inside out. Ingredients range from raw, alkalising and vibrant vegetables to crunchy nuts and seeds, to earthy gluten-free wholegrains and warming roast potatoes, all paired with a variety of dressings.

I often get asked for salad dressing ideas, so I have provided you with a variety in this chapter. Get creative and swap them around to use alongside any dish, or to simply liven up fresh seasonal produce.

I hope you enjoy these salads as much as I do. There are so many wonderful, crowd-pleasing recipes, over-flowing with beautiful flavours and vibrant colours, that will work amazingly for lunches, light dinners, pot lucks, barbecues and entertaining friends and family.

QUICK TIPS FOR HEARTY SALAD

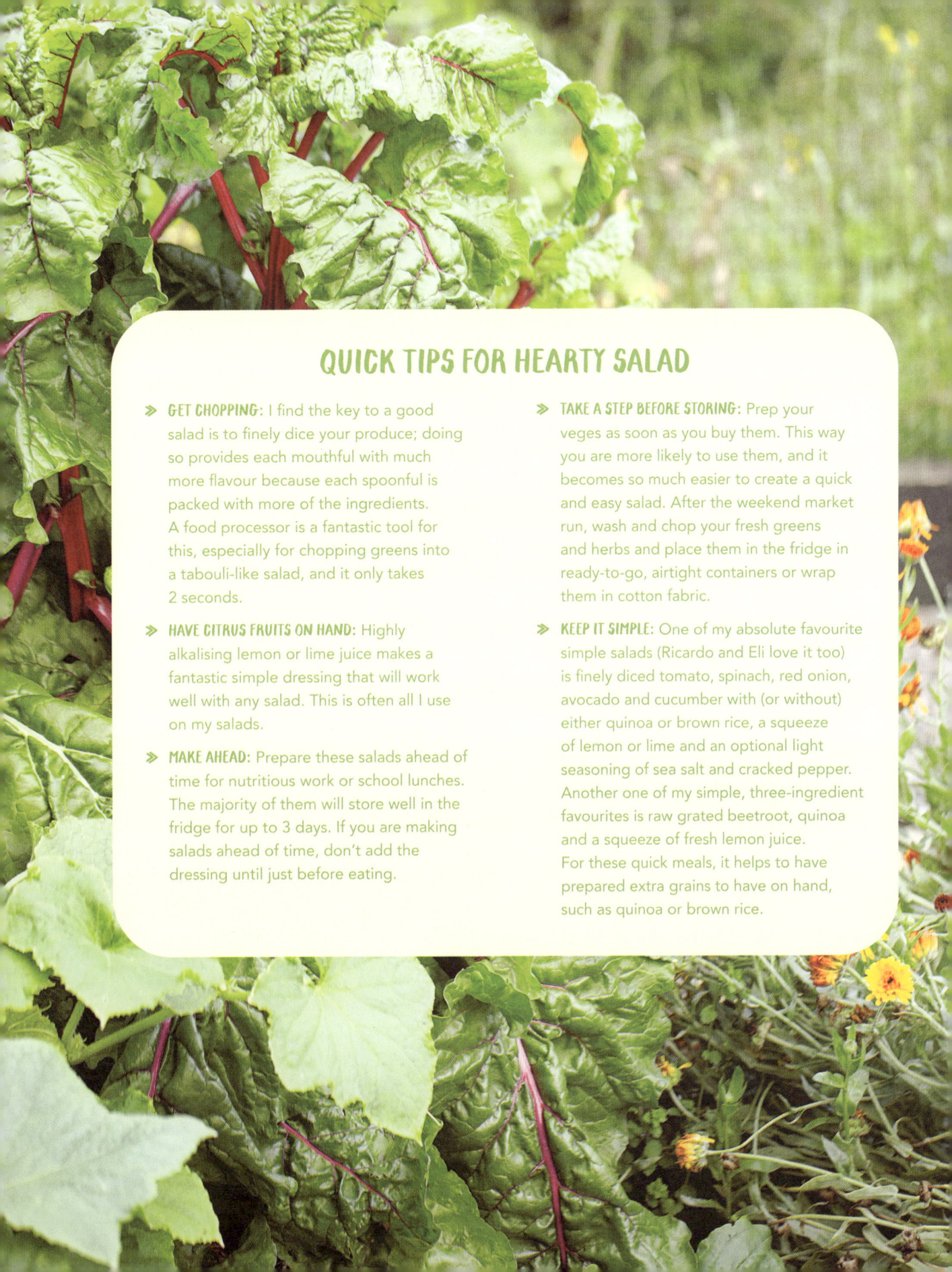

» **GET CHOPPING:** I find the key to a good salad is to finely dice your produce; doing so provides each mouthful with much more flavour because each spoonful is packed with more of the ingredients. A food processor is a fantastic tool for this, especially for chopping greens into a tabouli-like salad, and it only takes 2 seconds.

» **HAVE CITRUS FRUITS ON HAND:** Highly alkalising lemon or lime juice makes a fantastic simple dressing that will work well with any salad. This is often all I use on my salads.

» **MAKE AHEAD:** Prepare these salads ahead of time for nutritious work or school lunches. The majority of them will store well in the fridge for up to 3 days. If you are making salads ahead of time, don't add the dressing until just before eating.

» **TAKE A STEP BEFORE STORING:** Prep your veges as soon as you buy them. This way you are more likely to use them, and it becomes so much easier to create a quick and easy salad. After the weekend market run, wash and chop your fresh greens and herbs and place them in the fridge in ready-to-go, airtight containers or wrap them in cotton fabric.

» **KEEP IT SIMPLE:** One of my absolute favourite simple salads (Ricardo and Eli love it too) is finely diced tomato, spinach, red onion, avocado and cucumber with (or without) either quinoa or brown rice, a squeeze of lemon or lime and an optional light seasoning of sea salt and cracked pepper. Another one of my simple, three-ingredient favourites is raw grated beetroot, quinoa and a squeeze of fresh lemon juice. For these quick meals, it helps to have prepared extra grains to have on hand, such as quinoa or brown rice.

MIDDLE EASTERN RAW CAULIFLOWER TABOULI *with* SWEET ROAST CHICKPEAS

SERVES 4 OR 6–8 AS A SIDE SALAD

- 1 head cauliflower (approx. 1kg / 2 lb 4 oz), cut into large florets
- 1 cup dried apricots, diced
- 2 large spring onions, thinly sliced
- 2 teaspoons garam masala
- 1 teaspoon ground cumin
- 1 teaspoon onion powder
- 3 tablespoons lemon juice
- 1 tablespoon apple cider vinegar
- handful fresh coriander, roughly chopped
- handful fresh mint, roughly chopped
- sea salt and cracked pepper, to taste

Sweet roast chickpeas

- 400 g (14 oz) can chickpeas, drained and rinsed (or 1½ cups cooked chickpeas)
- 1 teaspoon coconut sugar
- ½ teaspoon ground cinnamon
- ½ teaspoon ground cumin
- ½ teaspoon olive oil
- herbs, for garnish

When I first created this recipe, I became so obsessed with it that I would eat it almost every day. The combination of the Middle Eastern spiced raw cauliflower, fresh mint and sweet apricots creates an addictively light and refreshing raw salad. Cauliflower is a great source of many vitamins and minerals, and makes for the perfect raw alternative to rice, especially if you're looking for a lighter option. The chickpeas add that extra crunch and protein, but I often omit them and serve the salad as a side with Sesame Baked Falafel Bites (see page 224), Cauliflower Kofta Balls (see page 206), roast potatoes or simply topped with a large sliced avocado.

Preheat the oven to 180°C (350°F) fan bake. Line a baking tray with baking paper.

For the chickpeas, place all the ingredients in a small bowl and mix to combine, ensuring all the chickpeas are coated in the mixture. Tip onto the prepared baking tray and spread out into a single layer. Bake for 30 minutes, until golden and crispy.

Place the cauliflower in a food processor. Blend for about 5–7 seconds, or until the cauliflower resembles rice. Be careful not to over-blend, as it will turn into a liquid mush.

Transfer the cauliflower to a large bowl and add all the other ingredients. Mix to combine and season to taste.

To serve, place the salad in a shallow serving bowl and scatter the chickpeas and herbs on top.

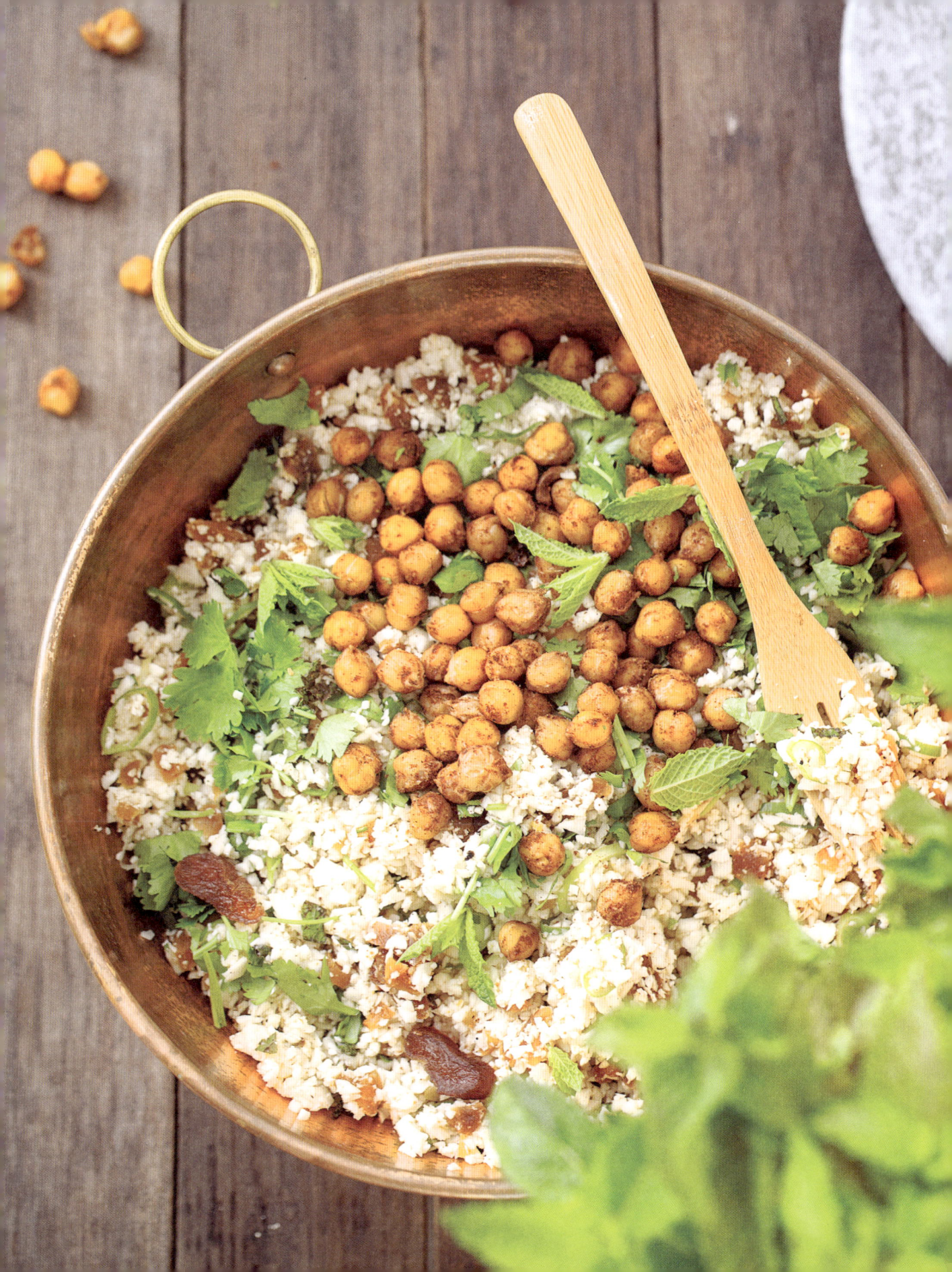

WILD RICE SALAD with LEMONGRASS, TURMERIC and COCONUT DRESSING

SERVES 4–6

1 cup wild rice mix (I use a combination of red, black and wild rice)

2 cups water

100 g (3½ oz) snow pea sprouts, chopped

handful coriander, plus extra to garnish

handful Thai basil leaves, plus extra to garnish

2 spring onions, chopped

1 small telegraph cucumber, diced

3 tablespoons sesame seeds, plus extra to serve

½ cup shredded coconut, plus extra to serve

Lemongrass, turmeric and coconut dressing

1 stalk lemongrass, tough shell removed and inner part chopped

¾ cup coconut milk

¼ cup water

1 packed tablespoon grated fresh ginger

½ teaspoon ground turmeric

1 tablespoon coconut sugar

1½ tablespoons coconut aminos (or tamari)

This large salad packs a punch in terms of both nutrients and epic flavours for an easy weekday Thai-inspired dinner or the perfect work lunch. The cucumber and snow pea sprouts provide a hydrating mouthful, while the wild rice makes it hearty. Lemongrass is one of my favourite ingredients for adding a fresh lemony kick to dips, dresses and sauces, and it truly shines through in the creamy turmeric and coconut dressing.

Place the rice and water in a saucepan, cover, and bring to a boil. Once boiling, reduce the heat to low and simmer for 25–30 minutes, or until the water has been absorbed and the rice is soft.

For the dressing, place all the ingredients in a blender and blend until smooth.

Place the cooked rice in a large bowl along with all the other salad ingredients, and toss to combine. Add the dressing to the bowl and mix well.

To serve, transfer to a serving bowl and top with a light sprinkle of shredded coconut and sesame seeds. Garnish with fresh coriander and Thai basil leaves.

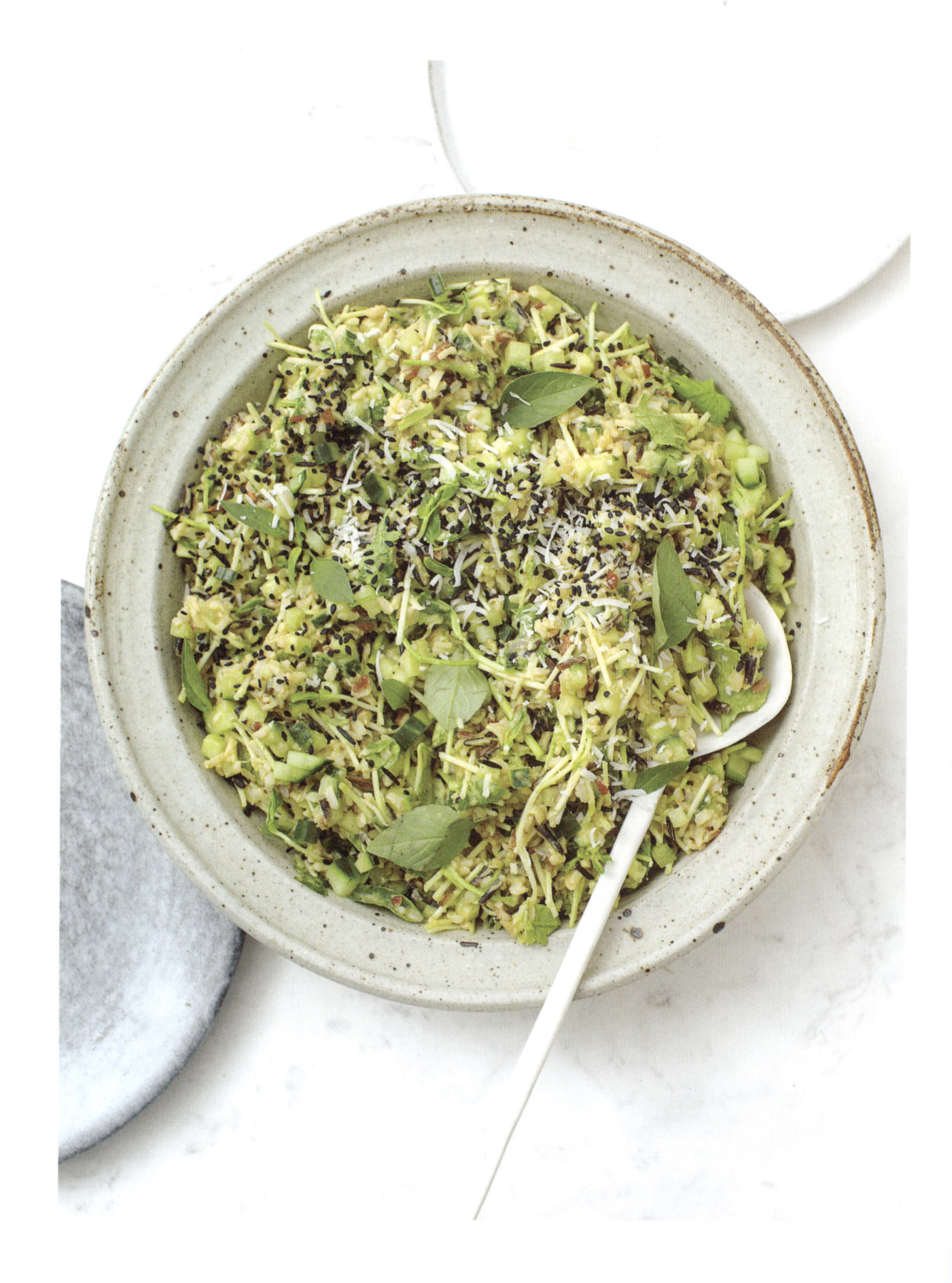

BUCKWHEAT, MESCLUN, ROAST HAZELNUTS and AVOCADO with APRICOT and GINGER DRESSING

SERVES 4

3 cups water
1 cup raw buckwheat groats, rinsed
½ cup raw hazelnuts
2 packed cups mesclun leaves
2 cups cherry tomatoes, cut into quarters
½ small red onion, thinly sliced
2 medium avocados, stoned and diced

Apricot and ginger dressing
½ cup dried apricots
2 tablespoons wholegrain mustard
2 tablespoons apple cider vinegar
1½ tablespoons hemp oil (or olive oil)
1 teaspoon finely grated fresh ginger
½ cup fresh orange juice
½ cup water

Buckwheat is a fantastic, gluten-free grain—well, technically it's a seed closely related to the rhubarb plant—with a somewhat nutty flavour. It's the perfect base for this salad, while the roast hazelnuts and the apricot and ginger dressing bring the whole plate to life. The dressing is also amazing with simple fresh greens, in a salad sandwich, or try it over lightly steamed vegetables, such as broccoli and cauliflower.

Preheat the oven to 180°C (350°F) fan bake. Line a baking tray with baking paper.

Place the water in a saucepan over medium-high heat and bring to a boil. Once boiling, add the buckwheat, cover, and cook for 12–15 minutes, until the buckwheat is soft and fluffy. Be careful not to cook for too long as it can become too soft with a mushy texture. Remove from the heat and place in a strainer. Rinse under cold water and drain well.

Place the hazelnuts on the prepared baking tray and spread out into a single layer. Bake for about 8 minutes, tossing twice, until slightly browned and fragrant. Watch closely for the last few minutes as they will burn quickly. Remove from the oven and set aside.

For the dressing, place all the ingredients in a blender and blend for 20–30 seconds, until mostly smooth. There may be a few remaining chunks of dried apricots.

Place the mesclun on a large serving plate and arrange the tomatoes and onion on top, followed by the buckwheat and avocado. Pour some dressing evenly over the salad and serve the rest on the side. Finish by scattering over the roasted hazelnuts.

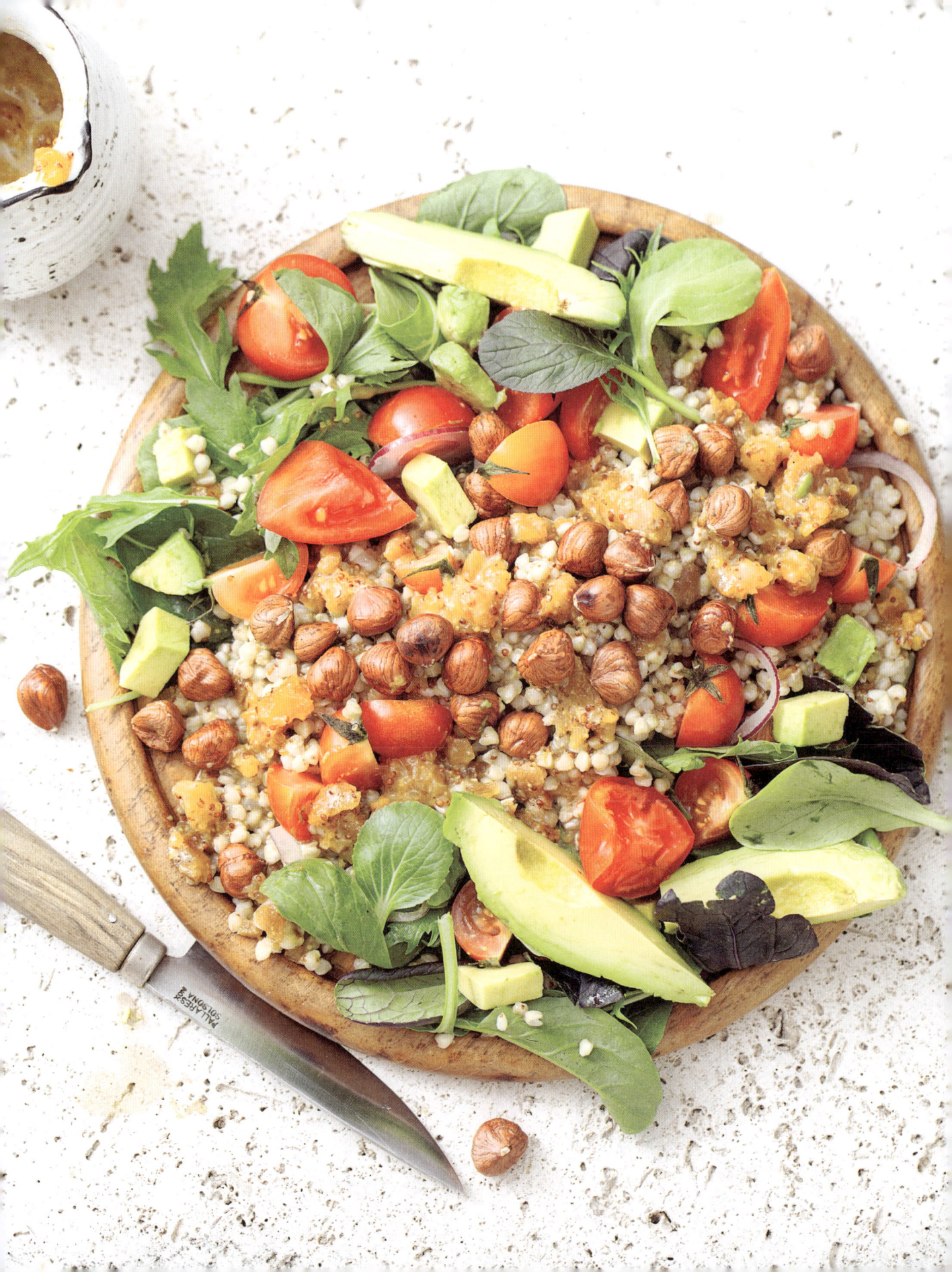

GREEN LENTIL, KALE, CAPER, MINT and HEMP SALAD with CHOPPED ALMONDS

SERVES 4–6

1 cup green lentils, rinsed
1 litre (35 fl oz) water
1 bunch cavolo nero or curly kale, stems removed and finely chopped
handful fresh mint leaves
¾ cup currants
¼ cup capers
1 large spring onion, sliced
⅛ teaspoon white pepper
¼ cup hempseeds
1 tablespoon balsamic vinegar
¾ cup raw almonds, chopped
1 large lemon, halved

To serve
fresh mint leaves
lemon wedges

This is one of those lively, nutrient-dense salads that I often crave for a wholesome dinner. I absolutely love the refreshingly sweet and zesty flavours with the crunchy texture to match. Green lentils, hempseeds, almonds and kale provide fantastic sources of protein, along with a stellar list of other essential nutrients, and pair wonderfully with the currants, capers, mint, lemon and balsamic to create a sensational salad your body will love you for.

Place the lentils and water in a saucepan, cover, and bring to a boil. Reduce the heat and simmer for 20–25 minutes, until soft. Drain.

Tip the lentils into a large bowl along with the kale, mint, currants, capers, spring onion, pepper, hempseeds, balsamic vinegar and half of the almonds. Squeeze over the lemon juice and toss to combine.

To serve, place the salad in a serving bowl and scatter over the remaining almonds. Garnish with mint and serve with lemon wedges.

NOTE: I blitz both the kale and the almonds separately in my food processor for this salad to create much quicker finely chopped kale and crushed almonds.

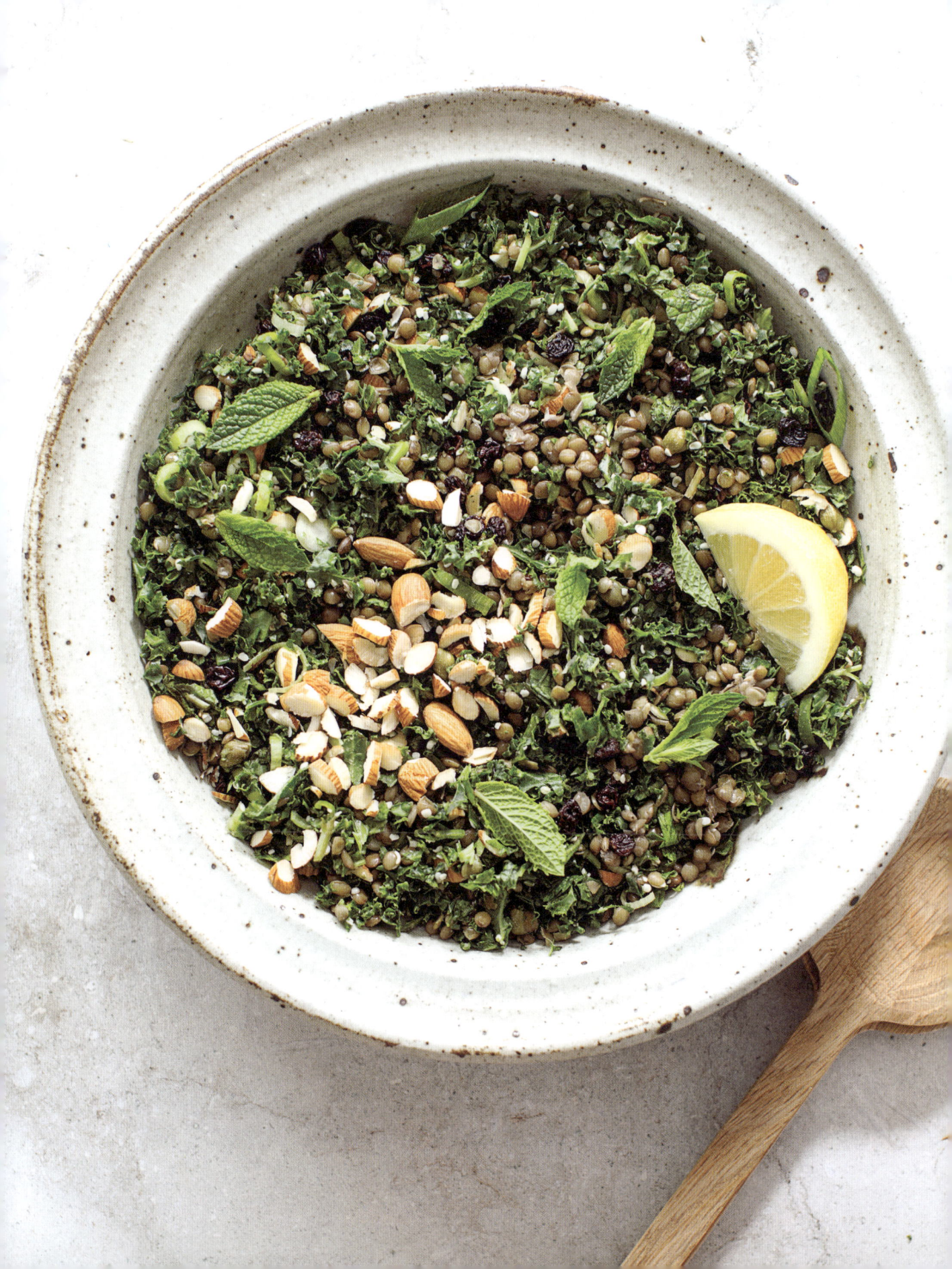

RAW CLEANSING BEETROOT, CARROT and WALNUT SALAD

SERVES 6–8 AS A SIDE SALAD

- 2 teaspoons cumin seeds
- 2 medium beetroot, trimmed, peeled and grated
- 2 large carrots, peeled and grated
- 2 spring onions, thinly sliced
- handful fresh parsley, roughly chopped
- handful fresh mint, roughly chopped, plus extra to serve
- ⅔ cup raisins (or sultanas)
- ½ cup walnuts, crushed
- ¼ cup raw sunflower seeds, plus extra to serve
- 2 tablespoons sesame seeds
- 1 teaspoon ground cumin
- 3 tablespoons balsamic vinegar

This antioxidant-packed salad was one of the first raw salads I made after transitioning to a plant-based lifestyle. Raw beetroot and carrot are two of my favourite daily staples. They provide an abundance of antioxidants, vitamins and minerals, especially when eaten in their raw and natural state. This juicy salad is the perfect combination of tangy balsamic vinegar, hints of cumin, fresh herbs and crunchy nuts and seeds for that added nutritional boost. Try it with my Cauliflower Kofta Balls (see page 206), or as a barbecue side salad on a summer's evening.

Heat a small frying pan over medium-high heat. Add the cumin seeds and toast for 2 minutes, swirling the pan almost constantly to avoid burning, until the seeds turn a shade darker and begin to pop.

Transfer to a large bowl and add all the other ingredients. Toss to combine.

To serve, transfer to a serving bowl and garnish with a light sprinkle of sunflower seeds and mint.

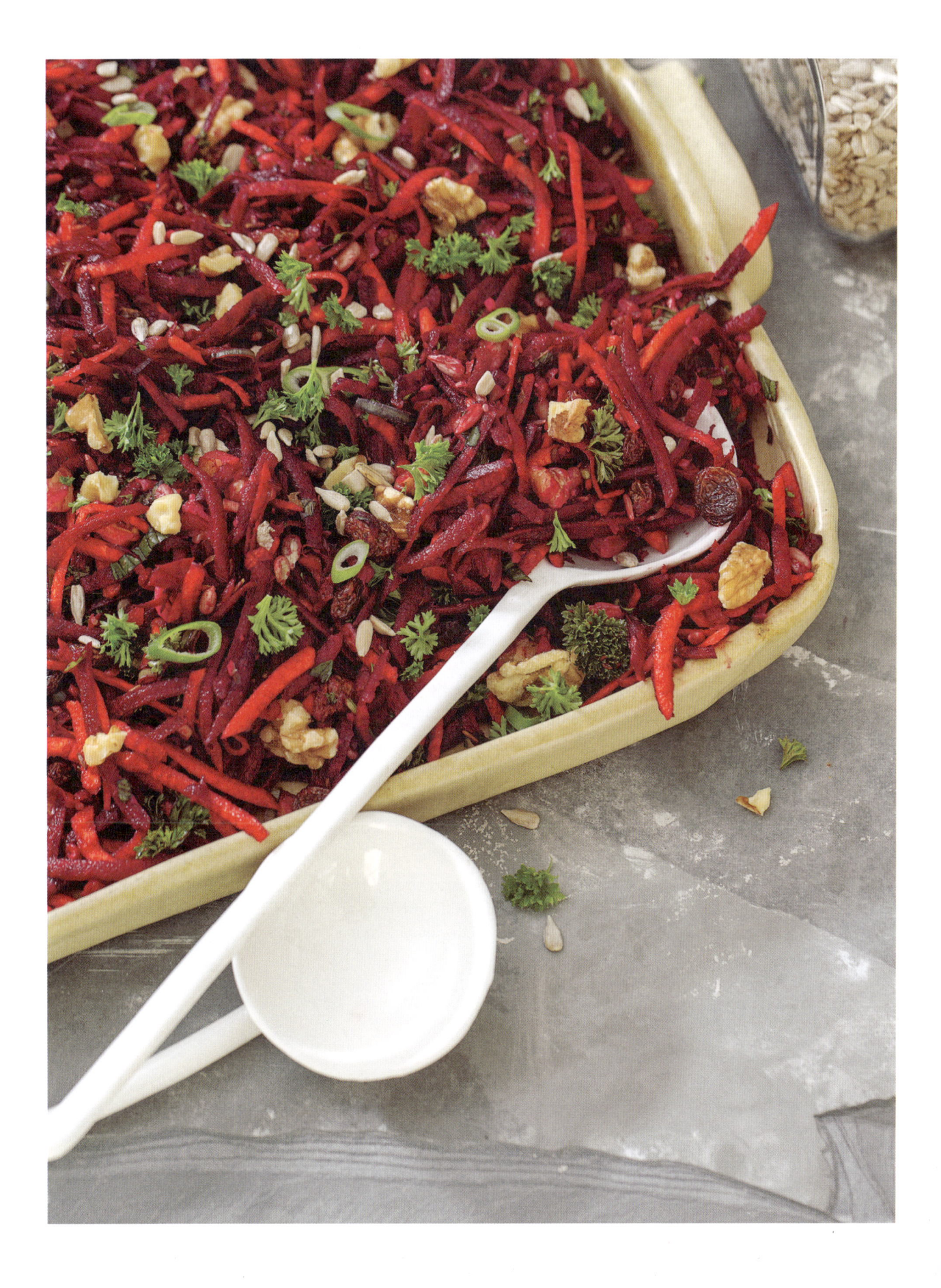

SPICED SORGHUM, GOJI BERRIES, PISTACHIOS, GREEN BEANS and LEMONY YOGHURT

SERVES 4

Spiced sorghum
1 cup sorghum (or buckwheat, millet or quinoa)
3 cups water
½ teaspoon ground cinnamon
½ teaspoon ground turmeric
¼ teaspoon mixed spice
¼ teaspoon sea salt

Salad
1 cup trimmed and sliced green beans
2 teaspoons cumin seeds
1 cup goji berries
handful fresh mint, chopped
handful fresh coriander, chopped
2 cups mesclun leaves
2 spring onions, sliced
2 tablespoons lemon zest
¼ cup lemon juice
⅛ teaspoon white pepper
½ cup raw unsalted pistachios

Lemony yoghurt
½ cup coconut yoghurt
2 tablespoons lemon juice
1 tablespoon lemon zest

To serve
fresh mint
½ sliced avocado (optional)

The story behind this beautiful salad began while in Portugal with my family. We had minimal kitchen utensils, a limited amount of ingredients and many of the spices were labelled in Portuguese—it made for a fun challenge. It resulted in a fresh, tangy, sweet and nutritious salad full of lightly spiced, beautiful Indian flavours; one I completely fell in love with and went on to perfect. The turmeric adds a touch of vibrance and earthy elements, complemented perfectly by the sweet-sour goji berries and the zingy yoghurt drizzle. Sorghum is another great gluten-free grain with a mild, earthy flavour.

For the sorghum, place all the ingredients in a saucepan, cover and bring to a boil. Once boiling, reduce the heat to low and simmer for 90 minutes, until the water has been absorbed. Remove from the heat and fluff with a fork.

For the salad, heat a small non-stick frying pan over medium heat. Add the beans and cumin seeds and cook, tossing frequently, for 3–5 minutes, until the beans are vibrant and slightly tender and the seeds are toasted and fragrant.

For the lemony yoghurt, place all the ingredients in a small bowl and mix to combine.

Place the sorghum, goji berries, mint, coriander, mesclun, spring onion, lemon zest and juice, and pepper into a large bowl. Toss to combine all the ingredients.

To serve, place the salad on a serving plate and scatter over the pistachios. Garnish with fresh mint, and finish with the avocado slices, if using. Serve with the lemony yoghurt on the side.

NOTE: Keep in mind that sorghum has a much longer cooking time than most other grains; if you're short on time, simply replace it with buckwheat, millet or quinoa.

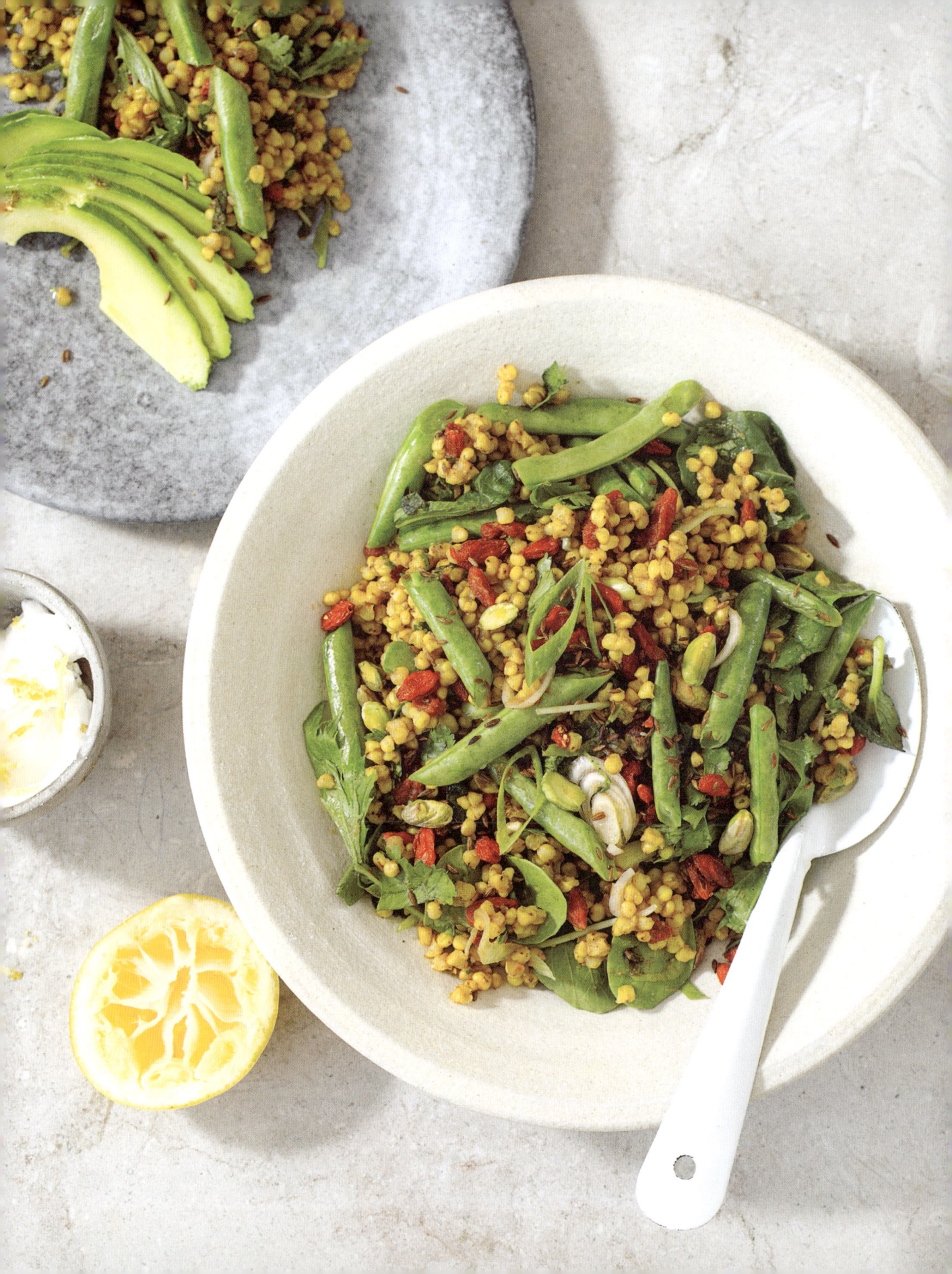

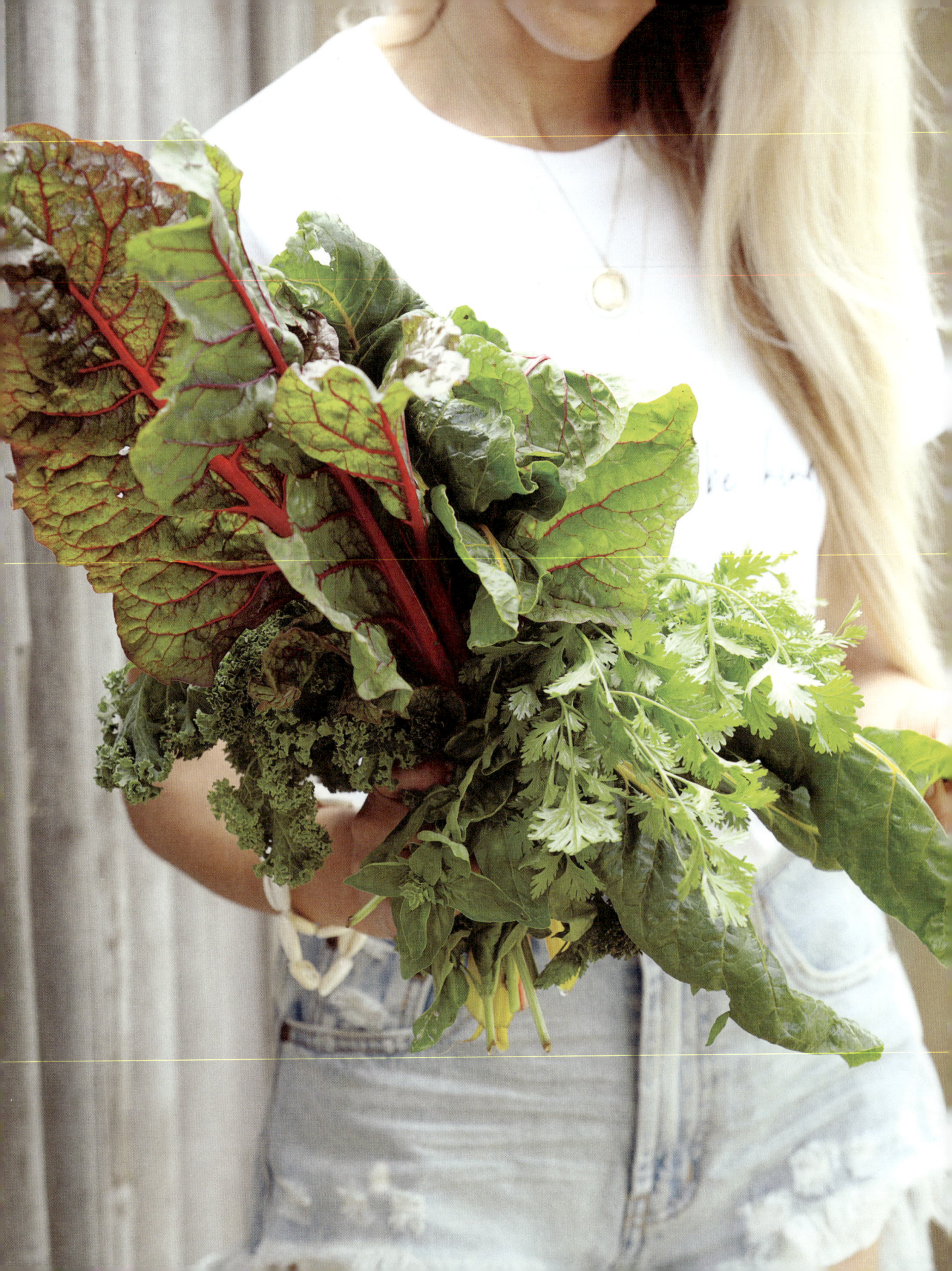

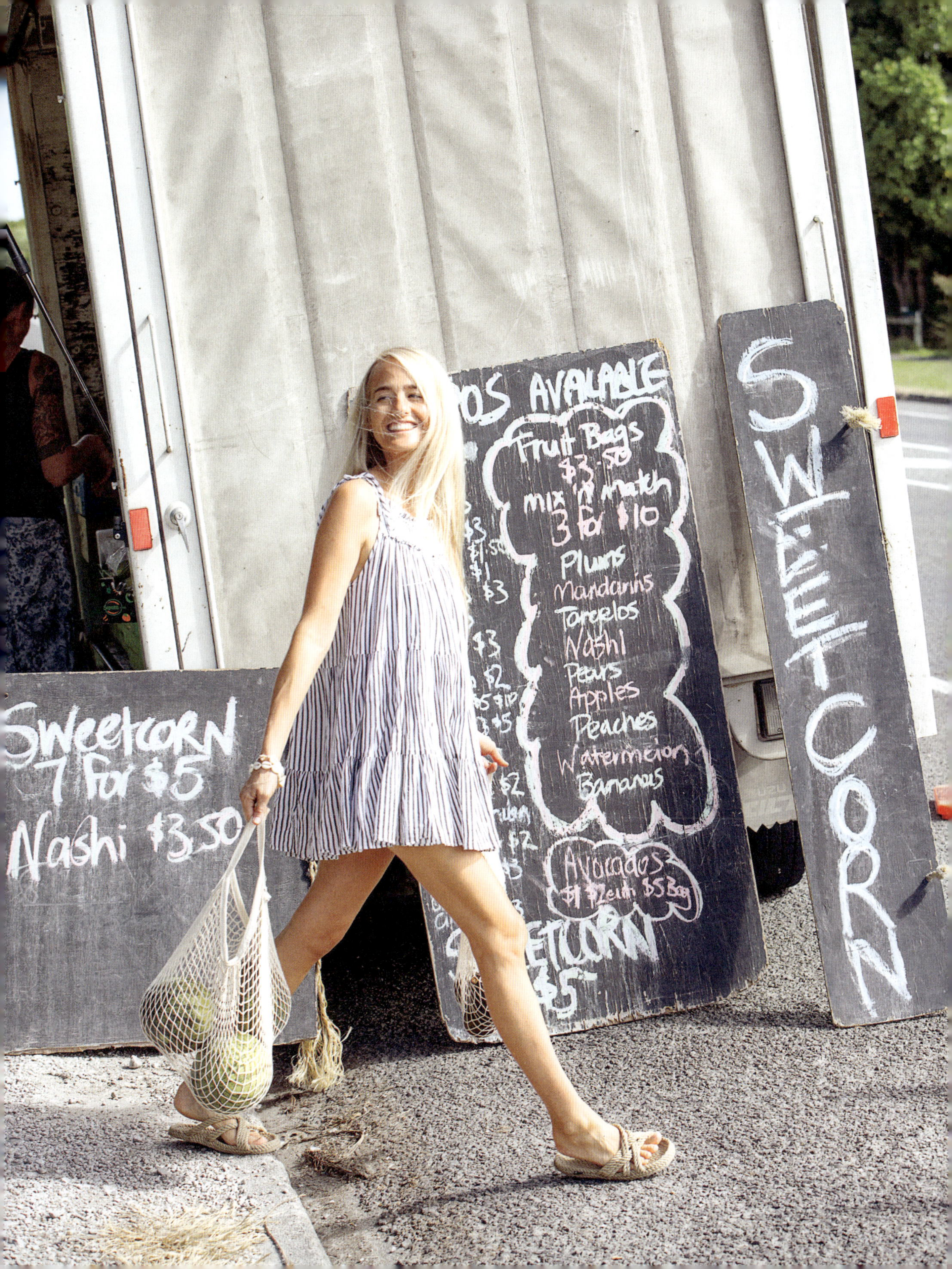
AVAILABLE
Fruit Bags
mix 'n match
3 for $10
Plums
Mandarins
Nashi
Pears
Apples
Peaches
Watermelon
Bananas
Avocados
SWEETCORN
Sweetcorn
7 For $5
Nashi $3.50

RAW BROCCOLI and SUNFLOWER SEED SALAD with CREAMY CASHEW DRESSING

SERVES 4, OR 6–8 AS A SIDE SALAD

2 medium heads broccoli, cut into bite-sized florets (approx. 6 cups)
1 cup raw sunflower seeds
½ cup raw sesame seeds
1 cup raisins (or sultanas)
½ red onion, thinly sliced
2 spring onions, thinly sliced, plus 1 tablespoon to serve)

Creamy cashew dressing
1 cup cashews, presoaked (see Recipe Notes page 47)
1½ tablespoons apple cider vinegar
1 tablespoon pure maple syrup
1 large clove garlic, diced
1 teaspoon wholegrain mustard
2 tablespoons lemon juice
⅓ cup water

I often make this salad for friends and family and have been asked for the recipe so many times. I originally created it for my Raw and Free blog, as it's a fantastic way to add raw broccoli into your diet, a cruciferous vegetable boasting many nutrients including vitamin C, fibre and potassium. The broccoli goes wonderfully with the sweet raisins, crunchy seeds and creamy cashew dressing to create a beautiful fusion of flavour, texture and raw nutrients.

Place the broccoli, seeds, raisins, red onion and most of the spring onion in a large bowl and toss to combine.

For the dressing, place all the ingredients in a blender and blend until smooth and creamy. Pour over the salad and mix to combine slightly.

To serve, transfer to a salad bowl and garnish with the remaining spring onion.

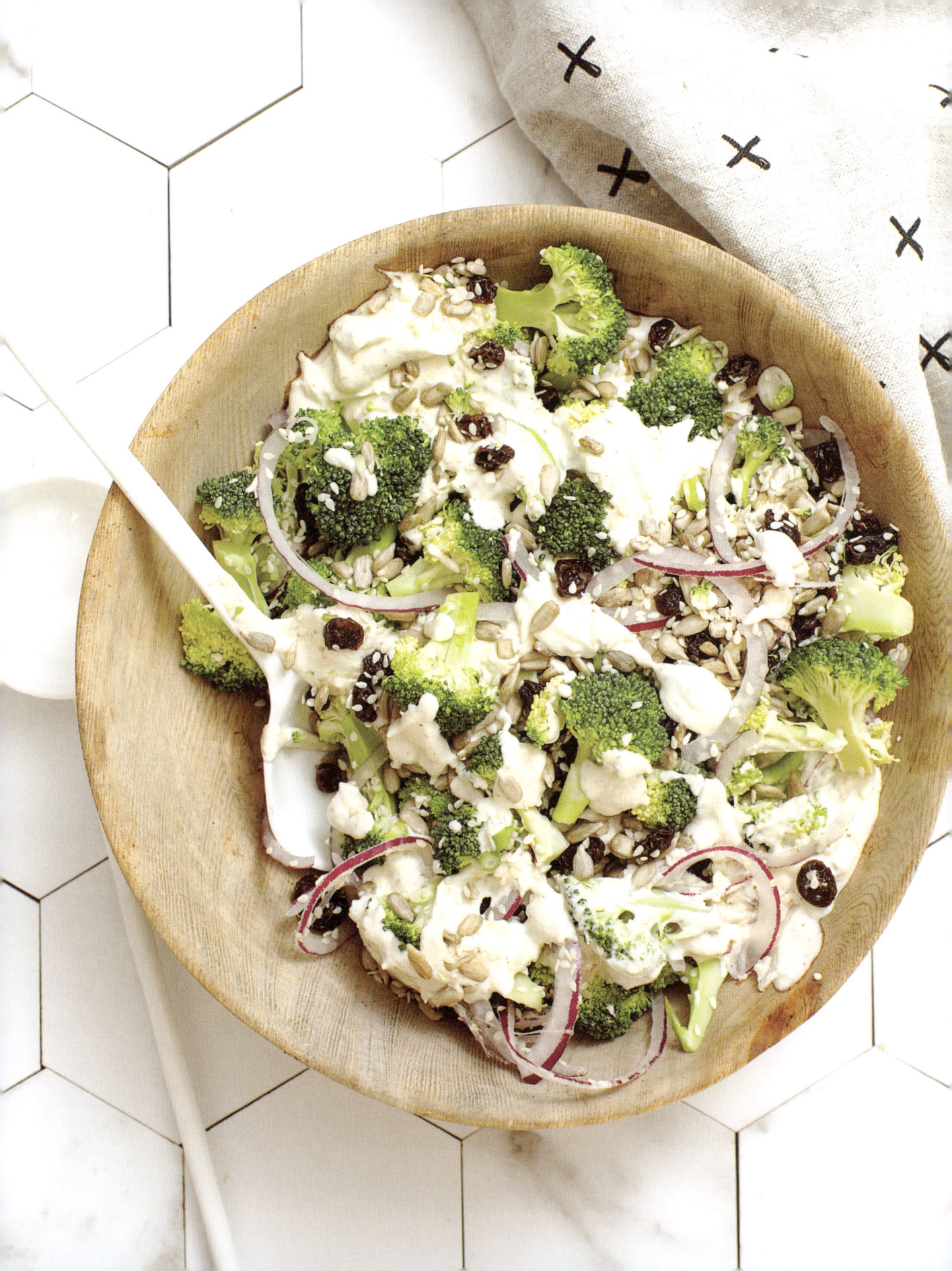

ROAST CAULIFLOWER TREES, CURRIED YOGHURT, PARSLEY and TOASTED ALMOND FLAKES

SERVES 4 OR 6–8 AS A SIDE SALAD

- 1 medium head cauliflower (approx. 1 kg / 2 lb 4 oz), cut into large florets then thinly sliced
- 1 teaspoon olive, avocado or coconut oil (optional)
- sea salt and cracked pepper, to taste
- 1 cup sliced almonds
- 1½ cups parsley, finely chopped
- 2 teaspoons coriander seeds, to serve

Curried yoghurt
- ¾ cup coconut yoghurt
- 2 tablespoons curry powder
- 3 tablespoons lemon juice
- 2 tablespoons water

This simple salad was inspired by one I fell in love with while on a trip to Bali. I love how it has minimal ingredients but still bursts with flavour. Parsley is one of the star ingredients; it's highly alkalising and one of my favourite herbs for adding a nutritional boost to almost any meal. Combined with roast cauliflower 'trees' and crunchy toasted almonds enrobed in a creamy Indian-spiced dressing, it's an incredibly tasty bite to eat.

Preheat the oven to 180°C (350°F) fan bake. Line a large baking tray with baking paper.

Place the cauliflower on the prepared baking tray and spread out into a single layer (you may need to use 2 trays). Drizzle over the oil, if using, and lightly season. Bake for 20–25 minutes, until tender.

Heat a frying pan over medium heat. Add the almonds and cook, tossing frequently to avoid burning, for about 2 minutes, until fragrant.

For the curried yoghurt, place all the ingredients in a bowl and whisk to combine.

Place the cauliflower, parsley, almonds and dressing in a large bowl and mix to combine.

To serve, transfer to a shallow serving bowl and scatter over the coriander seeds. Season with more cracked pepper.

NOTE: Depending on the thickness of your coconut yoghurt, you may need to add a little more water or lemon juice for a slightly thinner consistency.

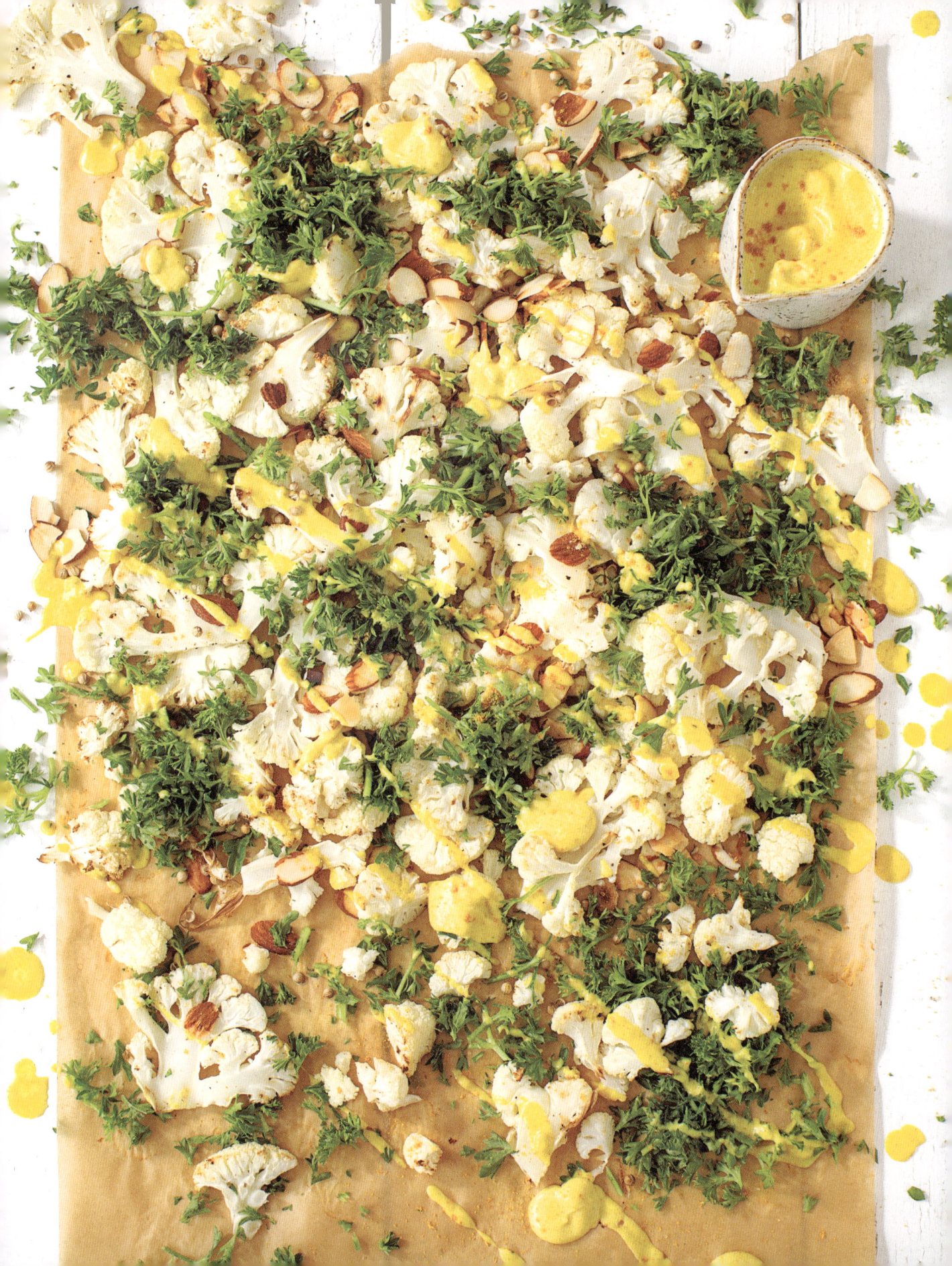

BLACK RICE, POMEGRANATE and MESCLUN with LEMON POPPYSEED DRESSING

SERVES 4

1 cup black rice
2 cups water
2 cups mesclun leaves (or rocket)
¼ cup mint, roughly chopped
¼ cup dill, roughly chopped
1 tablespoon balsamic vinegar
½ red onion, thinly sliced
sea salt and cracked pepper, to taste
½ cup pomegranate arils
⅓ cup pistachios

Lemon poppyseed dressing

⅓ cup lemon juice
1 tablespoon olive oil
1 tablespoon water
2 teaspoons pure maple syrup (or Date Syrup, see page 286)
1 teaspoon Dijon mustard
1 teaspoon poppyseeds
½ teaspoon onion powder

This is one of my favourite salads. Black rice is an iron-rich, gluten-free grain with antioxidant qualities, making it the perfect base for this light and simple salad. Dill and mint are two of my favourite herbs to use, as they provide a refreshing mouthful, and when paired with the pomegranates, crunchy pistachios and a zesty lemon and poppyseed dressing, the most beautiful salad is created. If you have the time, let this salad marinate so the black rice can soak up all the juicy flavours—I promise it's worth the wait.

Place the rice and water in a saucepan, cover, and bring to a boil. Once boiling, reduce the heat to low and simmer for about 25 minutes until the water has been absorbed and the rice is soft.

For the dressing, place all the ingredients in a bowl and whisk together.

Place the rice, mesclun leaves, mint, dill, balsamic vinegar, red onion and dressing in a bowl and toss to combine.

To serve, transfer to a shallow serving bowl or plate and season. Sprinkle over the pomegranate arils and pistachios.

NOTE: This dressing is amazing on just about any salad; it's a great one to make in advance and keep in the fridge for up to 5 days to quickly liven up your greens or roast veges.

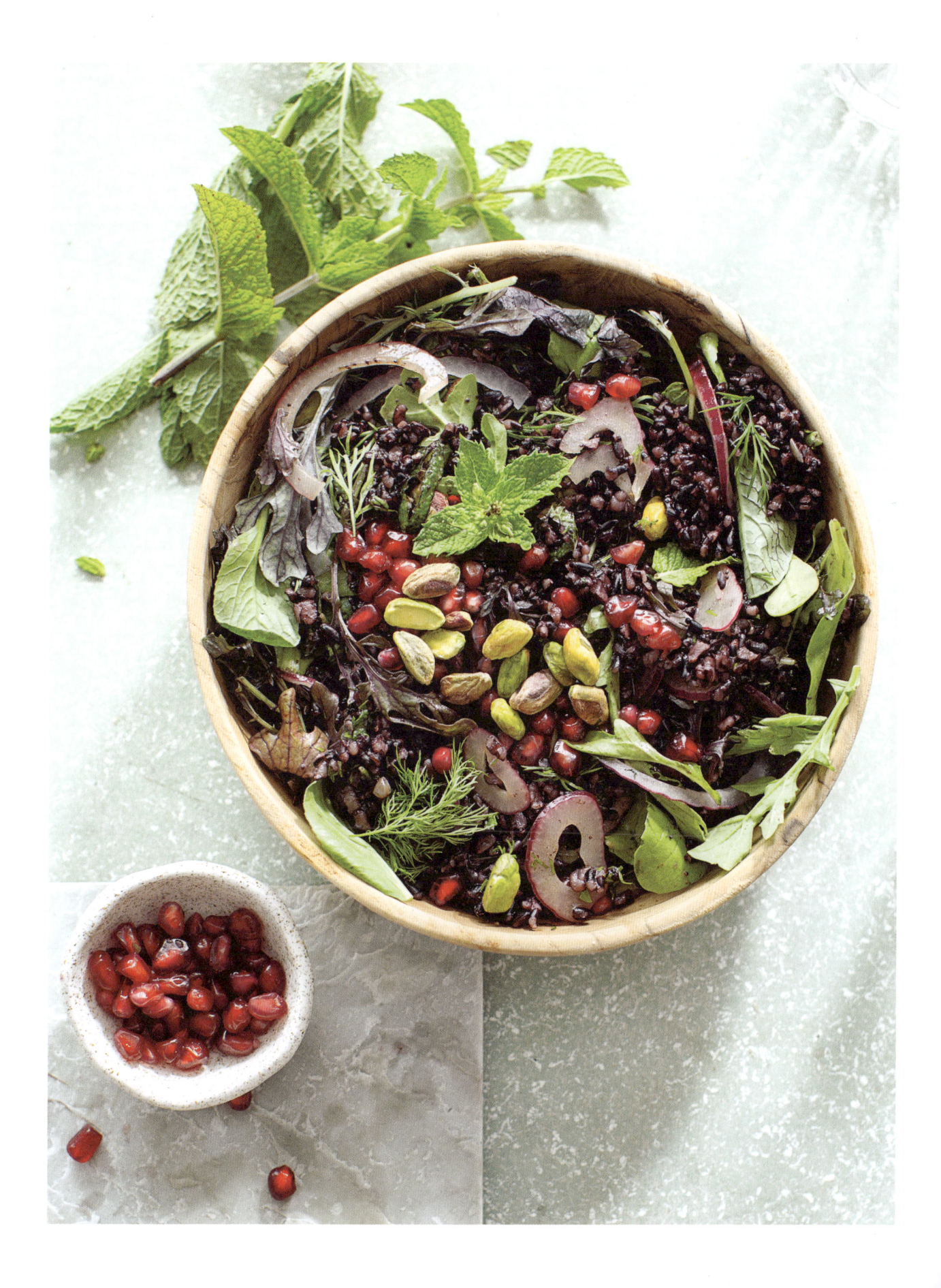

CREAMY KALE CAESAR SALAD with CHICKPEA CROUTONS and HEMP and CASHEW PARMESAN

SERVES 4

Chickpea croutons

400 g (14 oz) can chickpeas, drained and rinsed (or 1½ cups cooked chickpeas)
½ teaspoon olive oil
1 clove garlic, minced
¼ teaspoon garlic powder
¼ teaspoon sea salt
cracked pepper, to taste

Salad

1 small bunch cavolo nero or curly kale, stems removed and roughly chopped (approx. 4 cups)
1 head cos lettuce, finely shredded (approx. 4 cups)
Caesar Salad Dressing (see page 278)
⅓ cup Hemp and Cashew Parmesan (see page 282)

This mix of hearty greens, garlicky chickpeas and cheesy Hemp and Cashew Parmesan (see page 282) makes the most flavoursome, crowd-pleasing salad—perfect for a pot luck. The Caesar Salad Dressing (see page 278) is a super-tasty and versatile dressing: pour it over steamed potatoes and fresh herbs or enjoy it with just about anything. The garlicky chickpeas also make for a healthy snack idea, great for lunch boxes or a crunchy protein addition to any meal.

Preheat the oven to 180°C (350°F) fan bake. Line a baking tray with baking paper.

Place the chickpeas, olive oil, garlic, garlic powder and salt in a bowl, and season with cracked pepper. Mix to combine, ensuring all of the chickpeas are coated in the seasoning. Transfer to the prepared baking tray and spread out into a single layer. Bake for 25 minutes, until golden and crunchy.

Place the kale and lettuce in a large bowl. Pour over the dressing and mix to combine.

To serve, transfer to a large serving bowl or plate. Scatter over the chickpeas and sprinkle over the Hemp and Cashew Parmesan.

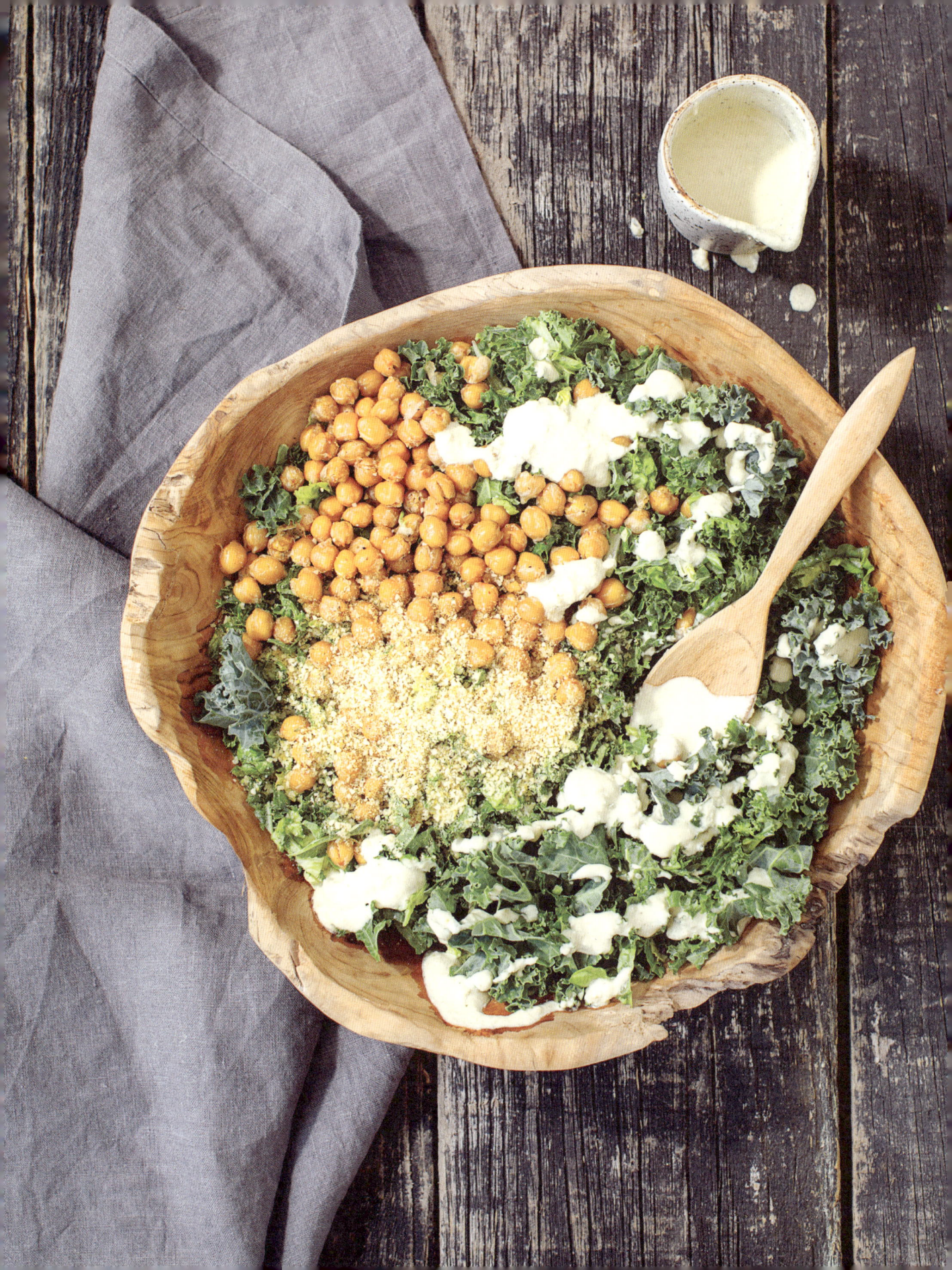

PEANUT SATAY POTATO SALAD
with RAW GREENS and BLACK SESAME

SERVES 4

1.2 kg (2 lb 10 oz) baby potatoes, washed and cut into bite-sized pieces
1 teaspoon olive, avocado or coconut oil (optional)
sea salt and cracked pepper, to taste
1 cup trimmed and halved beans
2 cups mung bean sprouts
½ small telegraph cucumber, diced
½ large green capsicum, diced
handful coriander, roughly chopped
1 spring onion, finely chopped
2 tablespoons crushed peanuts
1 tablespoon black sesame seeds

Peanut satay sauce
½ cup natural peanut butter
⅓ cup water
2 teaspoons pure maple syrup
2 cloves garlic, diced
2 tablespoons tamari (or coconut aminos)
1 tablespoon sesame oil
1 tablespoon apple cider vinegar
2 tablespoons lime juice

This plant-based take on the traditional Indonesian salad, Gado Gado, includes a mixture of crispy baby potatoes, raw fresh greens, crushed peanuts and black sesame seeds, all immersed in a creamy peanut satay sauce—need I say more? The peanut sauce is one of Eli and Milo's favourite dipping sauces; it's also the perfect accompaniment to raw vege sticks and rice paper rolls.

Preheat the oven to 180°C (350°F) fan bake. Line a large baking tray with baking paper.

Bring a saucepan of water to a boil. Place the potatoes in a colander over the water, cover, and steam for about 15–20 minutes until the potatoes are just tender. Drain. Add the oil, if using, and lightly season. Gently mix to combine. Tip onto the baking tray and spread out into a single layer. Bake for 25 minutes, or until golden and crunchy.

For the peanut satay sauce, place all the ingredients in a blender and blend for 20–30 seconds until smooth.

To serve, place the potatoes on a shallow serving plate and spread out evenly. Scatter over the green beans, mung bean sprouts, cucumber, capsicum, coriander and spring onion. Scatter over the nuts and seeds, and finish with a drizzle of peanut sauce. Serve the remaining sauce on the side.

NOTE: Store any leftover sauce in an airtight container in the fridge for up to 5 days.

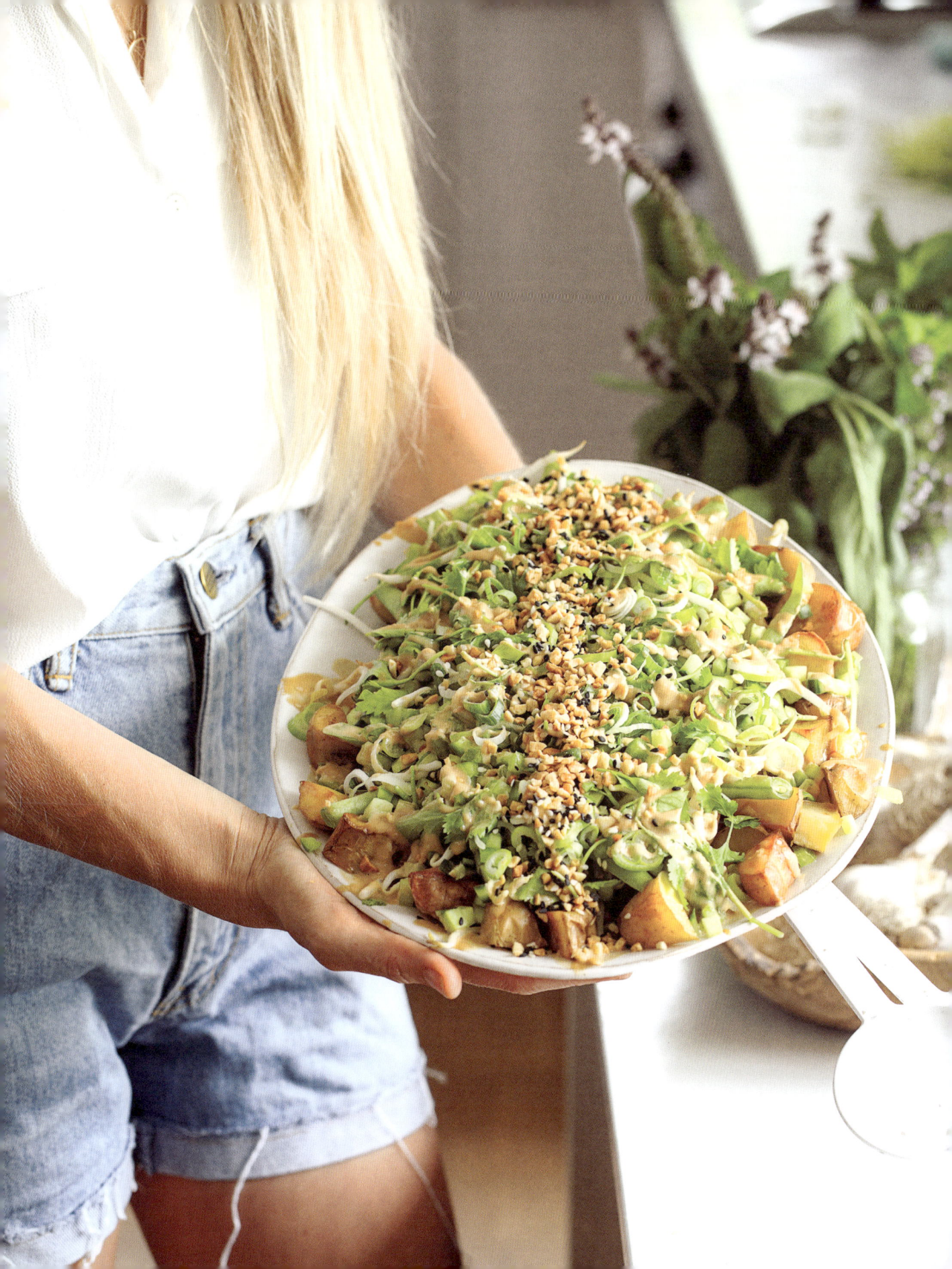

RAW RAINBOW THAI SALAD
with THAI BASIL and LIME DRESSING

SERVES 4

- 2½ cups thinly shredded red cabbage
- 2 carrots, peeled and julienned
- 2 zucchini, trimmed and spiralised
- 1 red capsicum, deseeded and sliced into thin strips
- 1 yellow capsicum, deseeded and sliced into thin strips
- 2 spring onions, thinly sliced
- handful fresh coriander, roughly chopped
- handful Thai basil leaves, plus extra sprig to garnish
- ¾ cup raw cashews (or almonds)
- 2 tablespoons black sesame seeds
- 2 tablespoons raw crushed peanuts

Thai basil and lime dressing
- ½ cup coconut milk (from a can)
- ⅓ cup fresh coriander leaves
- ⅓ cup Thai basil leaves
- 1 kaffir lime leaf
- 1 tablespoon pure maple syrup
- 2 teaspoons tamari (or coconut aminos)
- 1 tablespoon natural peanut butter
- 1 clove garlic, diced
- 1 cm (½ in) piece fresh ginger, peeled
- 2 tablespoons lime juice

When you eat healthy, raw plants you begin to feel the incredible benefits—a feeling that becomes highly addictive. This is the perfect meal for anyone wanting to eat the rainbow in vibrant raw veges, with one of the tastiest Thai dressings I've ever made. This lively salad makes a highly nutritious meal alone, but could easily be bulked up by adding an optional side of marinated tofu.

Place the cabbage, carrot, zucchini, capsicums, spring onion, fresh herbs and cashews, and half of the sesame seeds and peanuts, in a large bowl.

For the dressing, place all the ingredients in a blender and blend for 20–30 seconds until smooth.

Pour the dressing over the salad and mix to combine.

To serve, place the salad in a serving bowl and sprinkle the remaining sesame seeds and peanuts on top. Garnish with a sprig of Thai basil.

NOTE: This salad is best dressed directly prior to serving as the dressing will draw out the liquid in the vegetables.

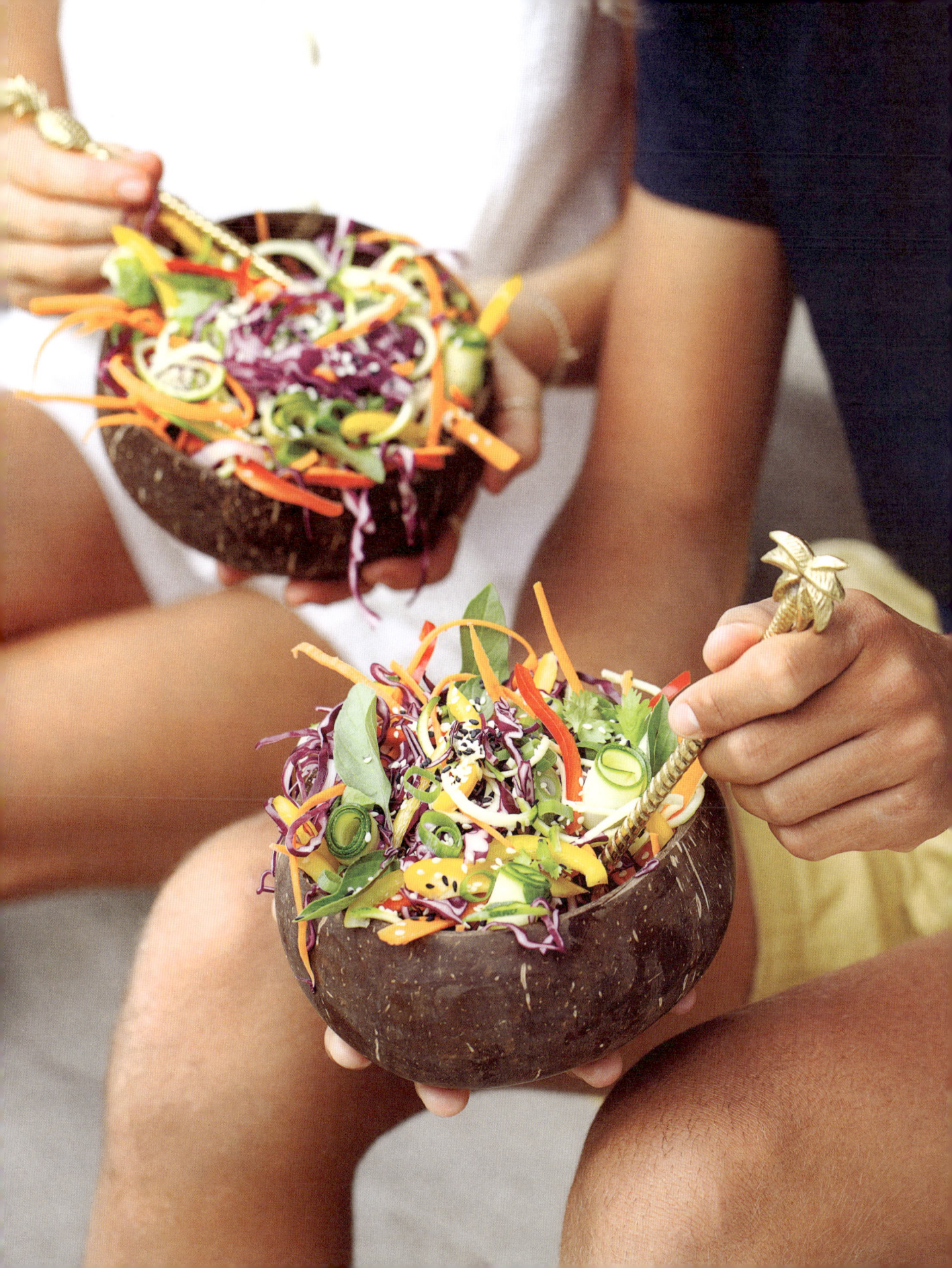

BROWN LENTIL, BEETROOT and AVOCADO SALAD with ORANGE VINAIGRETTE and SUMAC TAHINI

SERVES 4

1 large beetroot (approx. 500 g/1 lb 2 oz)
2 x 400 g (14 oz) cans brown lentils, drained and rinsed (or 3 cups cooked lentils)
handful coriander, roughly chopped
handful mint, roughly chopped
2 spring onions, thinly sliced
2 teaspoons ground sumac
1 teaspoon ground cumin
1 teaspoon fennel seeds
2 large avocados, halved and stoned
sea salt and cracked pepper, to taste
1 tablespoon hemp or sesame seeds, to garnish (optional)

Orange vinaigrette
⅓ cup freshly squeezed orange juice (approx. 1 large orange)
1 teaspoon mustard
1 tablespoon olive oil
½ teaspoon pure maple syrup
1 tablespoon water
1 tablespoon apple cider vinegar

Sumac tahini drizzle
2 tablespoons hulled tahini
2 tablespoons lemon juice
2 tablespoons water
1 clove garlic, crushed
1 teaspoon ground sumac
⅛ teaspoon dried thyme
1 teaspoon pure maple syrup

This salad ticks all the boxes and makes for the perfect pot-luck or barbecue salad. It's both nutritious and incredibly tasty, with tangy, slightly sweet and aromatic flavours. The soft beetroot and lentils are tossed through fresh herbs, spices and a simple orange vinaigrette and, for an extra flavourful flourish, I pair it with a drizzle of my creamy sumac tahini. Sumac is the star spice in this salad, a lemony flavoured spice commonly used in Middle Eastern dishes.

Bring a large saucepan of water (enough to cover the beetroot) to a boil. Once boiling, add the unpeeled beetroot, reduce the heat to low, cover and cook for 50–60 minutes, until the beetroot is fork tender. Drain and let cool for 5 minutes, or until the beetroot is cool enough to handle. Peel the skin off (it should come off easily), slice the beetroot in half, then cut into 1 cm (½ in) cubes. Wash your hands immediately to prevent staining.

Heat a small frying pan over medium-high heat. Add the fennel seeds and toast, tossing constantly to avoid burning, for 2 minutes. Set aside.

For the vinaigrette, place all the ingredients in a jar, seal the lid and shake to combine.

For the tahini drizzle, place all the ingredients in a bowl and whisk together. Set aside.

Place the beetroot, lentils, coriander, mint, spring onion, sumac, cumin, fennel seeds and vinaigrette in a large bowl and gently toss to combine. Season to taste.

To serve, transfer the salad to a round, shallow serving plate. Thinly slice one of the avocados widthways and arrange the slices into two separate sections over the salad. Repeat with the remaining avocado. Sprinkle with seeds to garnish, if desired, and serve with a bowl of the sumac tahini drizzle on the side.

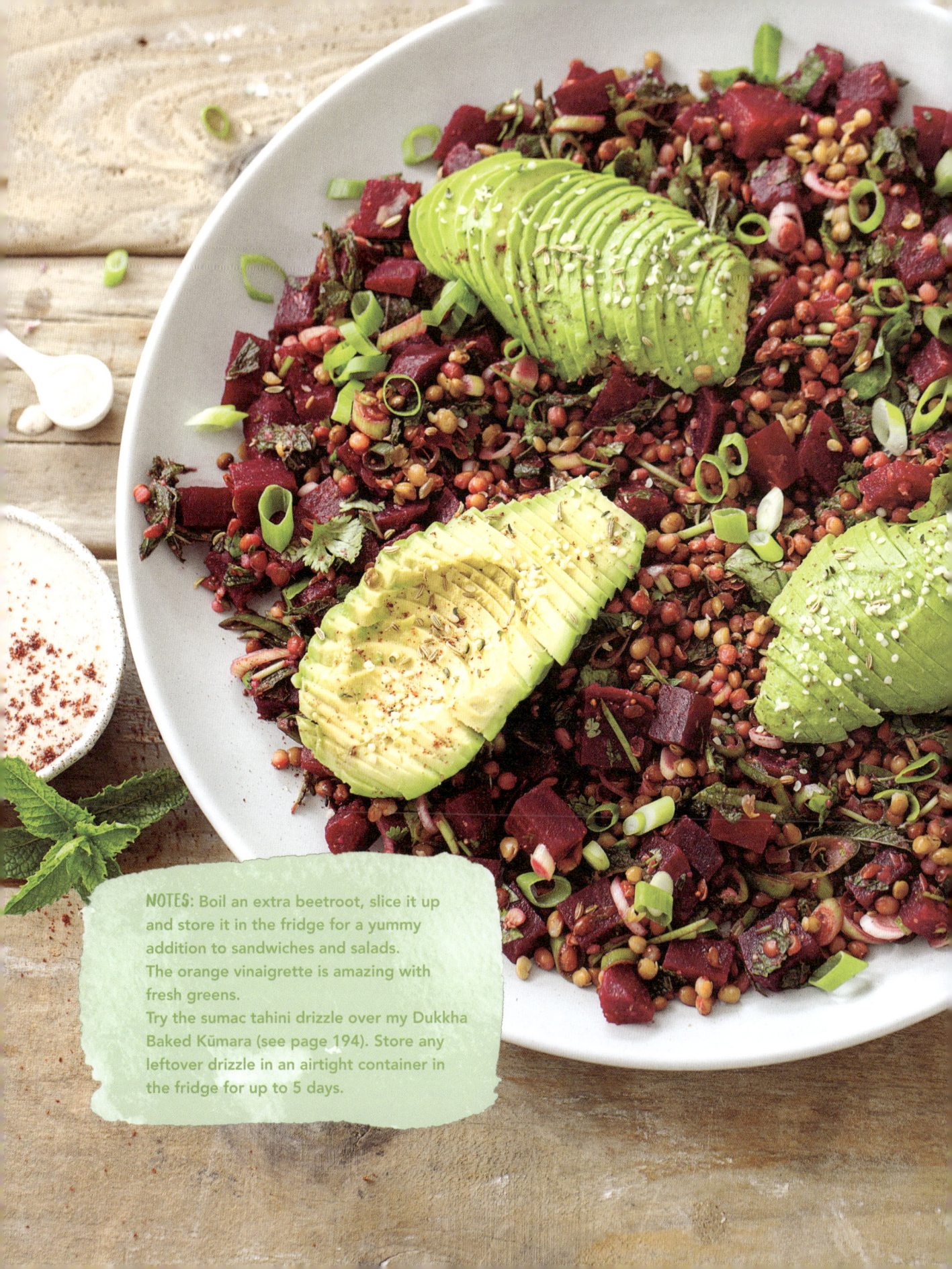

NOTES: Boil an extra beetroot, slice it up and store it in the fridge for a yummy addition to sandwiches and salads.

The orange vinaigrette is amazing with fresh greens.

Try the sumac tahini drizzle over my Dukkha Baked Kūmara (see page 194). Store any leftover drizzle in an airtight container in the fridge for up to 5 days.

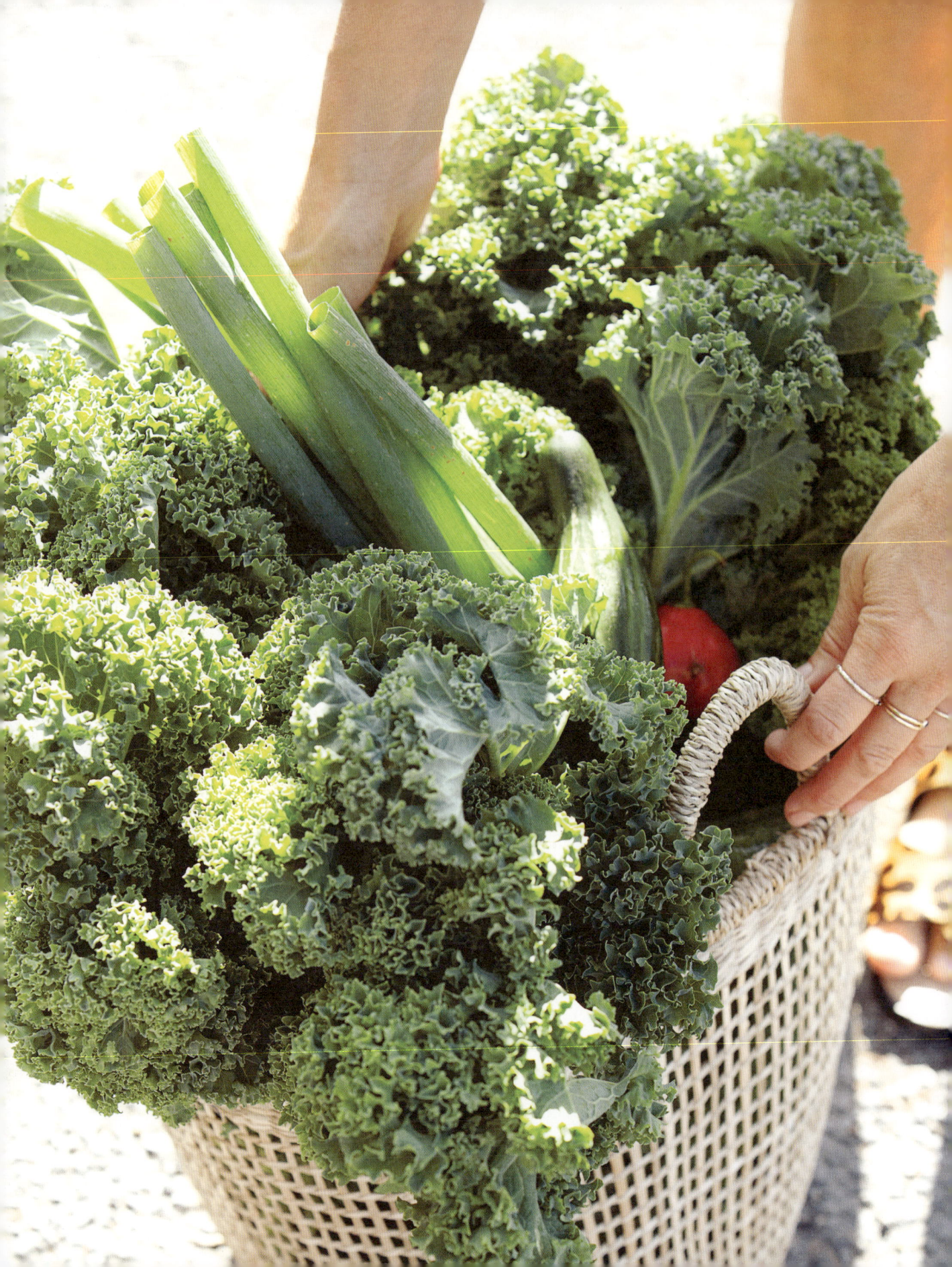

SPRAY FREE
HASS AVOCADOS
$1 each
4-5 days til ripe

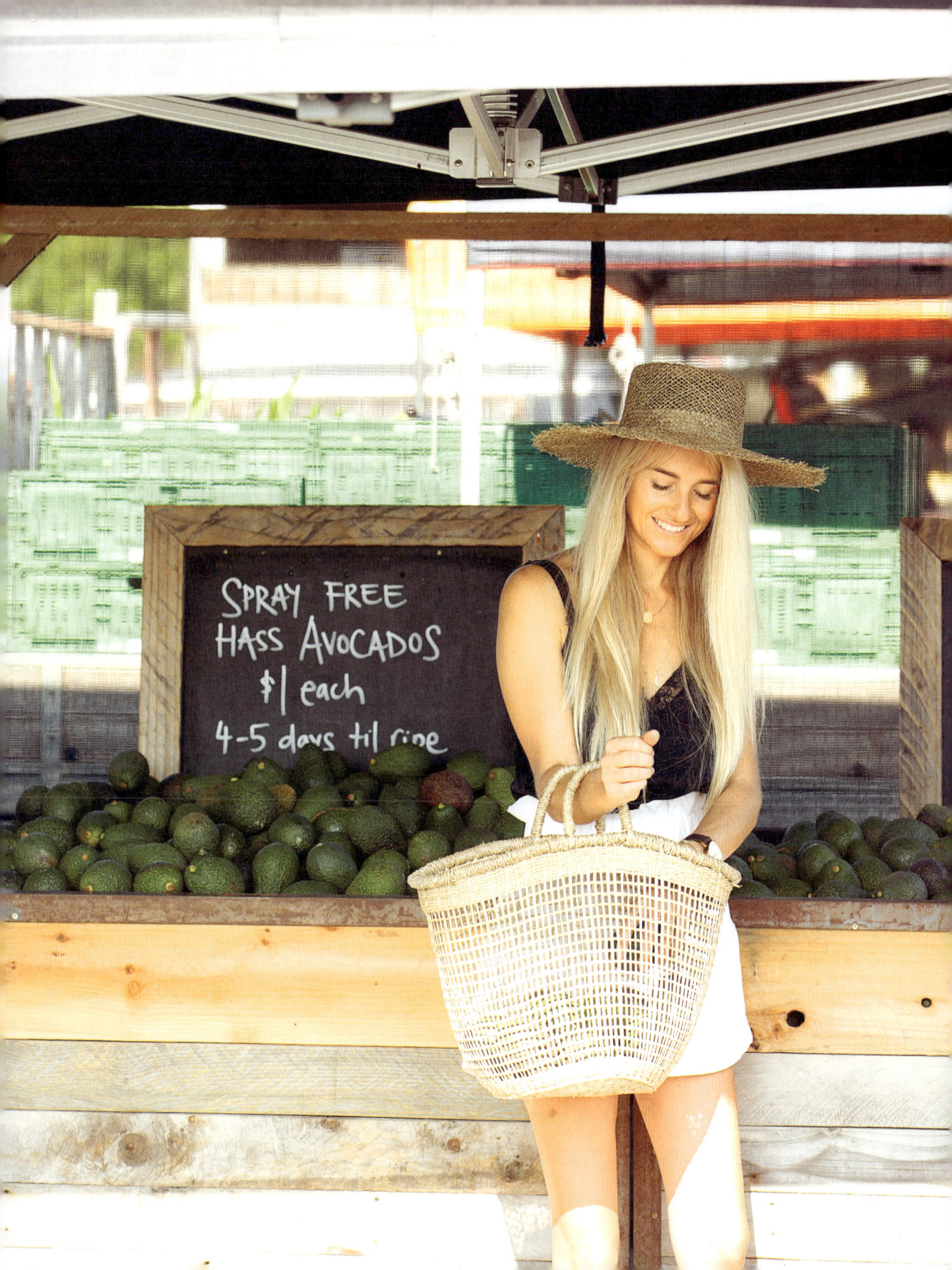

MEXI MUSHROOMS and SMASHED AVOCADO with CHIPOTLE YOGHURT DRIZZLE

SERVES 4

This one is for all the lovers of Mexican food. There are so many things to love about this salad; with the zesty lime and lettuce base, massaged in smashed avocado, garlic and black olives, then topped with crispy Mexican mushrooms and finished with a drizzle of chilli chipotle yoghurt, there are flavours galore. These mushrooms are little beauties; lightly coated in a lime and chilli seasoning and baked to perfection. Try adding them to pastas, soups or burgers for an epic flavour booster.

Preheat the oven to 180°C (350°F) fan bake. Line a large baking tray with baking paper.

For the Mexi mushrooms, place the mushrooms, buckwheat flour, oregano, lime juice, olive oil and chipotle in a large bowl. Season and mix to combine, ensuring all the mushrooms are coated in the mixture. Tip onto the baking tray and spread out in a single layer. Bake for 35–40 minutes, tossing 2–3 times. In the first 20 minutes of cooking it is normal for the mushrooms to produce a lot of liquid; this will be absorbed as the mushrooms continue to cook.

For the salad, place the lettuce, spring onion, lemon and lime juice, garlic and olives in a large bowl. Scoop out the avocado flesh and add to the bowl. Using your hands, massage the avocado into the lettuce leaves, leaving a few small chunks.

For the chipotle yoghurt drizzle, place all the ingredients in a bowl and whisk together. Depending on the thickness of your coconut yoghurt, you may need to add a little more (or less) lemon juice for a thinner/thicker consistency.

To serve, place the salad on a serving platter and top with the mushrooms. Drizzle over enough dressing to cover the salad and serve the rest on the side.

Mexi mushrooms
- 400 g (14 oz) button mushrooms, sliced
- 2 tablespoons buckwheat flour
- 1 tablespoon dried oregano
- 2 tablespoons lime juice
- ½ teaspoon olive oil
- ¼ teaspoon ground chipotle (or ⅛ teaspoon cayenne pepper)
- sea salt and cracked pepper, to taste

Salad
- 2 heads cos lettuce, roughly chopped
- 1 large spring onion, thinly sliced
- 2 tablespoons lemon juice
- ¼ cup lime juice
- 2 cloves garlic, crushed
- ½ cup pitted black olives, sliced
- 2 large avocados, halved and stoned

Chipotle yoghurt drizzle
- ½ cup coconut yoghurt
- 2 tablespoons lemon juice
- 1 teaspoon apple cider vinegar
- 1 tablespoon pure maple syrup
- ¼ teaspoon ground chipotle

NOTE: Replace the Mexi Mushrooms with my Balsamic Cajun Jackfruit (see page 200) for another totally moreish salad—one of my favourites. And swap out the jackfruit in the tacos for the mushrooms to create another epic taco spread.

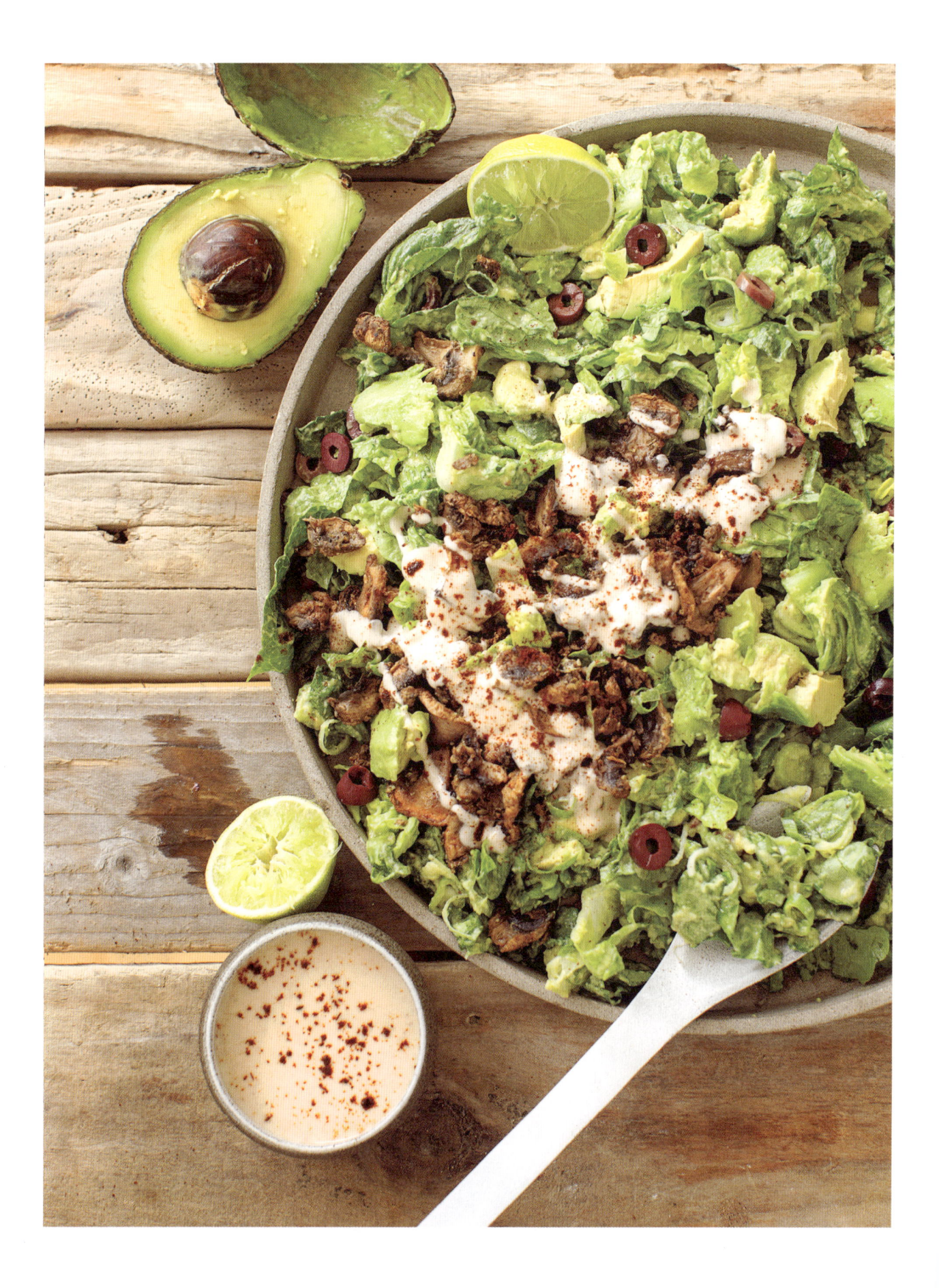

MOROCCAN MILLET and ROAST KŪMARA SALAD IN CREAMY LEMON and GINGER DRESSING

SERVES 4–6

500 g (1 lb 2 oz) orange kūmara, cut into small bite-sized cubes

sea salt and cracked pepper, to taste

1 teaspoon olive, avocado or coconut oil (optional)

½ cup millet

1 cup water

½ red capsicum, diced

½ cucumber, diced

2 spring onions, sliced

handful fresh mint, roughly chopped, plus extra sprig to garnish

handful fresh parsley, roughly chopped

½ cup dried dates, chopped

juice of 2 lemons

2 cups finely chopped cos lettuce

2 tablespoons Dukkha (optional, see page 282)

Creamy lemon and ginger dressing

⅔ cup cashews, presoaked (see Recipe Notes page 47)

½ cup water

1 tablespoon apple cider vinegar

1 clove garlic

1 tablespoon lemon zest

3 tablespoons lemon juice

⅛ teaspoon ground ginger

¼ teaspoon mixed spice

This is the perfect salad to make ahead and keep in the fridge for lunches or an easy weekday dinner. It's a beautiful mix of creamy, fresh, tangy, sweet and perfectly spiced Moroccan flavours. I like to finish it with a sprinkle of Dukkha (see page 282), a fantastic fusion of herbs, nuts, seeds and spices that adds a beautiful Egyptian crunch to any meal. Millet is a mild-tasting grain; it makes the perfect gluten-free replacement for couscous, and can be added to both sweet and savoury dishes.

Preheat the oven to 180°C (350°F) fan bake. Line a baking tray with baking paper.

Place the kūmara on the baking tray and spread it out evenly. Season to taste and lightly drizzle with oil, if using. Bake for 30–35 minutes, or until tender.

Place the millet and water in a saucepan, cover and bring to the boil. Reduce the heat and simmer for 10–12 minutes, or until the water has been absorbed and the millet is soft and fluffy.

For the dressing, place all the ingredients in a blender and blend for about 20–30 seconds, until smooth.

Place the kūmara, millet, capsicum, cucumber, spring onion, herbs, dates, lemon juice and lettuce in a large bowl. Add the dressing and gently mix to combine all the ingredients.

To serve, transfer the salad to a serving bowl, season and garnish with a large sprig of mint. Sprinkle with Dukkha, if desired.

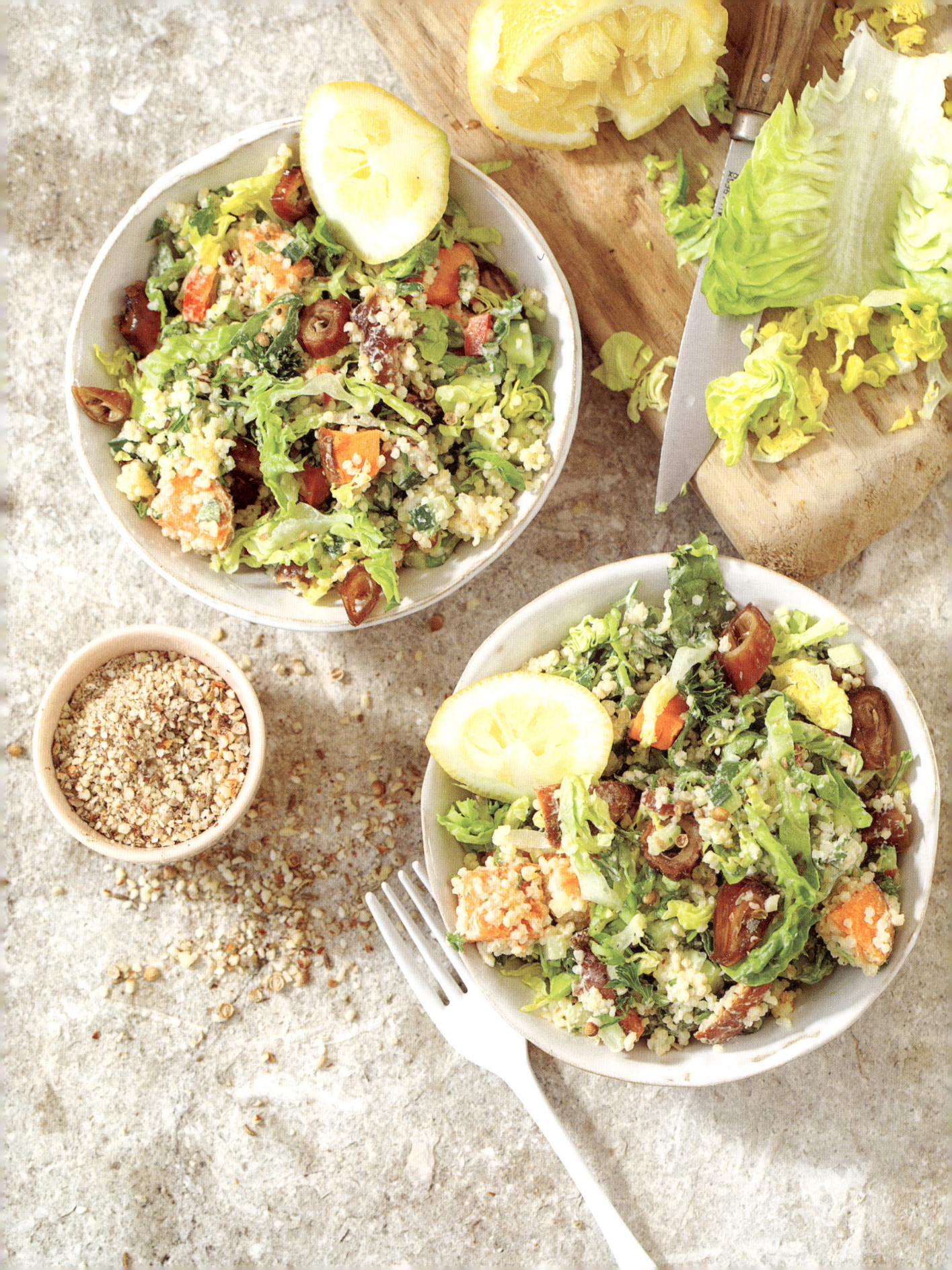

CARROT, COCONUT, CUMIN, ORANGE and BLACK QUINOA SALAD

SERVES 4, OR 6–8 AS A SIDE

⅓ cup black quinoa (optional)

4 medium-large carrots, peeled and grated

⅔ cup shredded coconut, plus 1 tablespoon extra to garnish

handful coriander, roughly chopped

⅓ cup raisins

1 teaspoon ground cumin

2 tablespoons lime juice

⅓ cup freshly squeezed orange juice (approx. 1 large orange)

1 tablespoon sesame seeds

⅛ teaspoon ground ginger

1 teaspoon pure maple syrup

These juicy raw carrots have the perfect balance of citrus from the oranges, tropical flavour from the coconut and earthy elements from the cumin. This is a slightly tweaked version of the original raw carrot salad I created for my Raw and Free blog, with the option of adding in the contrasting black quinoa for sustained energy or keeping it light and simple without it. This vitamin-C-packed salad works as a beautiful barbecue side, served in a burger or as a wholesome lunch or light dinner.

If using the quinoa, place it in a saucepan with ⅔ cup water, cover, and bring to a boil. Reduce the heat and simmer for 12–15 minutes, until the water has been absorbed and the quinoa is soft and fluffy.

To serve, place all the ingredients in a serving bowl and toss to combine. Garnish with a light sprinkle of shredded coconut.

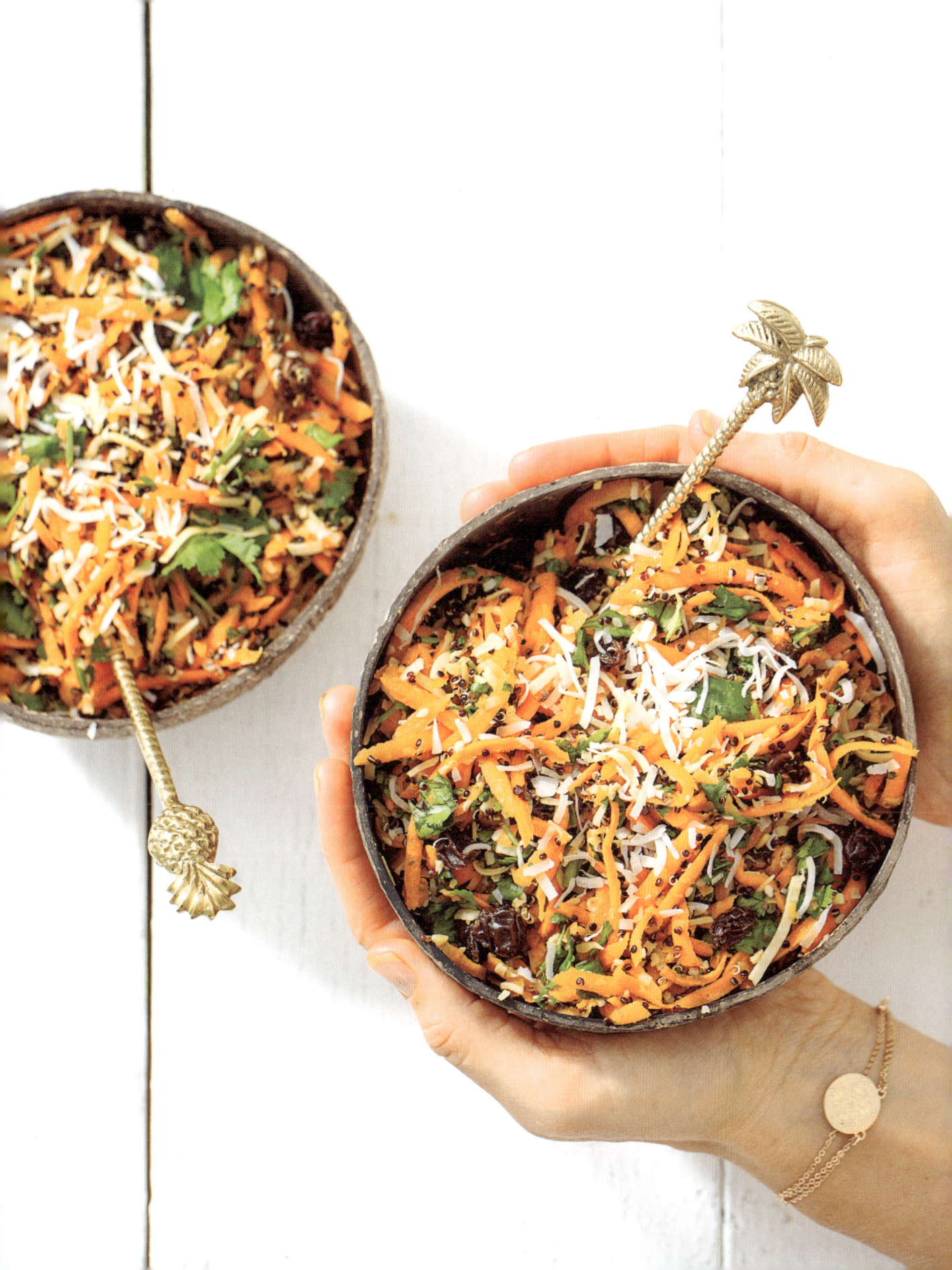

CITRUS CHILLI CARROTS, AVOCADO and PINE NUTS

SERVES 4

600 g (1 lb 5 oz) baby carrots
1 teaspoon olive oil
½ teaspoon chilli flakes, plus extra to serve
sea salt and cracked pepper, to taste
1 large lemon
1 large orange
¼ cup pine nuts
4 cups baby spinach leaves
2 medium avocados, stoned

My sister and I made this lovely salad for Christmas lunch a few years ago. I must admit, I've never been the biggest fan of cooked carrots. As with most veges, I prefer to eat them raw, but this salad completely won me over and I spent an entire summer eating it. The sweet and citrussy baby carrots taste divine topped with creamy avocado, toasted pine nuts and chilli flakes. It all makes for a beautifully simple and nutritious lunch or dinner.

Preheat the oven to 180°C (350°F) fan bake. Line a shallow baking tray with baking paper.

Place the carrots, oil and chilli flakes in a large bowl, season and mix. Tip onto the baking tray and spread out into a single layer. Cut the lemon and orange in half and place on top of the carrots, cut side down. Bake for 25–30 minutes, until the carrots are soft and cooked through.

Heat a small frying pan over medium-high heat. Add the pine nuts and toast for 2 minutes, swirling the pan almost constantly to avoid burning.

Remove the carrots from the oven and allow to cool for 10 minutes. Set the orange and lemon aside for dressing the salad at the end.

To serve, place the spinach leaves on a shallow serving plate. Dice one avocado, scoop out the pieces and arrange them over the spinach, followed by the carrots and pine nuts. Thinly slice the remaining avocado widthways and carefully scoop out the pieces with a large spoon. Arrange the slices into two sections over the salad. Finish by squeezing over the juice from the lemon and orange halves.

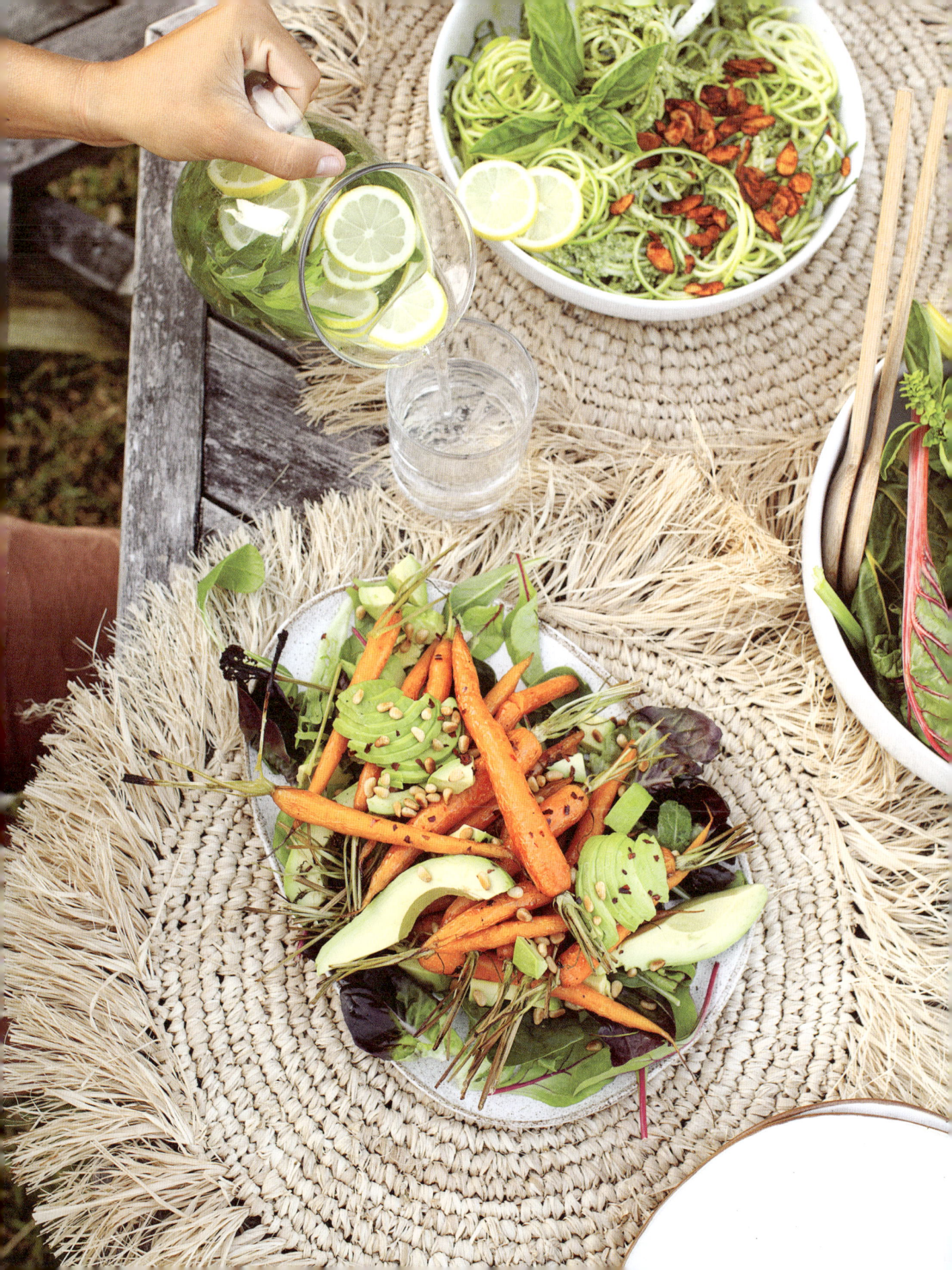

BASIL PESTO and ZUCCHINI PASTA SALAD with ALMOND BARBECUE TOPPERS

SERVES 4

- 150 g (5½ oz) quinoa pasta noodles (or any gluten-free noodles)
- 3 large zucchini, trimmed and spiralised
- 1 cup Hemp, Spinach and Basil Pesto (see page 222)
- handful fresh basil leaves, plus extra sprig to garnish
- sea salt and cracked pepper, to taste
- ½–¾ cup Almond Barbecue Toppers (see page 283)

I make this pasta salad quite often for my boys. It's a great way to sneak in lots of raw zucchini, and when tossed together with the Hemp, Spinach and Basil Pesto (see page 222) it creates a highly nutritious meal. For an added crunch and burst of flavour, the Almond Barbecue Toppers (see page 283) complete this salad perfectly, adding a cheesy, smoky pop into the mix. Spiralised zucchini is a fantastic alternative to pasta; a quick and easy raw meal I often whip up with a handful of cherry tomatoes, spinach and fresh basil.

Fill a large saucepan with water and bring to a boil. Add the pasta noodles and cook according to the packet instructions (usually around 10–15 minutes).

Place the quinoa noodles, zucchini, pesto and basil leaves in a large bowl. Season and mix to combine.

To serve, transfer the salad to a shallow serving bowl and top with the almond toppers. Garnish with a sprig of fresh basil.

NOTE: To make this a raw salad, simply replace the pasta with extra zucchini noodles.

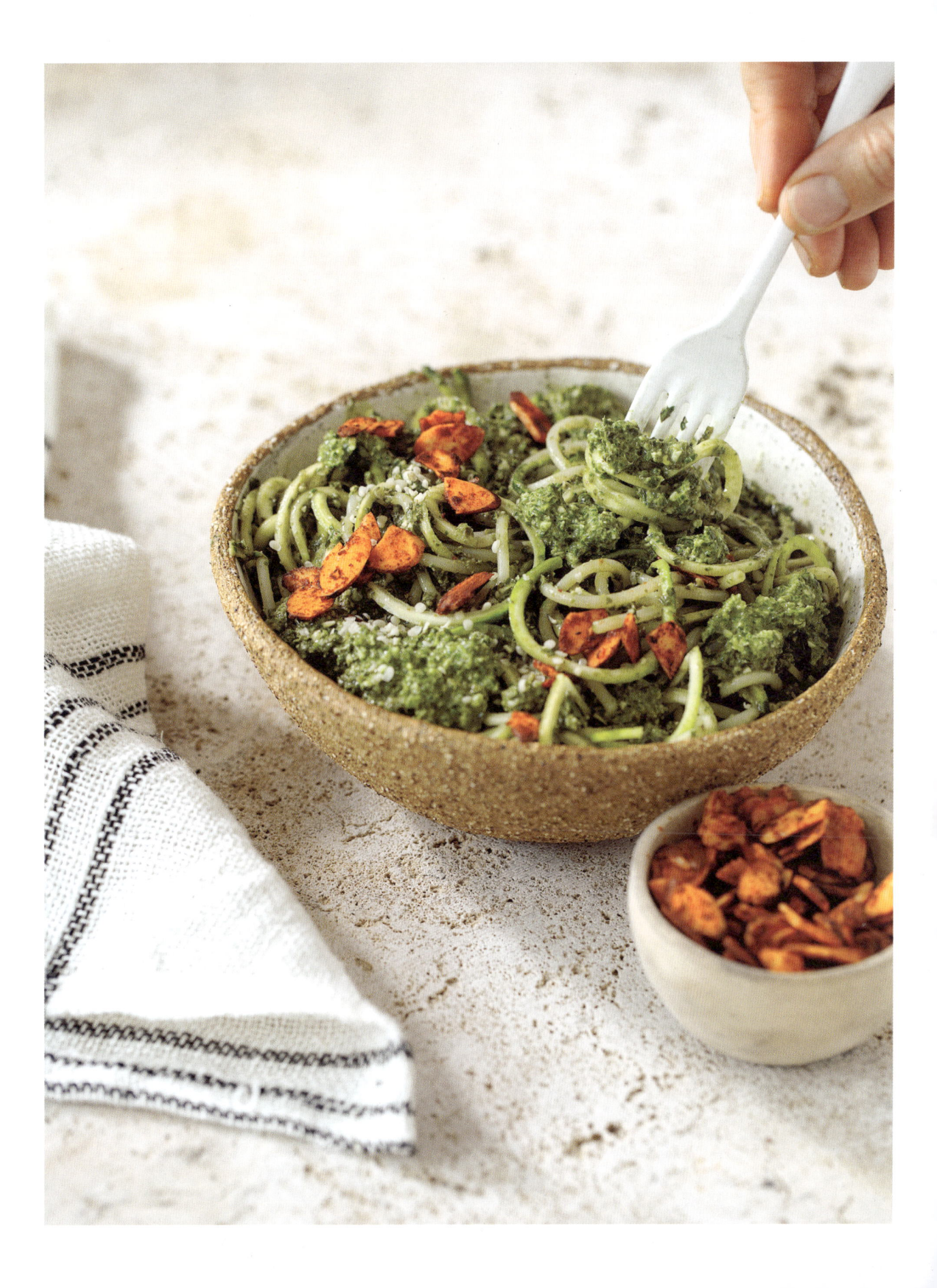

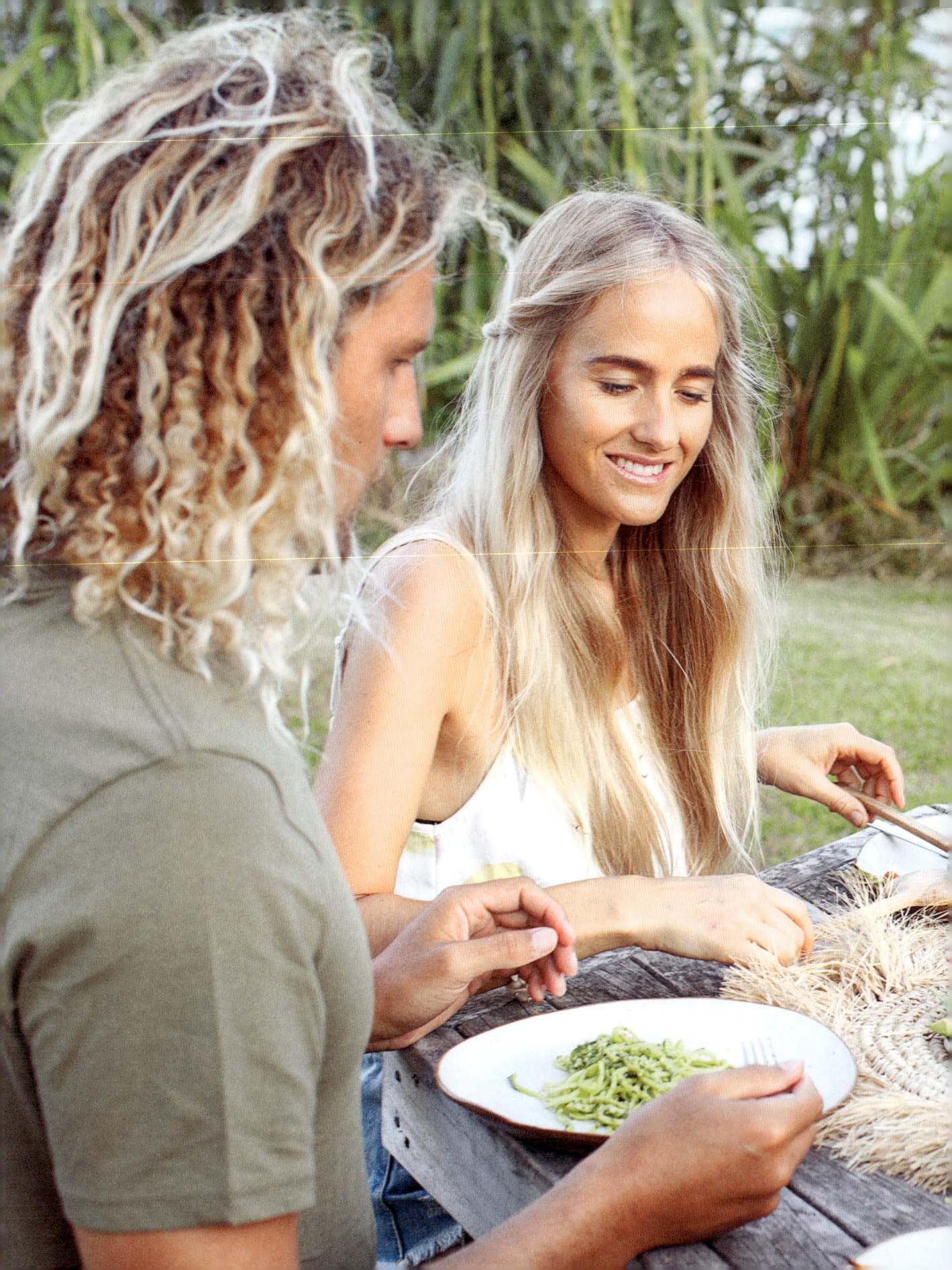

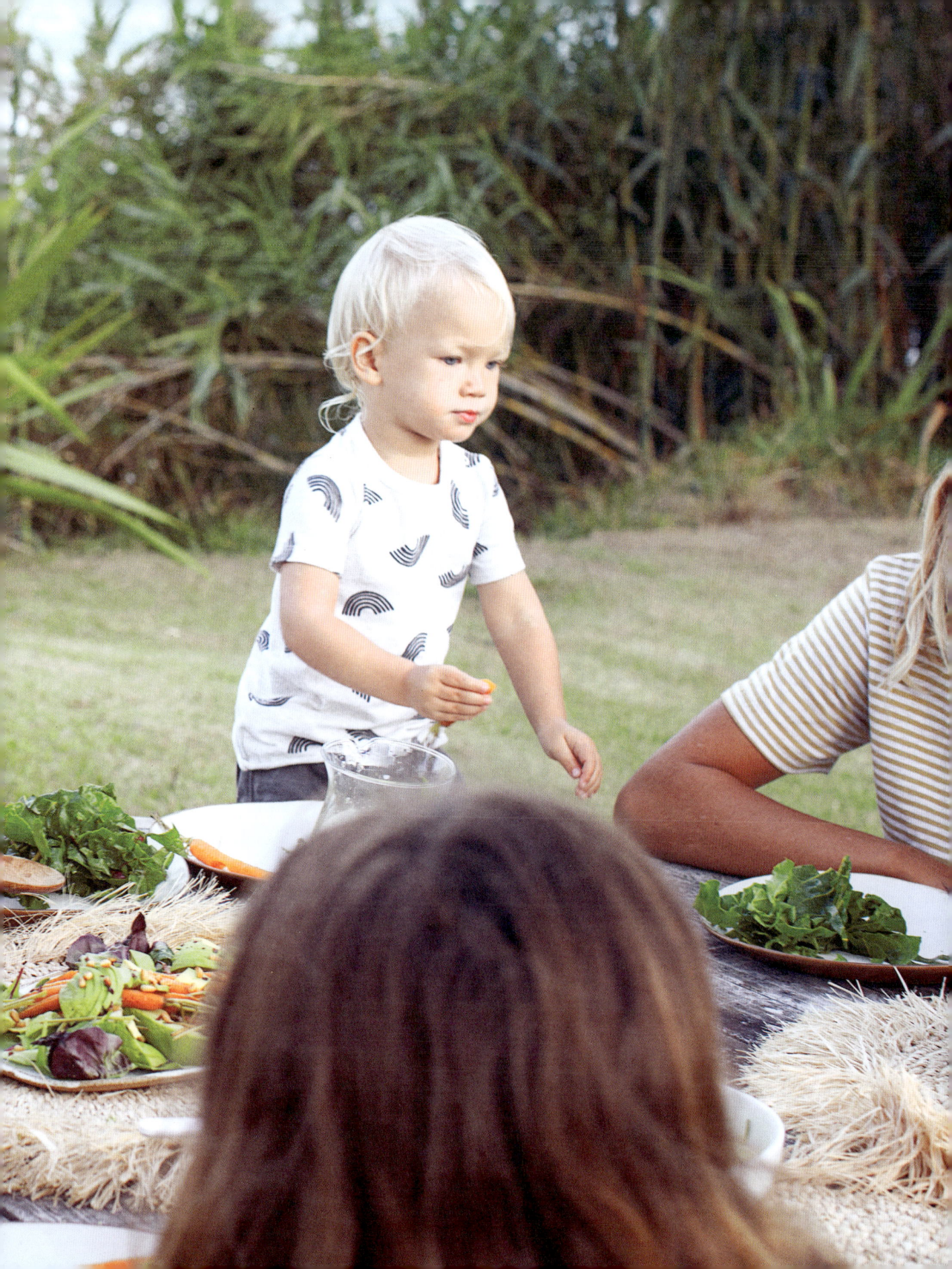

POTATO WEDGES, SWEETCORN and COS LETTUCE SALAD IN CREAMY CAESAR DRESSING

SERVES 4

6 large red-skin or agria potatoes, cut into wedges
olive oil, to drizzle (optional)
sea salt, to taste
3 cups finely chopped cos lettuce
1 small red onion, thinly sliced
2 spring onions, chopped
¾ cup cooked sweetcorn kernels
1 cup fresh parsley, chopped, plus extra finely chopped to serve
Caesar Salad Dressing (see page 278)
cracked pepper, to taste
2 tablespoons black olives, thinly sliced

You have to try this one, it's a definite hit with the kids. I created this salad a few years ago and almost ate the entire bowl in one sitting. It may sound a little different, but trust me, it's a winning combo. Potato wedges tossed through juicy sweetcorn, shredded lettuce, red onion, parsley, olives and black pepper and finished with a creamy Caesar Salad Dressing (see page 278) makes this salad totally moreish and impossible not to love.

Preheat the oven to 180°C (350°F) fan bake. Line a large baking tray with baking paper.

Place the potato wedges on the baking tray and spread out into a single layer. Lightly drizzle with olive oil, if using, and season with sea salt. Bake for 40 minutes, or until soft and golden.

To serve, place the potatoes, lettuce, red onion, spring onion, sweetcorn and parsley on a serving plate. Add the dressing and generously season with cracked pepper. Gently toss to combine. Scatter over the black olives and finish with a light sprinkle of parsley and more cracked pepper.

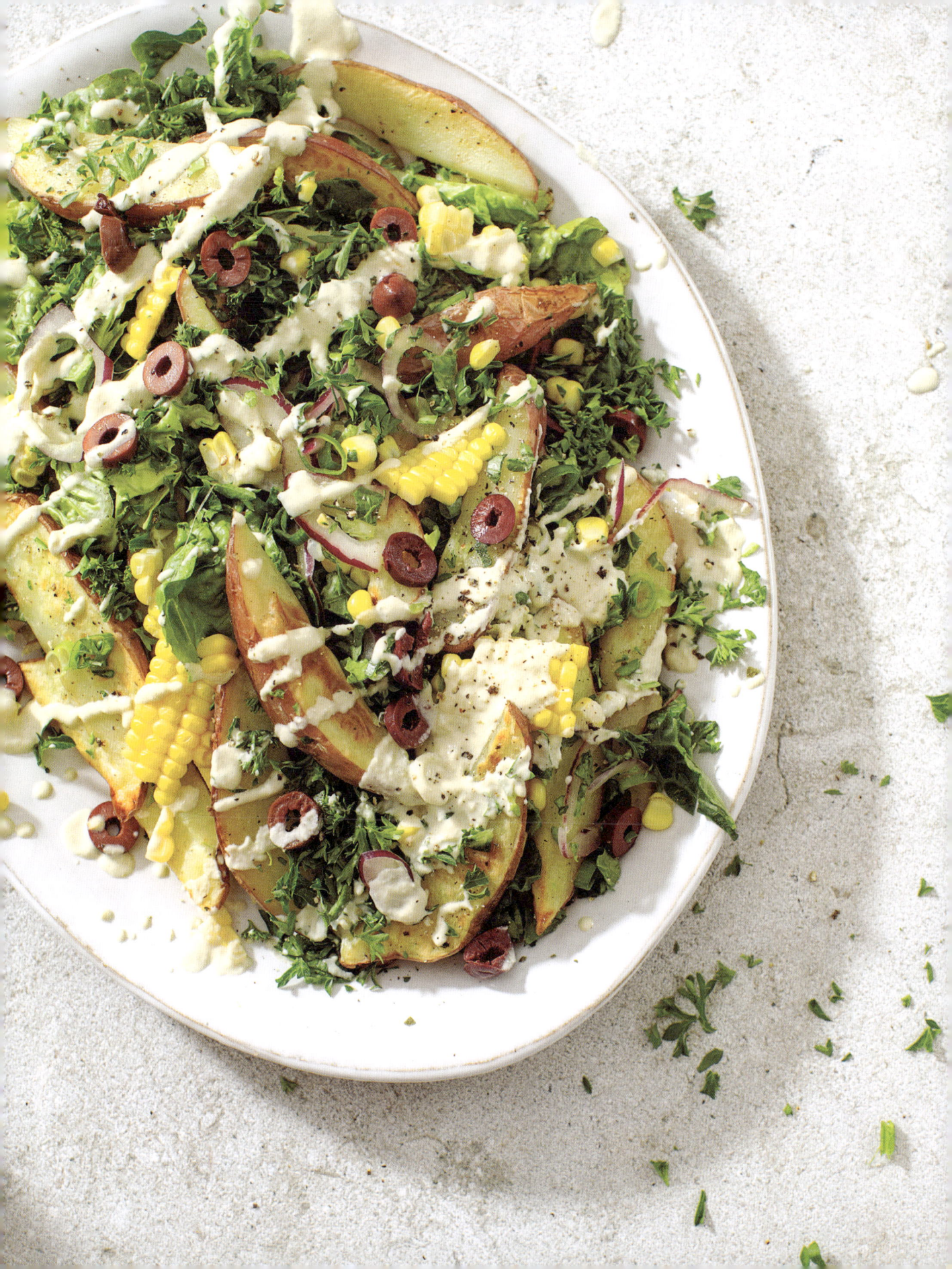

ROAST BUTTERNUT, RED QUINOA, ROCKET and CRANBERRY SALAD with MINT AÏOLI

SERVES 4

- 750 g (1 lb 10 oz) butternut pumpkin, skins on, cut into bite-sized cubes
- 1 teaspoon olive, avocado or coconut oil (optional)
- sea salt, to taste
- ¾ cup red quinoa
- 1½ cups water
- 1 small red onion, thinly sliced
- handful fresh mint, chopped
- ½ cup dried cranberries
- 2 cups baby rocket leaves
- 3 tablespoons lemon juice
- ⅛ teaspoon white pepper
- 1 tablespoon pomegranate molasses (optional)
- ½ cup Mint Aïoli (see page 276)

There's something addictive about these tender roasted butternut chunks, especially when they're tossed through fresh mint, peppery rocket and chewy cranberries for that bite of sweetness, then finished with a drizzle of creamy Mint Aïoli (see page 276). This is another awesome salad to have on hand for lunches or an easy weekday dinner. Red quinoa has a mild, earthy flavour and not only does it add a pop of colour to your meal, it also contains many nutrients including fibre, protein, iron and magnesium.

Preheat the oven to 180°C (350°F) fan bake. Line a baking tray with baking paper.

Place the pumpkin on the baking tray and spread out into a single layer. Drizzle over the oil, if using, and season with sea salt. Bake for 35–40 minutes, or until tender.

Place the quinoa and water in a saucepan, cover, and bring to a boil. Once boiling, reduce the heat to low and simmer for 12–15 minutes, until the water has been absorbed and the quinoa is soft and fluffy.

To serve, place the pumpkin, quinoa, onion, mint, cranberries and rocket leaves in a serving bowl. Add the lemon juice and white pepper, and pomegranate molasses, if using, and gently toss through the salad to combine. Finish by drizzling over the Mint Aïoli.

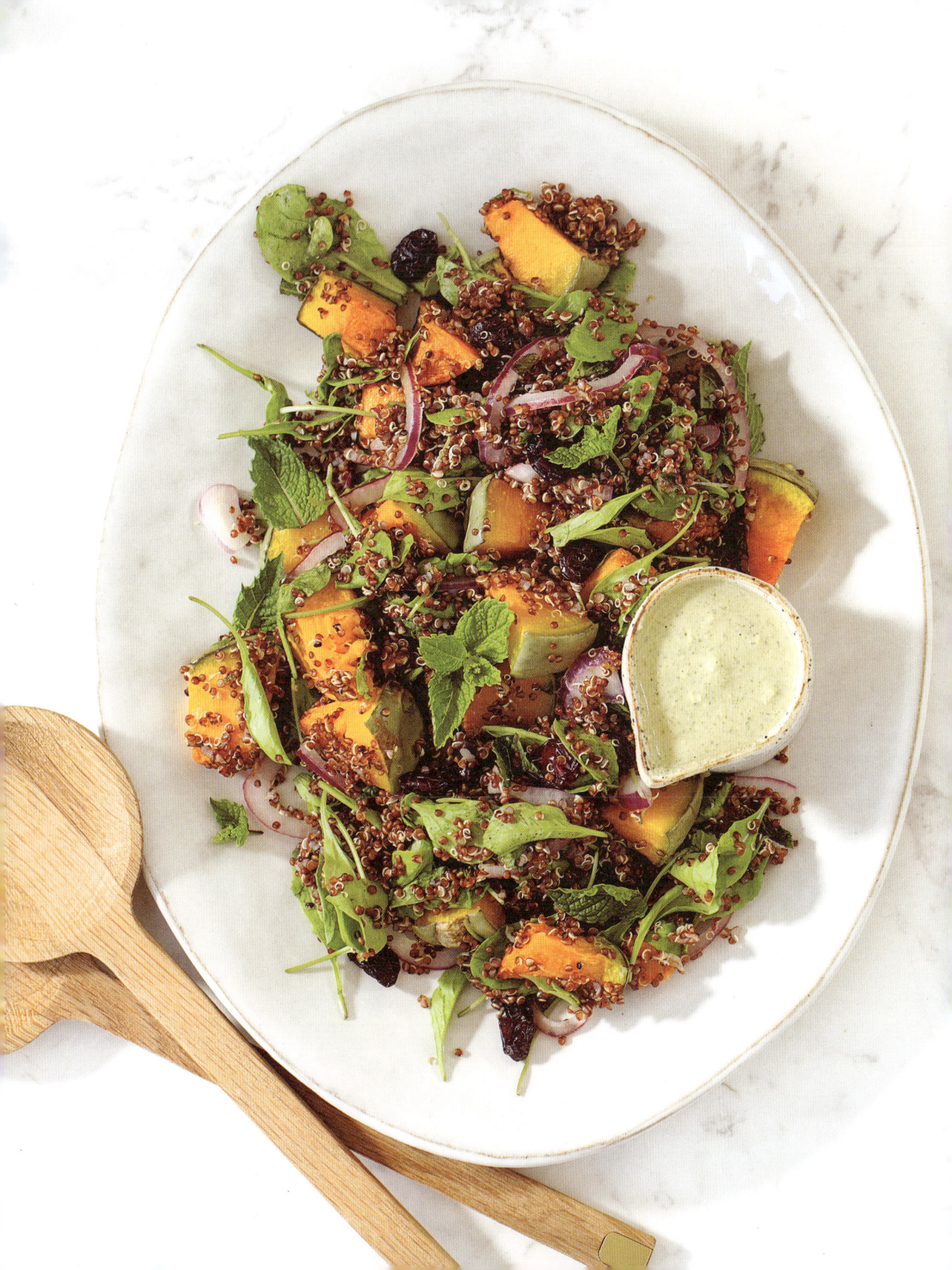

EVERYDAY SUPERFOOD SALAD with SWEET LEMON TAHINI DRIZZLE

SERVES 4

¾ cup raw mixed nuts and seeds (almonds, walnuts, pumpkin, sunflower)
2 cups fresh spinach, finely chopped
2 cups cavolo nero or curly kale, stems removed and finely chopped
1 cup sprouts (alfalfa, broccoli etc.)
1 small beetroot, peeled and julienned
1 carrot, peeled and julienned
1 cup finely chopped red cabbage
1 small red onion, thinly sliced
handful fresh parsley, roughly chopped
¼ cup hempseeds, plus extra to serve
1 large firm avocado, stoned and cut into small cubes
1 lemon, halved

Sweet lemon tahini drizzle
½ cup tahini
½ cup lemon juice
3 tablespoons pure maple syrup

This salad is a staple in my life: a true powerhouse of nutrients full of the goodness we need to create a strong foundation within our bodies and to feed our cells the nourishment they need to thrive. You can adjust it with any fresh, seasonal produce you have on hand, add in a gluten-free grain or try it as a side with just about any recipe in this book. With only three ingredients and taking 30 seconds to make, the tahini dressing is my go-to for adding a sweet, creamy and zesty flavour to any salad.

Preheat the oven to 180°C (350°F) fan bake. Line a shallow baking tray with baking paper.

Place the nuts and seeds on the baking tray and spread out in a single layer. Bake for 8–10 minutes, or until golden. Watch closely for the last few minutes, tossing once or twice to avoid burning, as they will burn quickly.

For the sweet lemon tahini drizzle, place all the ingredients in a bowl and whisk together until smooth and creamy.

To serve, place the spinach, kale, sprouts, beetroot, carrot, red cabbage, onion, fresh parsley, hempseeds and half of the avocado in a serving bowl and gently toss to combine. Scatter over the remaining avocado, the toasted nuts and seeds and a light sprinkle of hempseeds.

Serve with a bowl of the tahini drizzle and lemon on the side.

NOTE: You can blitz the spinach, kale and parsley in a food processor to easily create super-fine greens.

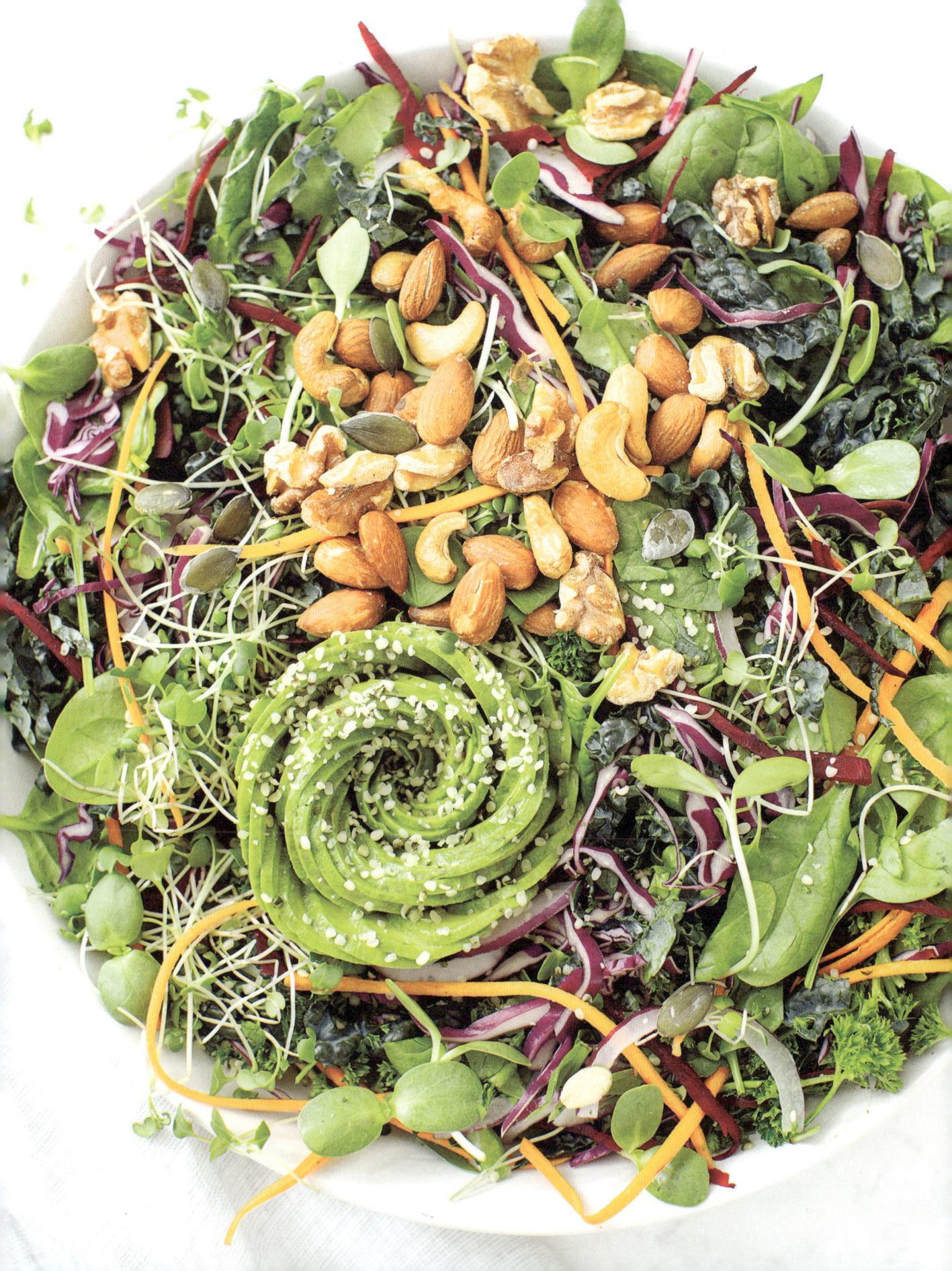

BROWN RICE ASIAN NOODLE SALAD with SESAME LIME DRESSING

SERVES 4

- 200 g (7 oz) brown rice noodles (or other gluten-free noodles)
- 3 cups finely shredded red cabbage
- 1 cup fresh coriander, roughly chopped, plus extra to serve
- 1 cup frozen shelled edamame beans
- 3 spring onions, thinly sliced
- 3 tablespoons sesame seeds
- lime wedges, to serve

Sesame lime dressing
- juice of 2 limes
- 1 tablespoon lime zest
- 3 tablespoons sesame oil
- 1 tablespoon pure maple syrup
- 1 tablespoon tamari
- 1 clove garlic, crushed

I'm always that person who chooses the Asian noodle option when selecting a variety of salads from a salad bar. I love the zesty freshness of it, absorbed in all the Asian flavours with the crunchy, soft and silky textures to match. This is another family favourite, with crunchy raw red cabbage, fresh coriander, edamame beans and sesame seeds, tossed through a zesty sesame and lime dressing.

Bring a large pot of water to a boil. Once boiling, add the noodles and cook according to the packet instructions (usually about 4–6 minutes, until soft). Be careful not to cook for too long as the noodles can become too soft and mushy. Drain and immediately rinse in cold water to stop the noodles from cooking any further.

For the sesame lime dressing, place all the ingredients in a bowl and whisk together.

Place the noodles, cabbage, coriander, edamame beans, spring onion and 2 tablespoons of the sesame seeds in a large bowl. Pour over the dressing and toss to combine well.

To serve, transfer the noodle mixture to a serving plate. Scatter over the remaining sesame seeds and coriander leaves. Arrange the lime wedges on the side.

NOTE: I buy my brown rice noodles from a health food store. I find they work the best in this salad as they have a mild flavour and texture, but they could easily be substituted for another gluten-free option if you struggle to find them, such as buckwheat or quinoa noodles.

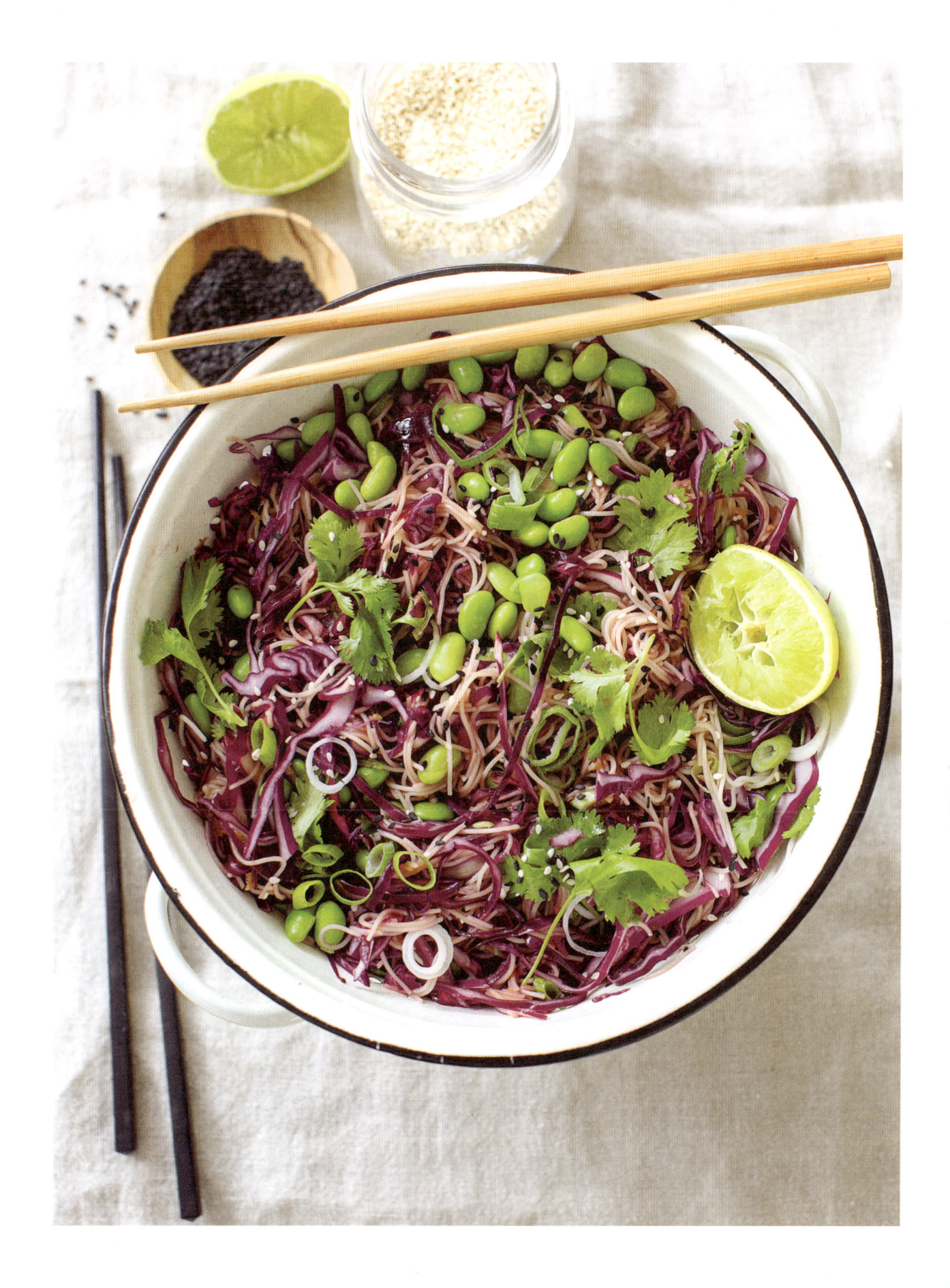

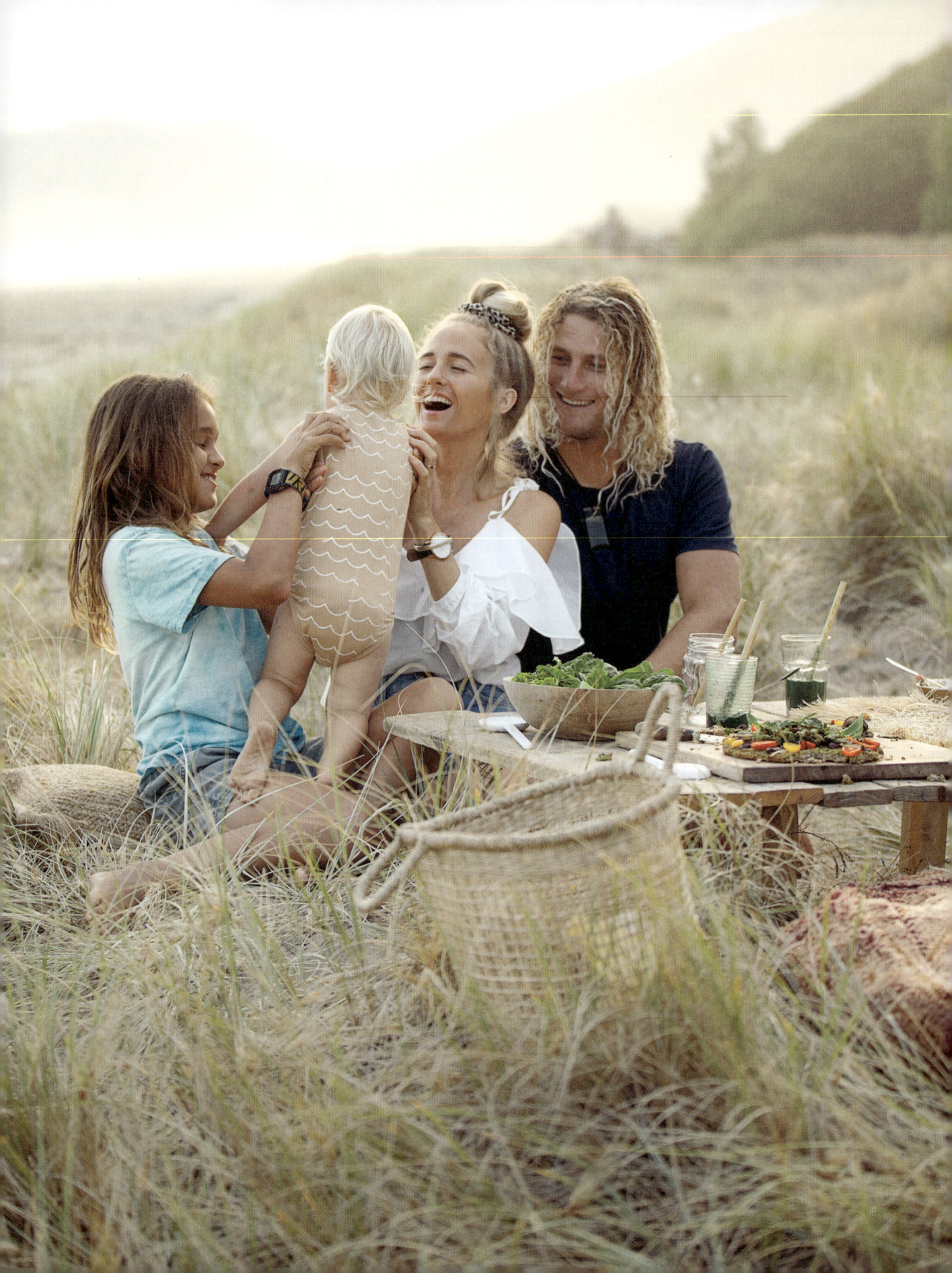

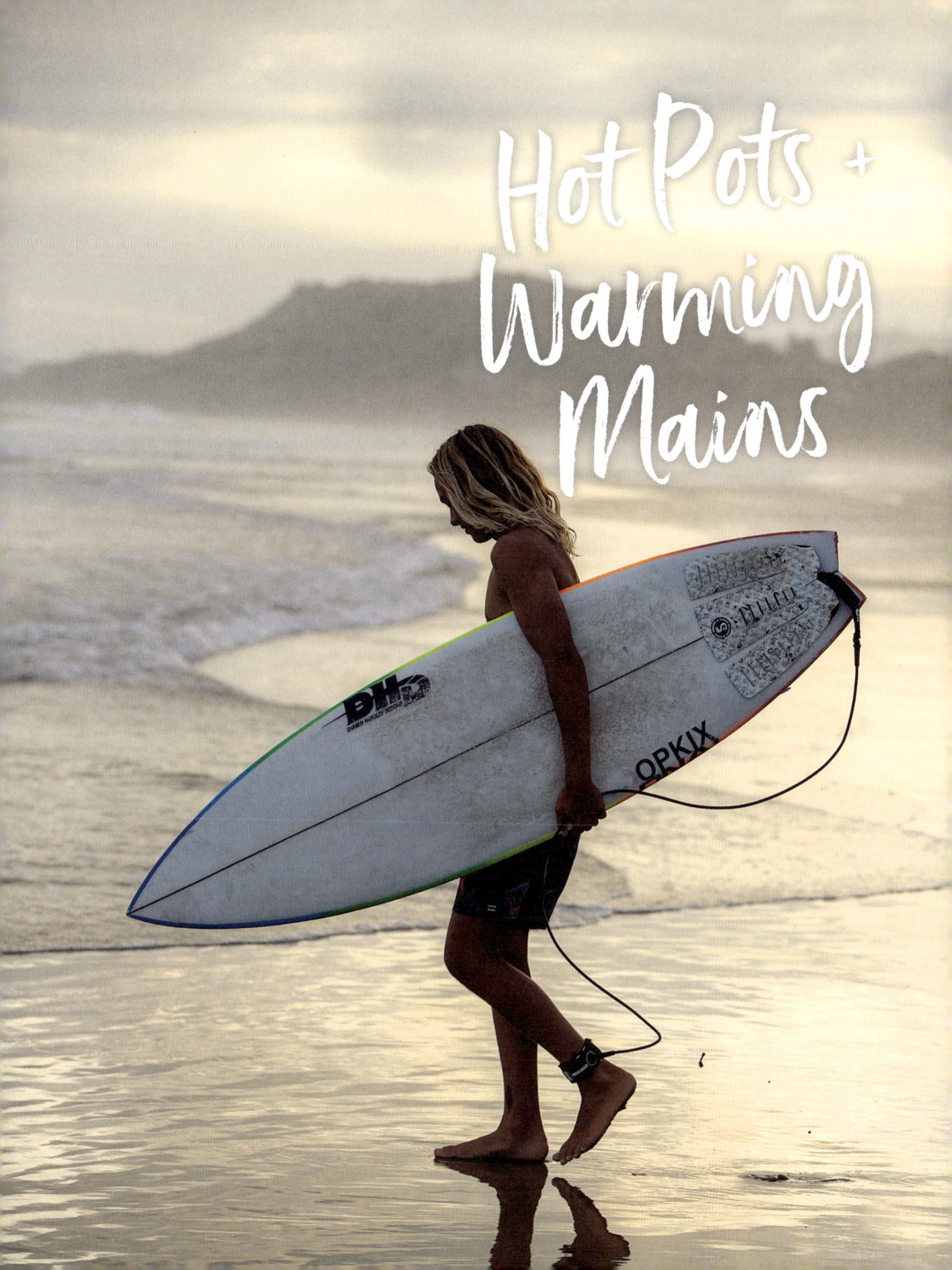

Hot Pots + Warming Mains

Hot Pots + Warming Mains

In this chapter I've created a variety of the most flavourful, belly-warming, plant-based mains, some of which have become our family favourites. From aromatic curries to moreish potato bakes, and juicy stuffed capsicums to nourishing Buddha bowls, all the recipes are enriched with a variety of herbs and spices and inspired by many different cuisines including Mexican, Indian, Asian, Italian, Greek and Thai.

Most of these recipes use basic herbs, spices and vegetables. My goal was to use plant-based staples as ingredients to make it easier and more cost-effective for you to recreate the dishes. Feel free to substitute any of the vegetables with the fresh seasonal produce locally grown in your area.

QUICK TIPS FOR HOT POTS AND WARMING MAINS

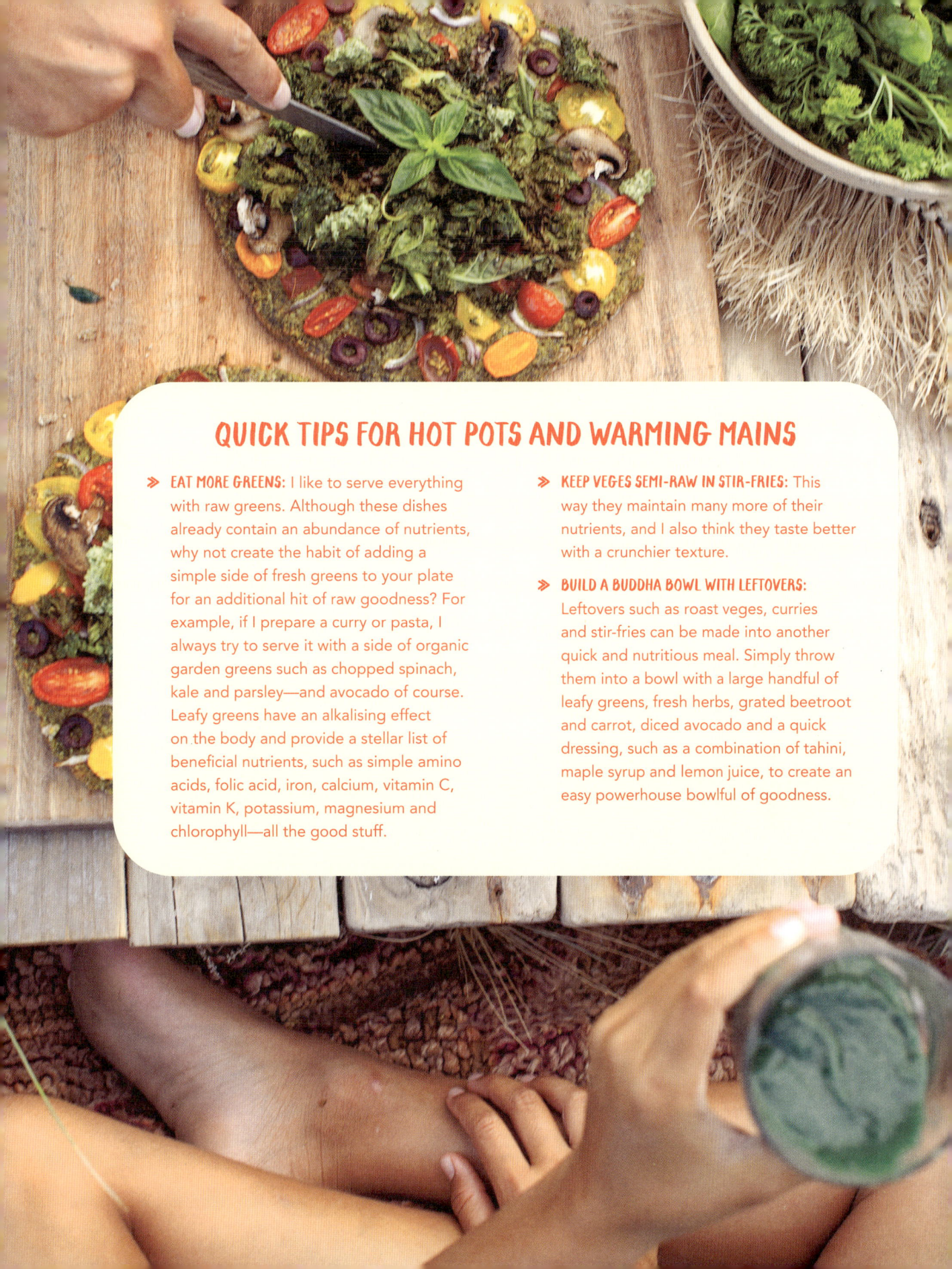

» **EAT MORE GREENS:** I like to serve everything with raw greens. Although these dishes already contain an abundance of nutrients, why not create the habit of adding a simple side of fresh greens to your plate for an additional hit of raw goodness? For example, if I prepare a curry or pasta, I always try to serve it with a side of organic garden greens such as chopped spinach, kale and parsley—and avocado of course. Leafy greens have an alkalising effect on the body and provide a stellar list of beneficial nutrients, such as simple amino acids, folic acid, iron, calcium, vitamin C, vitamin K, potassium, magnesium and chlorophyll—all the good stuff.

» **KEEP VEGES SEMI-RAW IN STIR-FRIES:** This way they maintain many more of their nutrients, and I also think they taste better with a crunchier texture.

» **BUILD A BUDDHA BOWL WITH LEFTOVERS:** Leftovers such as roast veges, curries and stir-fries can be made into another quick and nutritious meal. Simply throw them into a bowl with a large handful of leafy greens, fresh herbs, grated beetroot and carrot, diced avocado and a quick dressing, such as a combination of tahini, maple syrup and lemon juice, to create an easy powerhouse bowlful of goodness.

INDIAN JACKFRUIT MAKHANI

SERVES 4–6

Sauce
400 ml (14 fl oz) can coconut milk
⅓ cup tomato paste
2 kaffir lime leaves
1 teaspoon curry powder
1 teaspoon mixed spice
1 teaspoon ground ginger
½ teaspoon fenugreek seeds
2 tablespoons tamari (or coconut aminos)
2 tablespoons coconut sugar (or pure maple syrup)
2 tablespoons water

Curry
1 teaspoon olive, avocado or coconut oil (optional)
1 brown onion, sliced
4 cloves garlic, diced
1 cinnamon stick
2 carrots, peeled and thinly sliced
1 red capsicum, diced
1 tablespoon poppyseeds
400 g (14 oz) can young jackfruit, drained

To serve (optional)
brown rice
garden greens
fresh coriander or parsley, chopped
sliced avocado

This take on the popular butter chicken will fast become a family favourite in your home. It's loaded with juicy jackfruit in a rich, sweet and creamy tomato-based sauce, using aromatic Indian spices. The inspiration for this curry came from Eli and Milo, as 'vege butter chicken' had always been one of their favourite Indian mains. They also made the perfect taste-testers, and after many attempts we finally nailed a beautifully flavoursome vegan Indian makhani. This curry can easily be adapted with any other veges you have on hand or by adding in a protein, such as chickpeas or tofu.

For the sauce, blend all the ingredients until smooth and creamy. Set aside.

Heat the oil in a large frying pan over medium-high heat. Add the onion and garlic and cook for 5–7 minutes, stirring frequently, until soft and fragrant. Add the cinnamon stick, carrots, capsicum, poppyseeds and jackfruit. Reduce the heat to low.

Pour over the sauce and stir through. Simmer, stirring occasionally, for about 15 minutes, until the sauce has thickened and the veges are just tender.

Serve over brown rice or garden greens, and garnish with lots of fresh herbs. Top with avocado, if desired.

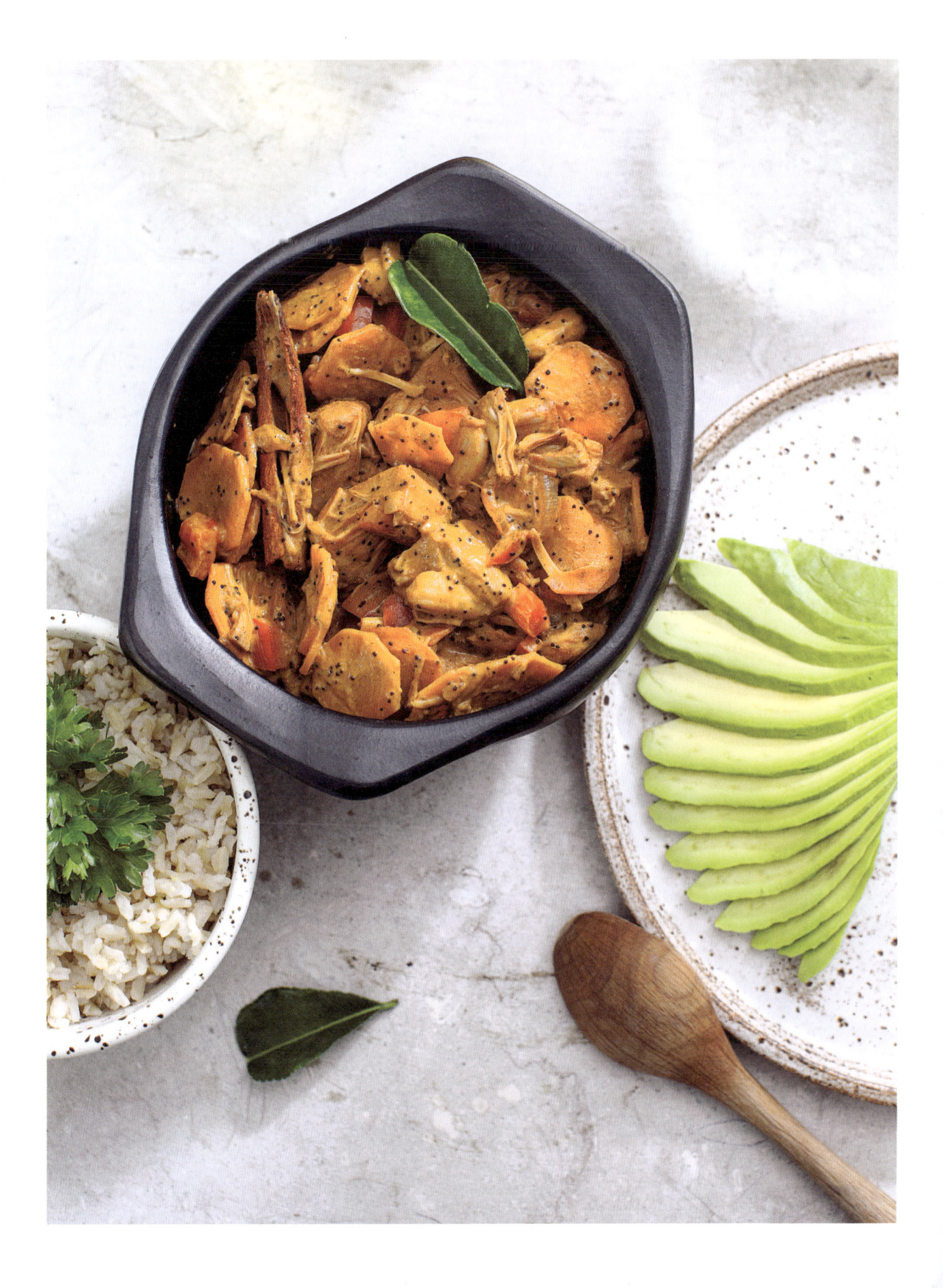

ROAST CAULIFLOWER, CAPSICUM and CHICKPEA YELLOW CURRY

SERVES 4

- 1 head cauliflower, cut into small florets
- 3 red capsicums, cut into 1 cm (½ in) strips
- olive, avocado or coconut oil (optional)
- ⅓ cup shallots, chopped
- 2 tablespoons finely grated fresh ginger
- 4 cloves garlic, diced
- 2 cups canned coconut milk
- 400 g (14 oz) can chickpeas, drained and rinsed (or 1½ cups cooked chickpeas)
- 2 tablespoons curry powder
- 1½ teaspoons ground turmeric
- 1 tablespoon maple syrup
- 2 tablespoons tamari (or coconut aminos)
- 2 cups baby spinach leaves
- fresh coriander, to garnish

To serve (optional)
- brown rice
- leafy greens
- Garlic Chickpea Flatbread (see page 291)

In this beautiful bowlful of goodness, the roast cauliflower is paired with chickpeas and juicy charred capsicums in a creamy, gingery turmeric sauce. It makes a delicious meal served over a bed of fresh crispy greens, or with a side of brown rice or quinoa. This vibrant, warming curry was originally created by my mum and sister, who enjoy it served more like a chunky soup with a side of sourdough.

Preheat the oven to 180°C (350°F) fan bake. Line a baking tray with baking paper.

Place the cauliflower and capsicum on the baking tray. Drizzle with oil, if desired. Bake for 20–25 minutes, turning halfway through, until lightly browned.

Heat the oil in a large frying pan over medium-high heat, if using. Add the shallots, ginger and garlic, and cook for 5–7 minutes, stirring frequently, until soft and fragrant. Add the coconut milk, chickpeas, curry powder, turmeric, maple syrup and tamari and stir to combine. Mix through the cauliflower and capsicum, reduce the heat to low and continue to simmer for 12–15 minutes, or until thickened. Mix through the spinach leaves and garnish with coriander just before serving.

Serve over brown rice, fresh greens or with a few slices of my Garlic Chickpea Flatbread.

NOTE: You'll need to open two 400 ml (14 fl oz) cans of coconut milk for 2 cups worth, so you'll have leftover coconut milk. Store it in an airtight container in the fridge for up to 5 days; it makes a great creamy addition to smoothies or nice cream.

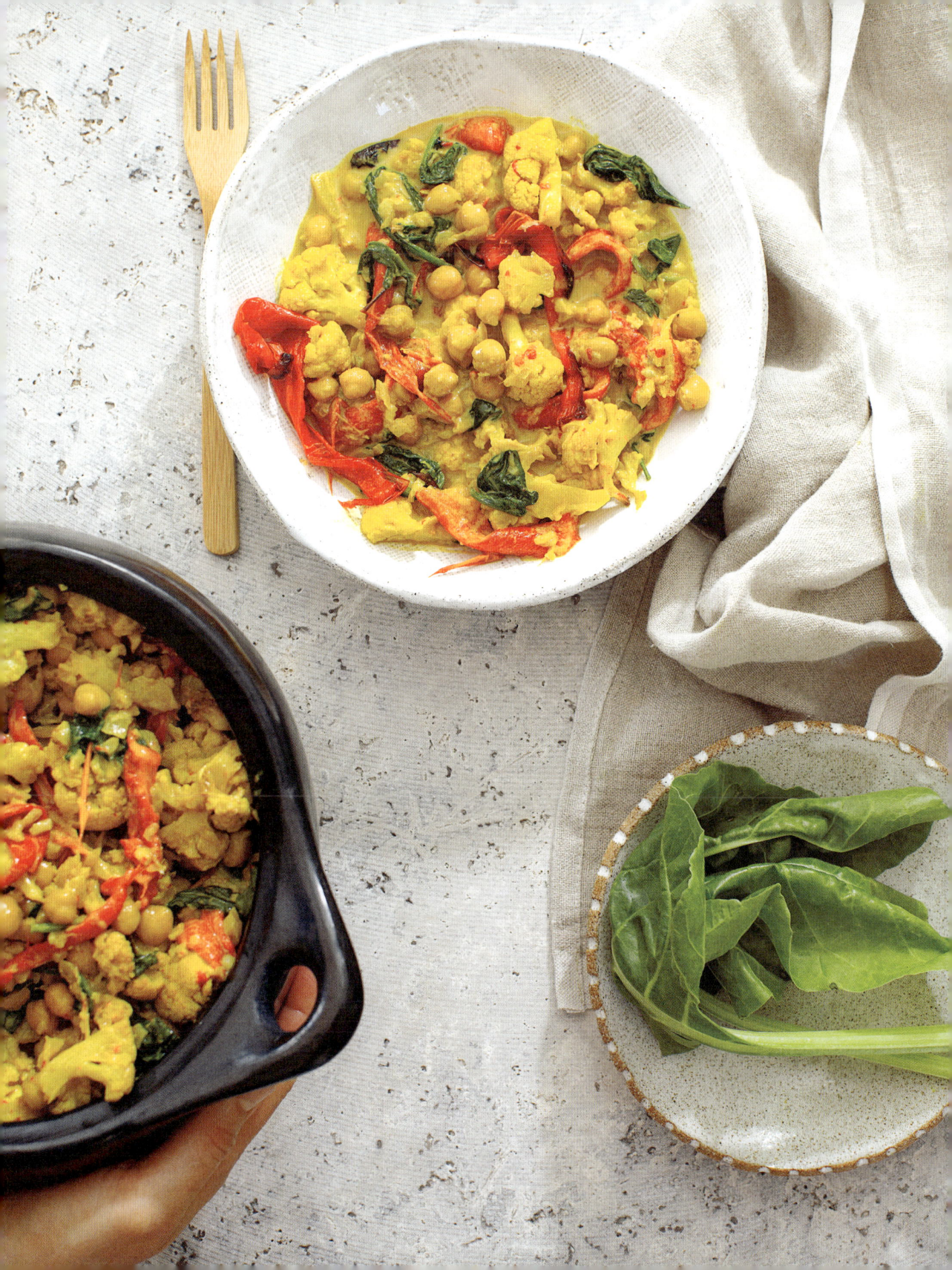

ITALIAN LENTIL BOLOGNAISE with RAW ZUCCHINI NOODLES

SERVES 4–6

Lentil Bolognaise
1 teaspoon olive, avocado or coconut oil (optional)
1 large brown onion, diced
4 cloves garlic, diced
2 large carrots, peeled and grated
2 cups button mushrooms, sliced
2 cans brown lentils, drained and rinsed (or 3 cups cooked lentils)
2 cups tomato passata
⅓ cup coconut milk (from a can)
2 tablespoons tamari (or coconut aminos)
1 tablespoon balsamic vinegar
1½ teaspoons ground cumin
1 tablespoon dried oregano
⅔ cup whole black olives
2 teaspoons pure maple syrup
⅛ teaspoon cayenne pepper
½ cup fresh dill

Raw zucchini noodles
4 large zucchini, trimmed

To serve (optional)
coconut yoghurt
fresh dill

An oldie but oh such a goodie. This one-pot hearty main is definitely a staple in our home and one of Ricardo's long-time favourites. Prior to going vegan I was vegetarian for many years, so I've had the time to perfect these lentils—Ricardo and I often joke about who makes it better. The olives are one of the star ingredients as they give it that true authentic Italian flavour. It's packed with protein, and can be eaten alone with a dollop of coconut yoghurt or served over a bed of fresh greens, raw zucchini noodles or gluten-free spaghetti.

For the Bolognaise, heat the oil in a large frying pan over medium-high heat. Add the onion and garlic and cook for 5–7 minutes, stirring frequently, until soft and fragrant. Add the carrots and mushrooms and cook for an additional 2 minutes.

Add the lentils, passata, coconut milk, tamari, balsamic vinegar, cumin, oregano, olives, maple syrup and cayenne pepper. Reduce the heat to low and simmer for 8–10 minutes, stirring occasionally, until fragrant. Mix through the fresh dill just before serving.

For the zucchini noodles, use your chosen device to spiralise the zucchini.

Serve the bolognaise on a bed of zucchini noodles, with a dollop of coconut yoghurt and fresh dill if desired.

NOTE: If making this meal for little ones, leave out the cayenne pepper or only add a tiny pinch.

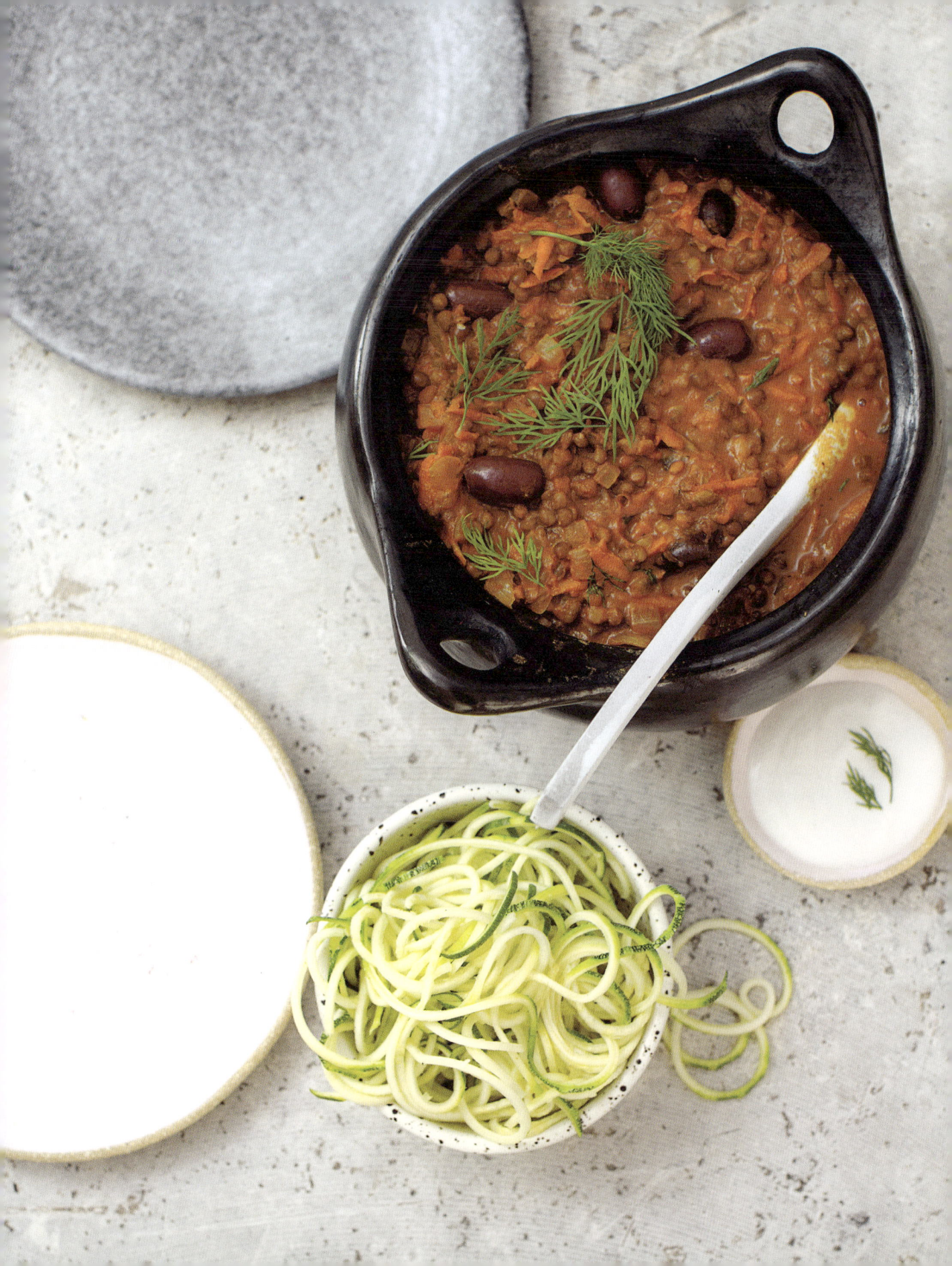

EGGPLANT, JACKFRUIT and BLACK SESAME IN LIME-INFUSED ALMOND GRAVY

SERVES 4–6

1 teaspoon olive, avocado or coconut oil (optional)
½ red onion, sliced
4 cloves garlic, diced
1 large eggplant (or 2 small), cut into bite-sized cubes
250 g (9 oz) mushrooms, sliced
4 spring onions, sliced
1 green capsicum, deseeded and sliced lengthways into 1 cm (½ in) strips
1 tablespoon dried thyme
400 g (14 oz) can young jackfruit, drained
¼ cup black sesame seeds
½ teaspoon chilli flakes (optional)
1 cup coriander, chopped

Gravy
⅔ cup almond butter
1½ cups water
¼ cup tamari
½ cup nutritional yeast
2 tablespoons balsamic vinegar
1 tablespoon sesame oil
1 tablespoon coconut sugar
2 cloves garlic, diced
2 cm (¾ in) piece fresh ginger, peeled
zest and juice of 2 limes

To serve (optional)
quinoa
chopped fresh herbs, such as coriander and parsley
lime wedges

There are two things to love about this beautiful stew-style mingle. One, it's seriously delicious, and two, it's something a little different. The eggplant is amazing as it soaks up all the creamy flavours like a sponge, and as for the jackfruit, well, I'm a tad obsessed to say the least. This dish is one you'll want to keep on the weekly menu, and after the flavours have been left to marinate overnight it also makes for an epic bowlful of leftovers for lunch with sliced avocado.

Heat the oil in a large frying pan over medium-high heat. Add the red onion and garlic and cook for 5–7 minutes, stirring frequently, until soft and fragrant.

Add the eggplant, mushrooms, spring onion, capsicum and thyme, and mix to combine. Reduce the heat to low, cover and simmer for 10 minutes, stirring occasionally.

Meanwhile, for the gravy, place all the ingredients in a blender and blend until smooth and creamy.

Add the gravy to the pan, along with the jackfruit, and stir to combine. Simmer for 8–10 minutes, stirring occasionally, until the gravy has thickened and the veges are tender.

Add the black sesame seeds, chilli flakes, if using, and coriander, and gently mix to combine.

Serve over a warm bed of quinoa and top with fresh garden herbs such as coriander and parsley. Place lime wedges on the side.

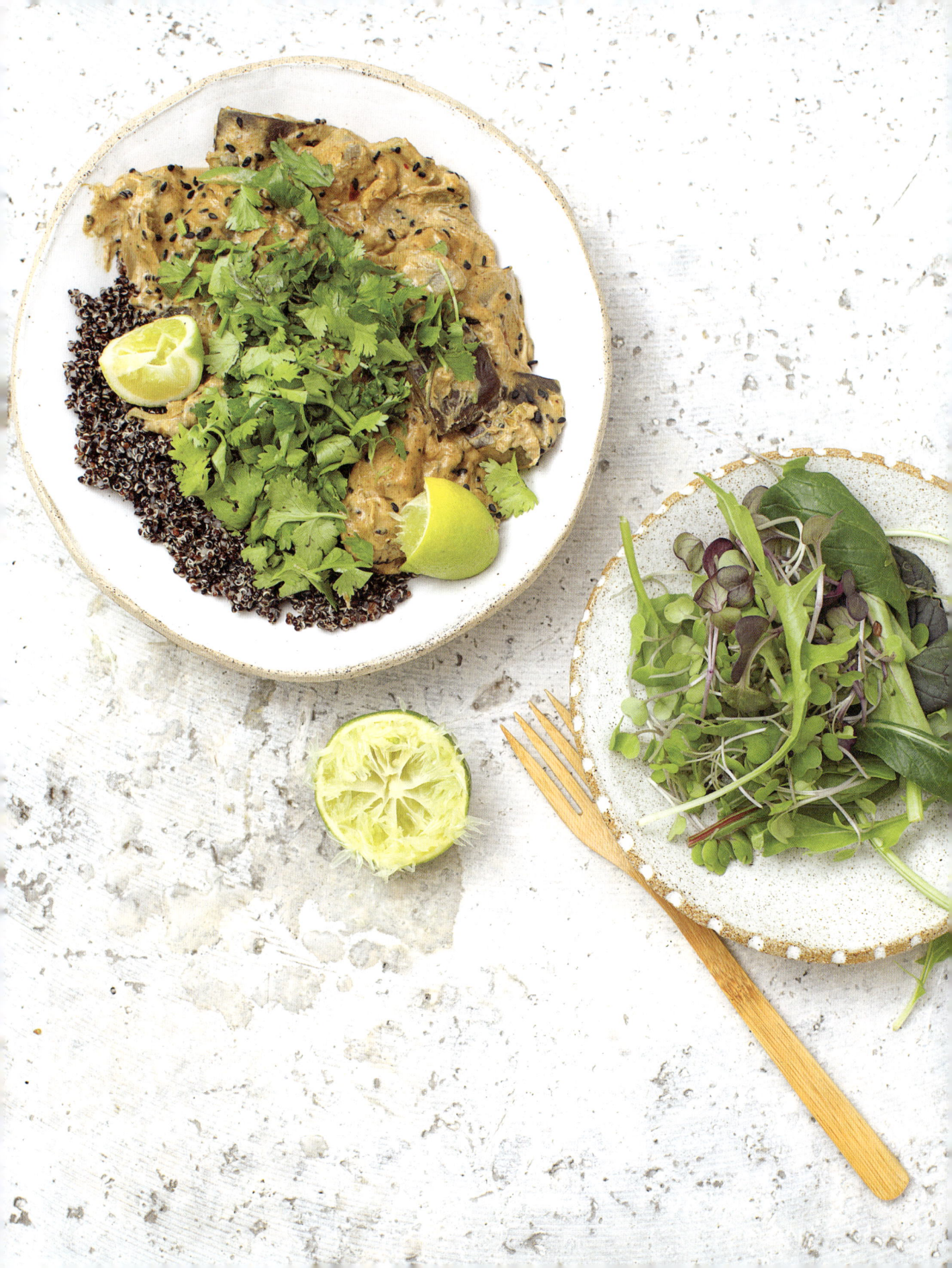

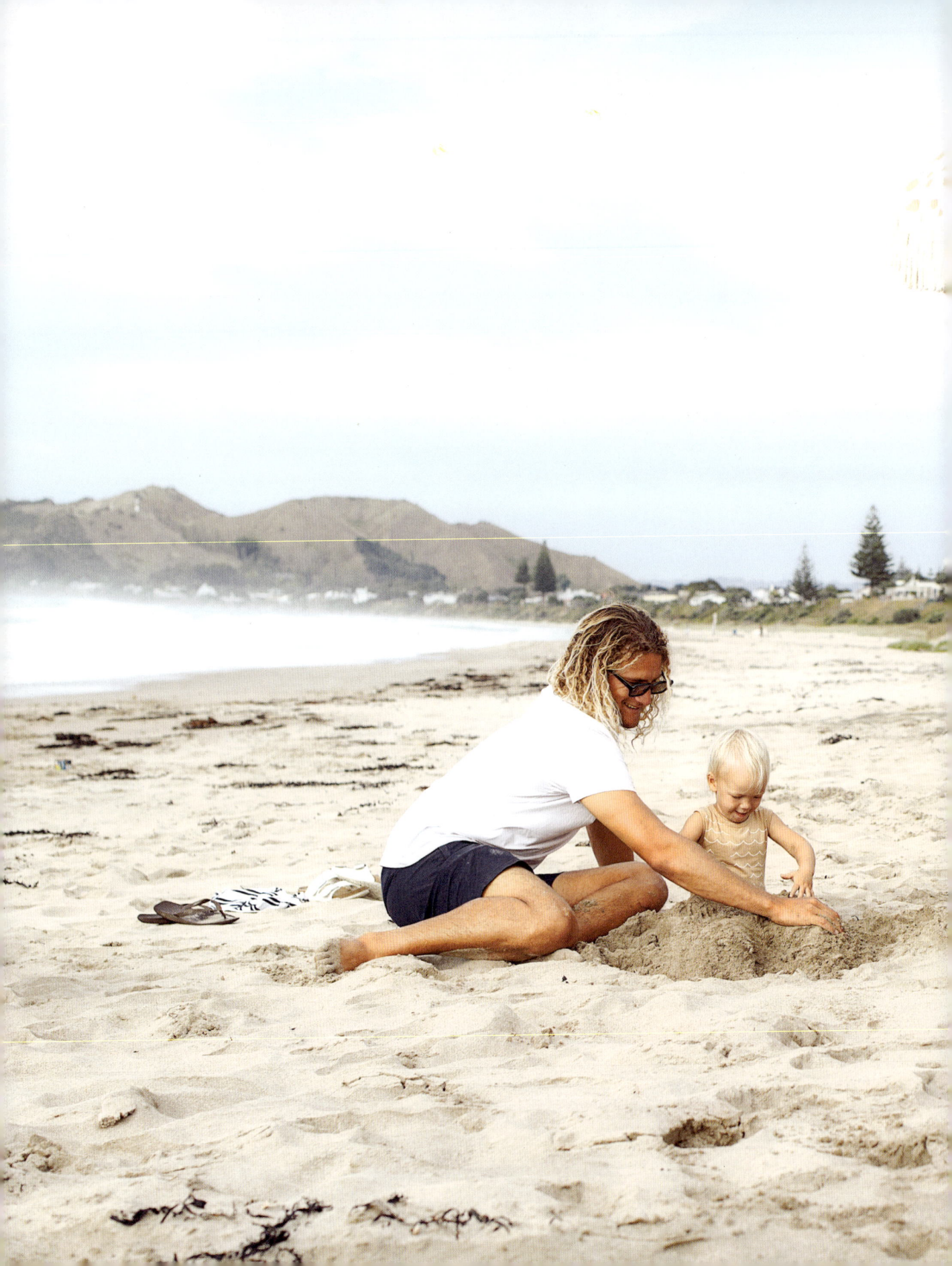

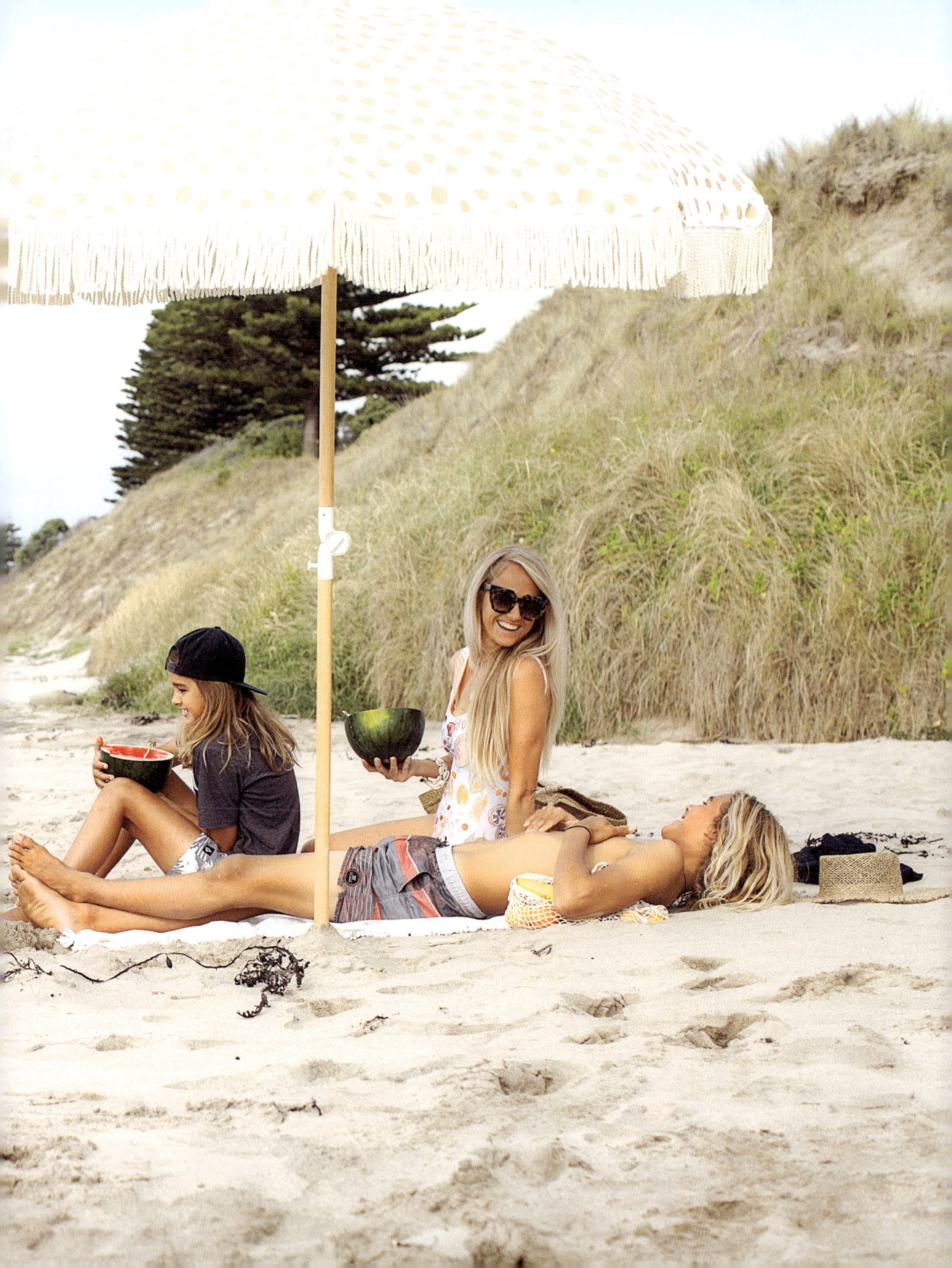

LEMONGRASS, LIME and COCONUT THAI CURRY with CRISPY POTATOES

SERVES 4–6

2 medium-large agria potatoes, cut into large cubes
1 teaspoon olive, avocado or coconut oil (optional)
1 brown onion, diced
3 cloves garlic, diced
1 zucchini, trimmed and sliced
1 green capsicum, sliced lengthways into 1 cm (½ in) strips
1 cup green beans, trimmed and sliced
1 bunch broccolini, trimmed
2 teaspoons black mustard seeds

Curry sauce
400 ml (14 fl oz) can coconut milk
2 packed cups fresh spinach
3 large kaffir lime leaves
1 stalk lemongrass, sliced
½ cup fresh coriander leaves
¼ cup tamari
1 tablespoon curry powder
1 teaspoon ground coriander
1 teaspoon ground cumin
1 tablespoon coconut sugar (or pure maple syrup)
½ small green chilli (omit for children)

To serve (optional)
brown rice or black quinoa
fresh basil or Thai basil leaves
shredded coconut

This would have to be one of my favourite curries. It's packed with perfectly balanced flavours and loaded with lots of green garden goodness—even the sauce has a few sneaky cups of iron-rich spinach in it. When I was first transitioning into a plant-based lifestyle, this was one of the first curries I experimented with. I love the combination of lemongrass, lime and coconut, mixed with crunchy greens. Whether you're a curry-lover or not, I think you'll love this recipe—hopefully as much as I do.

Preheat the oven to 180°C (350°F) fan bake. Line a baking tray with baking paper.

Bring a saucepan of water to a boil. Place the potatoes in a colander over the water, cover, and steam for about 15–20 minutes until just tender. Tip onto the baking tray and spread out into a single layer. Bake for about 25 minutes, or until golden and crunchy.

For the curry sauce, blend all the ingredients in a blender until smooth. Set aside.

Heat the oil in a large frying pan over medium-high heat. Add the onion and garlic and cook for 5–7 minutes, stirring frequently, until soft and fragrant. Add the zucchini, capsicum, green beans, broccolini and black mustard seeds. Gently stir through the sauce and reduce the heat to low. Simmer for 8–10 minutes, stirring occasionally, until the sauce has slightly thickened and the veges are just tender, but not overcooked.

Remove the potatoes from the oven and gently mix through the curry.

Serve over a bed of brown rice or quinoa, and garnish with fresh herbs and coconut.

NOTE: This curry is much quicker to make when you have leftover potatoes in the fridge, or, to save time, simply leave the potatoes out. They are great for bulking it up but it's still delicious without them.

Hot Pots + Warming Mains

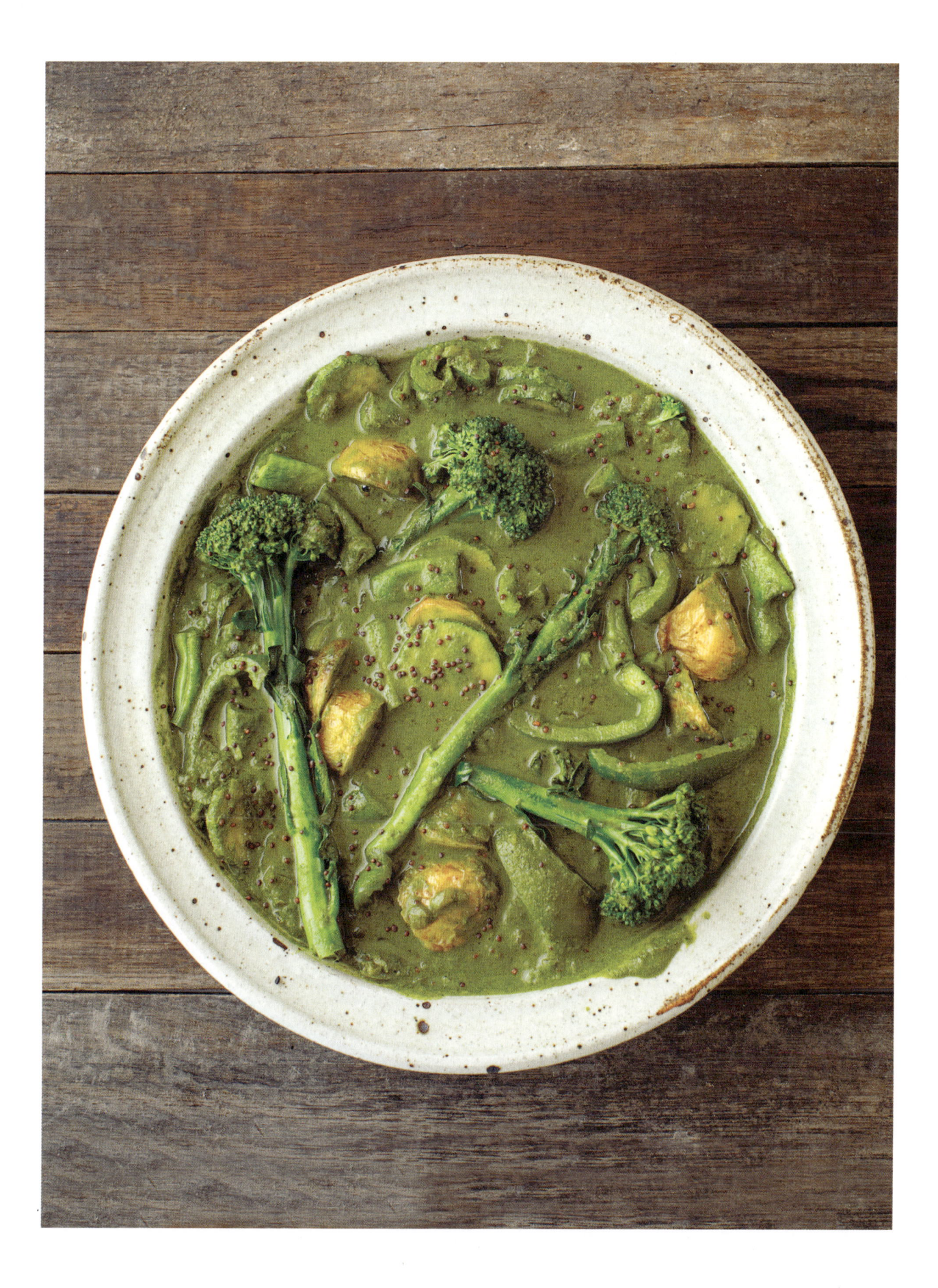

TERIYAKI RAINBOW QUINOA

SERVES 4–6

1 cup quinoa, rinsed
2 cups water
1 teaspoon olive, avocado or coconut oil (optional)
3 spring onions, sliced
2 cups button mushrooms, sliced
1 red capsicum, deseeded and cut into 1 cm (½ in) strips
1 cup snap peas, trimmed
1 bunch broccolini, ends trimmed
¾ cup frozen shelled edamame beans
½ cup raw cashews
¼ cup pine nuts

Teriyaki sauce
3 tablespoons tamari
2 tablespoons coconut sugar
2 tablespoons water
2 tablespoons apple cider vinegar
2 tablespoons lime juice
1 teaspoon sesame oil
1 teaspoon grated fresh ginger, grated
1 clove garlic, crushed

To serve (optional)
finely chopped fresh coriander
sesame seeds

This is a really quick, easy and nutritious lunch or dinner, packed with lots of protein and vibrant, rainbow veges. I like to keep the veges semi-raw so that they maintain a crunchy texture and also retain more of their nutrients. The teriyaki sauce is one of Eli's favourite kitchen specialities, he's become a whizz at making it for sushi rolls and it's also a fantastic addition to Asian-style Buddha bowls.

Place the quinoa and water in a saucepan, cover, and bring to a boil. Once boiling, reduce the heat to low and simmer for 12–15 minutes, until the water has been absorbed and the quinoa is soft and fluffy.

For the teriyaki sauce, place all the ingredients in a bowl and whisk together.

Heat the oil in a large frying pan over medium-high heat. Add the spring onions and mushrooms and cook, stirring frequently, for 5–7 minutes, until soft and fragrant. Add the capsicum, snap peas, broccolini, edamame beans, cashews and pine nuts and cook, stirring occasionally, for 3–5 minutes, until the veges are brighter in colour and just tender.

Add the quinoa and teriyaki sauce to the pan and mix to combine all the ingredients.

Serve with fresh coriander leaves and a sprinkle of sesame seeds.

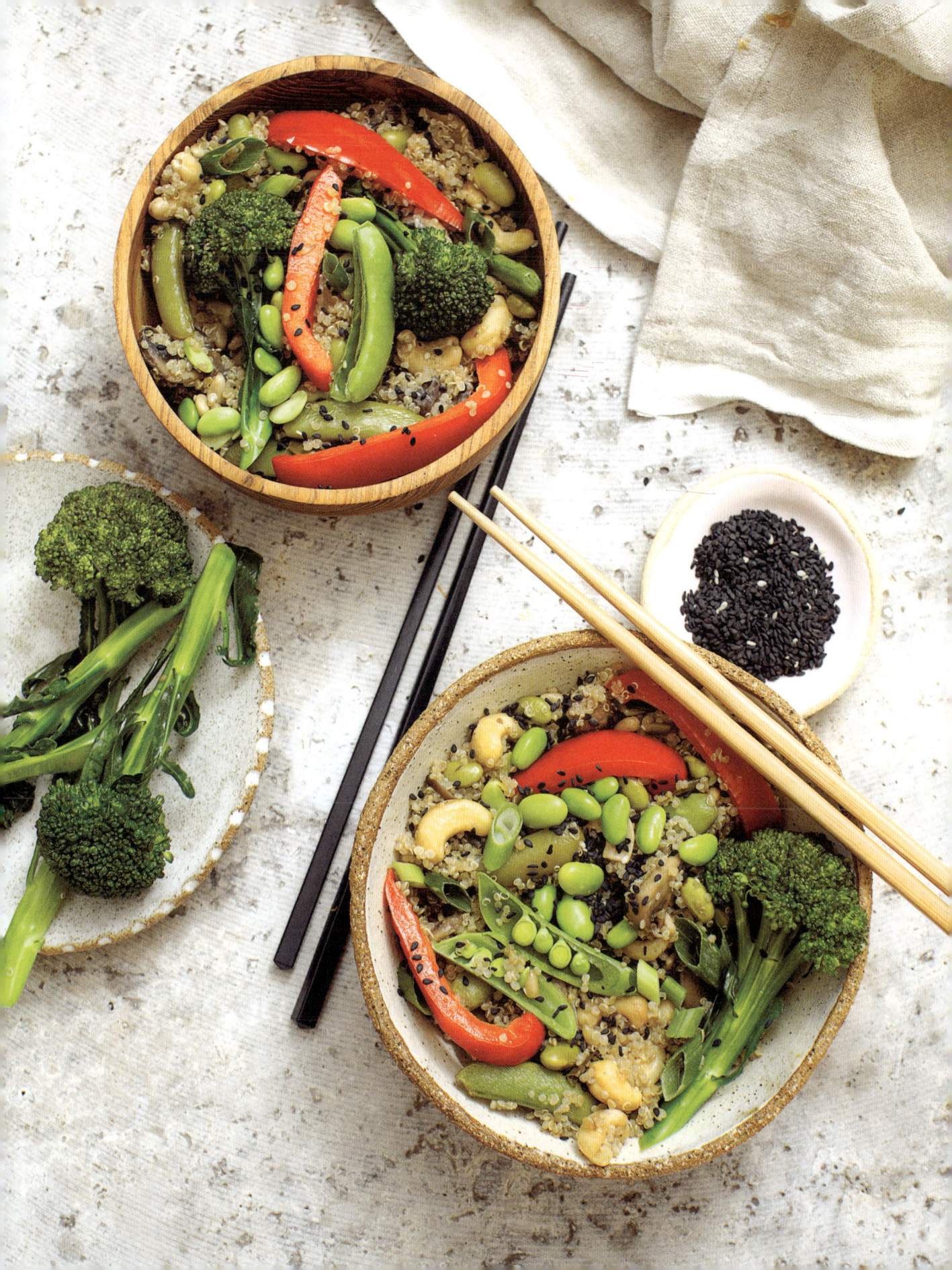

MOREISH POTATO and CHIVE BAKE

SERVES 4–6

5 medium-large agria potatoes (approx. 1 kg / 2 lb 4 oz), cut into bite-sized cubes

½ head cauliflower (approx. 500 g / 1 lb 2 oz), cut into bite-sized florets

½ head broccoli, cut into bite-sized florets

1 teaspoon olive, avocado or coconut oil (optional)

1 brown onion, thinly sliced

3 cloves garlic, diced

½ cup chopped fresh chives, plus extra for serving

1 tablespoon dried rosemary

1 teaspoon dried thyme

2 teaspoons caraway seeds

3 tablespoons pumpkin seeds

2 cups Cashew Cheese Sauce (see page 279)

sea salt and cracked pepper, to taste

To serve (optional)

fresh mixed greens (spinach, kale, rocket, etc.)

There really is no better word to describe this dish, it truly is moreish. I made it for a friend who was quick to describe it as 'sour cream and chives', with its rich Cashew Cheese Sauce (see page 279). It's a versatile dish that can easily be adapted by adding in any other seasonal veges you have on hand—such as pumpkin, kūmara, spinach or zucchini—and is also the perfect way to disguise them, especially for little people.

Preheat the oven to 180°C (350°F) fan bake.

Bring a large saucepan of water to a boil. Place the potatoes in a large colander over the water, cover, and steam for 20 minutes until fork tender. Add the cauliflower and broccoli to the potatoes for the last 5–7 minutes. Set aside.

Heat the oil in a small frying pan over medium-high heat. Add the onion and garlic and cook, stirring frequently, for 5–7 minutes, until soft and fragrant. Remove and place in a large bowl along with the chives, dried herbs, caraway seeds and pumpkin seeds. Add the potatoes, cauliflower, broccoli and cheese sauce, and gently mix to combine all the ingredients.

Tip the mixture into a large baking dish and spread out evenly. Season to taste. Bake for 25–30 minutes, until golden brown.

Once cooked, remove from the oven and sprinkle over extra chives. Serve with a side of fresh garden greens, if desired.

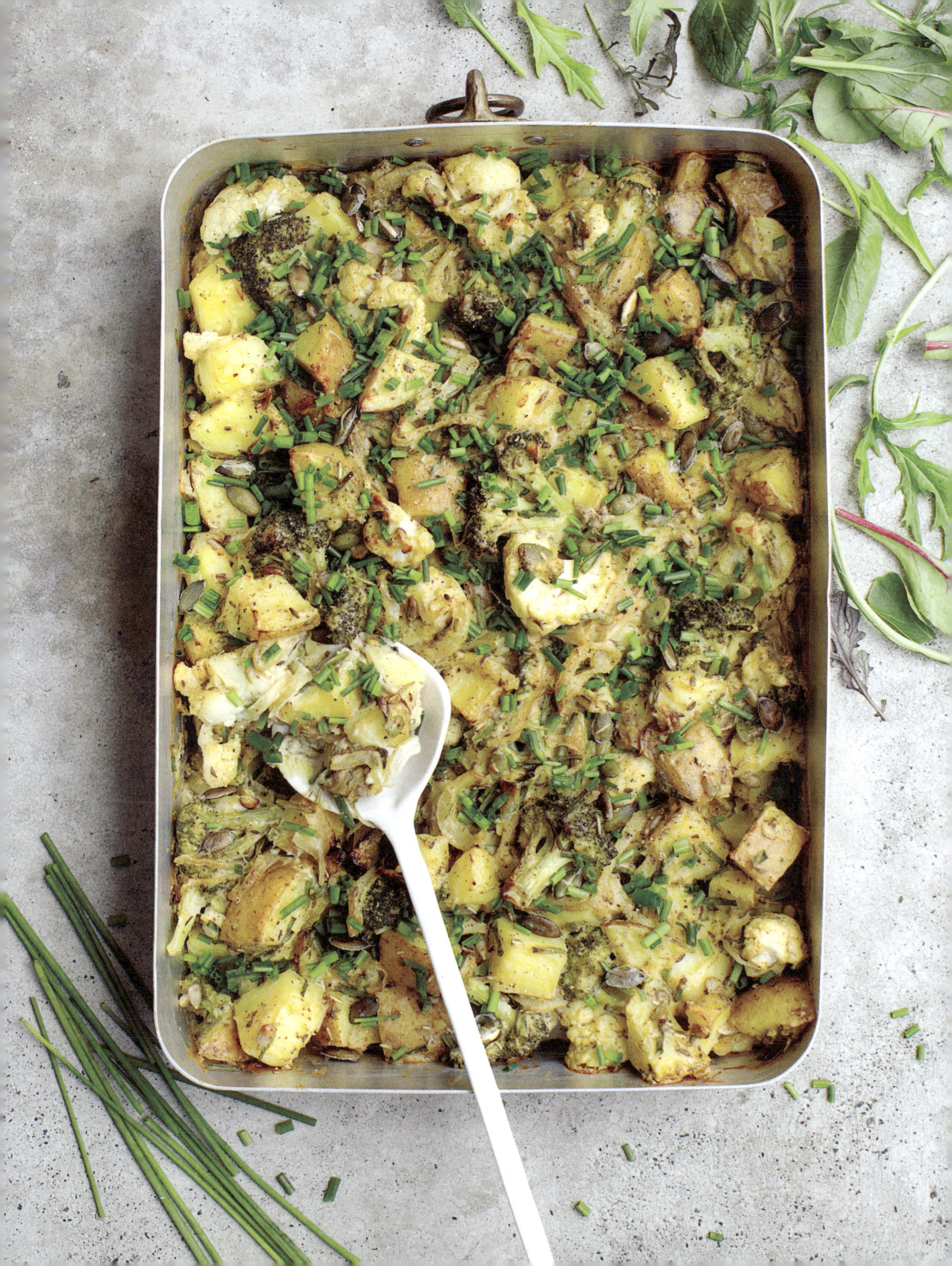

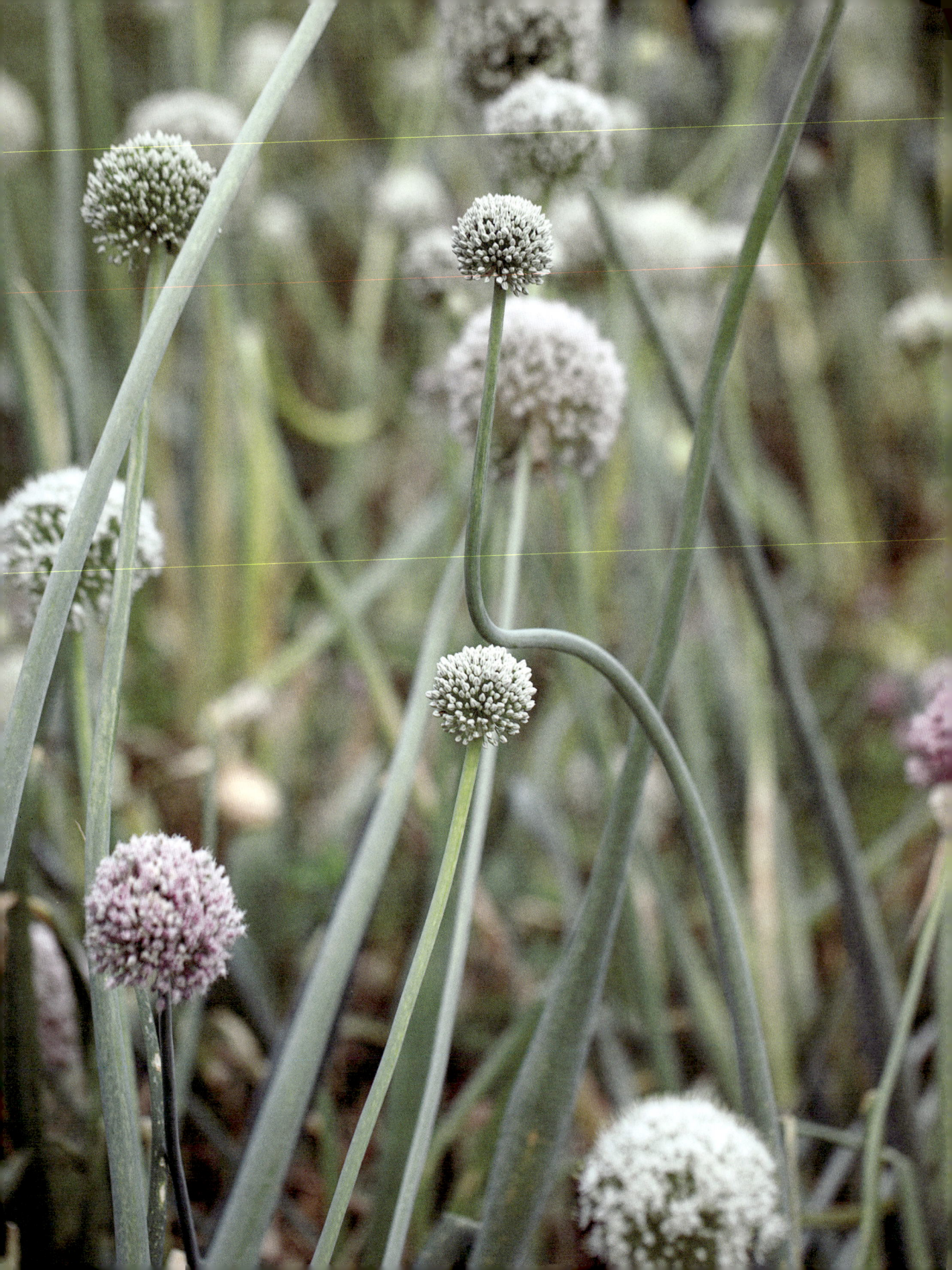

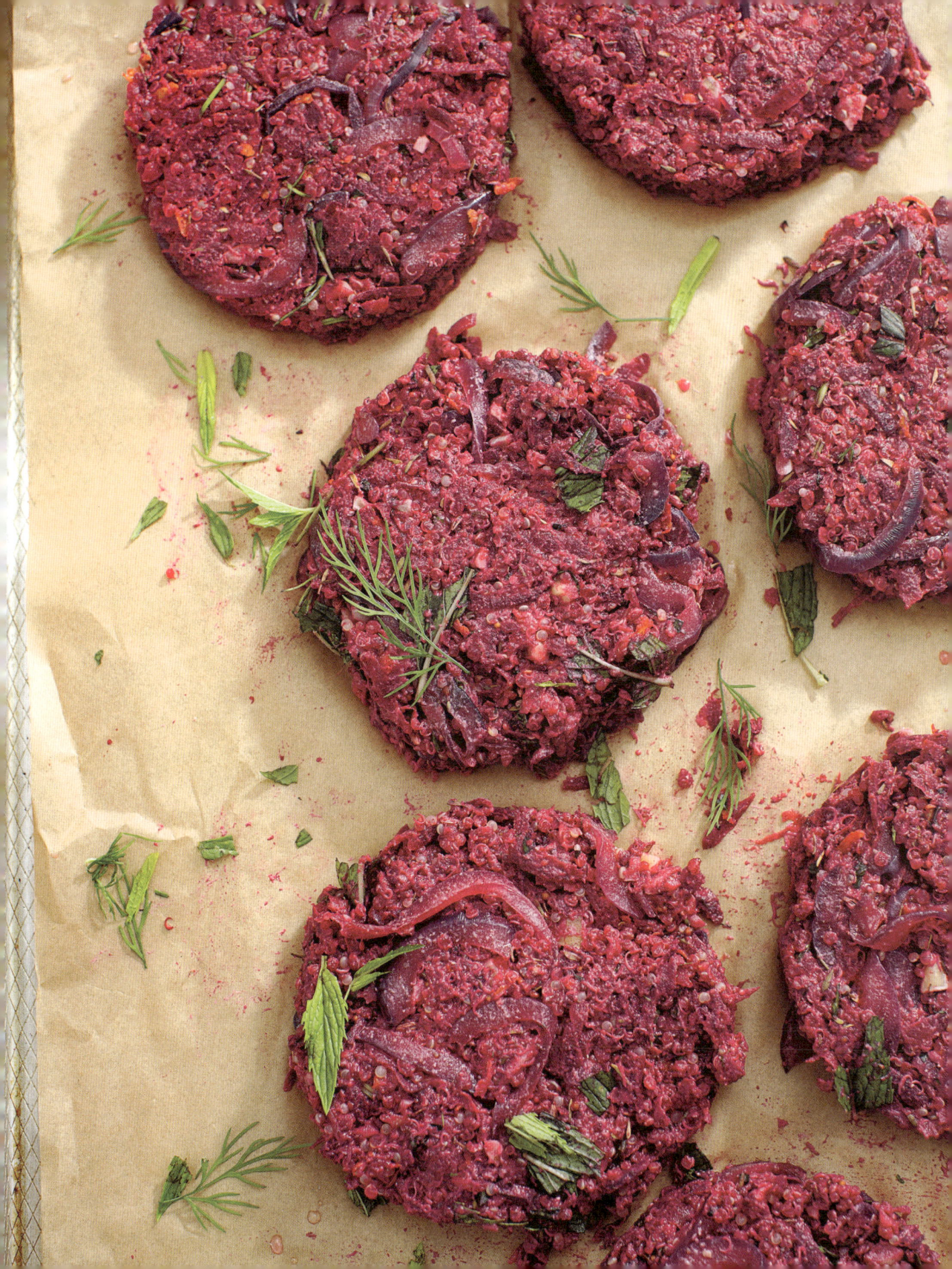

PAPRIKA ALFREDO PASTA
with HEMP and CASHEW PARMESAN

SERVES 6

500 g (1 lb 2 oz) gluten-free pasta (rice, quinoa, etc.)
1 teaspoon olive, avocado or coconut oil (optional)
1 red onion, diced
3 cloves garlic, diced
1 red capsicum, deseeded and cut into small cubes
3 packed cups baby spinach leaves
½ cup Hemp and Cashew Parmesan (see page 282)

Paprika Alfredo pasta sauce
1½ cups cashews, presoaked (see Recipe Notes page 47)
½ large red capsicum
2 cloves garlic
½ cup nutritional yeast
1½ cups rice milk (or Almond Milk or Hemp Milk, see page 290)
1 tablespoon white miso paste
1 tablespoon pure maple syrup
2 teaspoons smoked paprika
1 tablespoon sweet paprika

To serve (optional)
fresh parsley
sliced avocado
chilli flakes

A good wholesome pasta dish has always been one of my go-to comforting family dinners, especially when it comes to feeding three hungry boys. This gluten-free version is super-easy, nutritious and so incredibly tasty. I highly recommend it topped with my seriously addictive Hemp and Cashew Parmesan (see page 282). I always make a large batch, as any leftovers will freeze well or will make for an easy lunch the next day, served cold with sliced avocado.

Bring a large saucepan of water to a boil. Add the pasta and cook according to the packet instructions (usually around 15 minutes).

Heat the oil in a large frying pan over medium-high heat. Add the red onion and garlic and cook, stirring frequently, for 5–7 minutes, until soft and fragrant. Add the capsicum and cook for another 2–3 minutes. Set aside.

For the sauce, place all the ingredients in a blender and blend for 20–30 seconds, until smooth and creamy.

Drain the pasta. Place in a bowl, add the cooked onion mixture and the spinach, and pour the sauce over. Mix everything until well combined. If needed, reheat the pasta before serving.

Serve with a sprinkle of Hemp and Cashew Parmesan, and fresh parsley, avocado and chilli flakes, if desired.

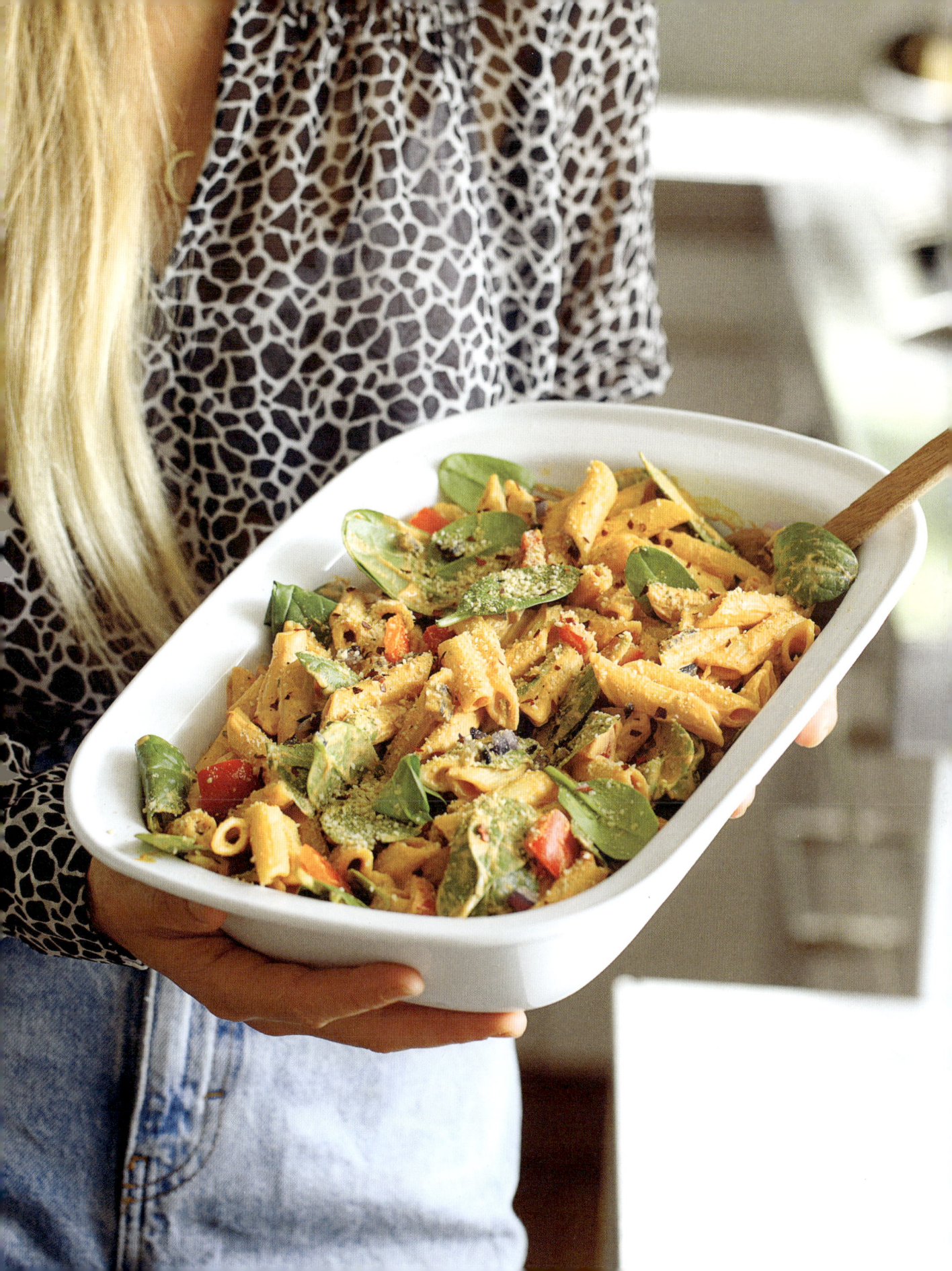

ROSEMARY and THYME HASSELBACKS with THE BEST EVER CREAMY COLESLAW

SERVES 4–6

Hasselback potatoes
8 small–medium potatoes (agria, russet, red, etc.; approx. 1.5 kg / 3 lb 5 oz)
1 tablespoon olive, avocado or coconut oil
1 teaspoon dried rosemary
1½ teaspoons dried thyme
½ bunch fresh rosemary (15 g)
sea salt and cracked pepper, to taste

Coleslaw
3 cups thinly shredded red cabbage
2 cups grated carrots
1½ cups roughly chopped parsley
1 spring onion, sliced
¼ cup finely diced red onion
½ cup sliced almonds
½ cup raisins

Creamy cashew tahini dressing
1 cup cashews, presoaked (see Recipe Notes page 47)
2 tablespoons tahini
2 tablespoons wholegrain mustard
3 tablespoons lemon juice
2 cloves garlic
1 tablespoon pure maple syrup
¼ cup water

The obsession is real—this simple combination of herby potatoes and creamy coleslaw is amazing. If you're looking for something different to try with your potatoes or kūmara, hasselbacks make for beautifully tender potatoes that soak up all the herby flavours I've added in this recipe. The creamy coleslaw is an absolute staple in our family, enjoyed as a side to almost any main. The sweet and creamy dressing is so versatile and also works perfectly with steamed potatoes, parsley, celery and red onion to create a beautiful potato salad.

Preheat the oven to 180°C (350°F) fan bake. Line a baking tray with baking paper.

Hold the end of one potato and use a sharp knife to make 1–2 mm (approx. 1/16 in) cuts across the width of the potato, all the way along, slicing about two-thirds of the way down into the flesh. Be careful not to slice all the way through. Repeat with the remaining potatoes.

Place the oil and dried herbs in a large bowl. Add the potatoes and gently toss them until they are evenly coated in the herby oil. Place them on the baking tray cut side up.

Pick the fresh rosemary leaves and stuff them sporadically into the cuts of the potatoes. Season, then bake for 50–60 minutes, or until the largest potato is soft and the edges are crispy.

For the coleslaw, place all the ingredients in a large bowl.

For the dressing, place all the ingredients in a blender and blend for 20–30 seconds, until smooth and creamy. Pour over the coleslaw and mix to combine.

Serve the hasselbacks with coleslaw on the side.

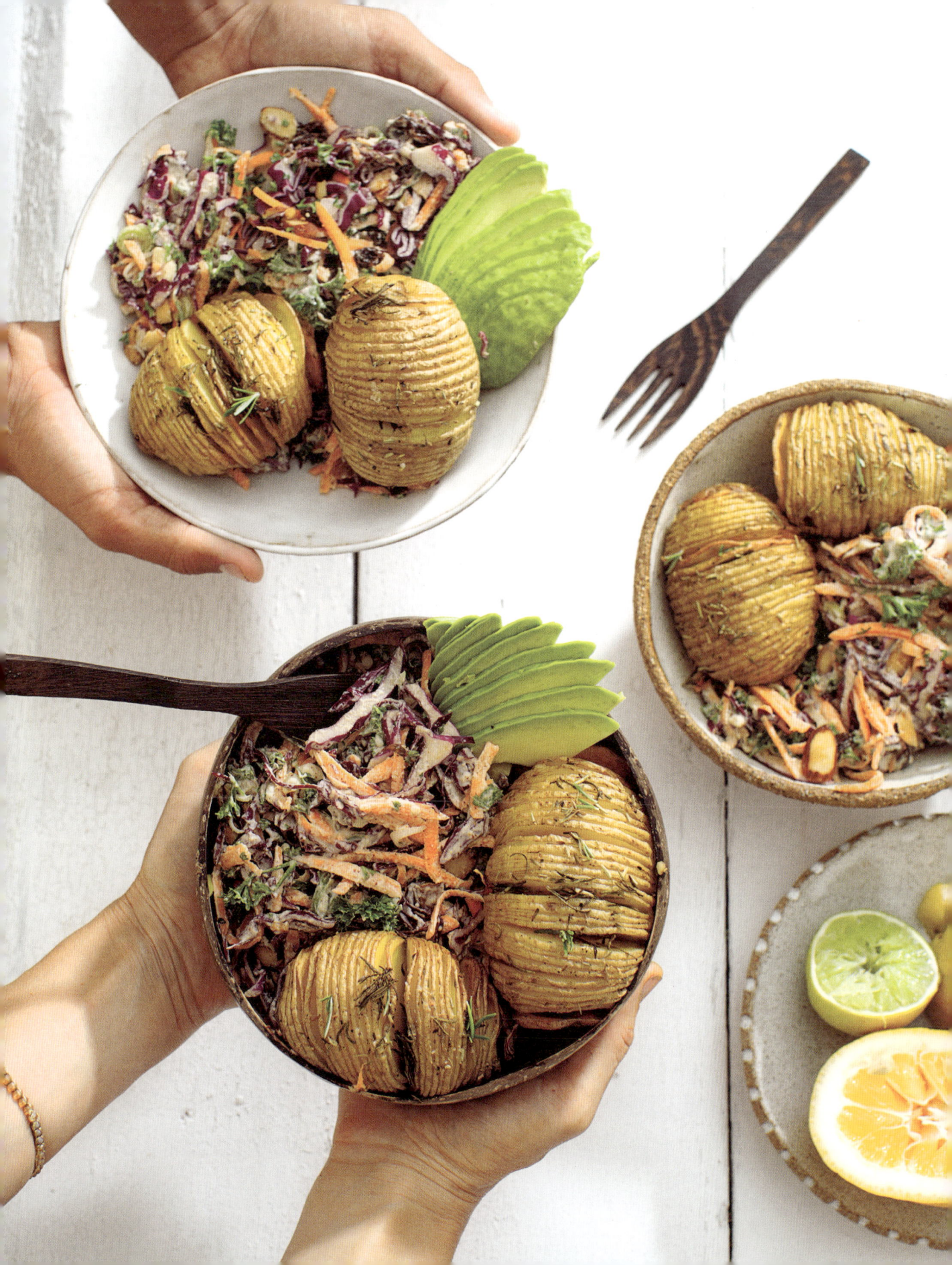

BASIL PESTO POTATO TOP PIE

SERVES 4–6

6 medium-large agria potatoes (approx. 1 kg–1.2 kg/2 lb 4 oz–2 lb 10 oz), washed, peeled and cut into large cubes
1 teaspoon olive, avocado or coconut oil (optional)
1 onion, diced
3 cloves garlic, diced
250 g (10½ oz) mushrooms, sliced
1 red capsicum, deseeded and diced
1 zucchini, trimmed and sliced
⅓ cup pine nuts
2 cups chopped spinach, fresh or frozen
400 g (14 oz) can cannellini beans, drained and rinsed (or 1½ cups cooked beans)
1 cup Hemp, Spinach and Basil Pesto (see page 222) or store-bought vegan basil pesto
1-2 tablespoons miso paste, optional
½ cup fresh basil leaves, chopped
½–¾ cup rice milk (or Almond Milk or Hemp Milk, see page 290)
½–1 teaspoon sea salt
⅛ teaspoon ground white pepper

If you love a good traditional shepherd's pie, you'll love this guilt-free plant-based version made with my nutritious Hemp, Spinach and Basil Pesto (see page 222). When I first created this recipe, I shared it with my mum and let's just say one bowl wasn't enough. It's a flavourful family meal; full of warm and comforting cannellini beans, fresh basil, crunchy pine nuts, creamy pesto and packed with lots of nutritional goodness.

Preheat the oven to 180°C (350°F).

Bring a large saucepan of water to a boil. Place the potatoes in a colander over the saucepan and steam for about 25 minutes, or until fork tender.

Heat the oil in a large frying pan over medium-high heat. Add the onion and garlic and cook, stirring frequently, for 5–7 minutes, until soft and fragrant. Add the mushrooms, capsicum, zucchini, spinach, pine nuts and cook, stirring occasionally, for another 8 minutes, until tender.

Remove from the heat and add the pesto, miso, if using, cannellini beans and basil leaves to the pan. Mix to combine and season to taste.

Transfer to a deep pie dish and spread out evenly.

Drain the potatoes. Transfer to a bowl with the rice milk, salt and pepper, and mash until the potatoes are smooth and creamy, adjusting the seasoning to taste.

Spread the potatoes out evenly over the pesto veges.

Bake for 40 minutes, or until the potatoes are beginning to brown. Garnish with extra pine nuts if you like.

NOTE: For faster preparation, pre-make the pesto. The miso boosts the flavour but can be left out.

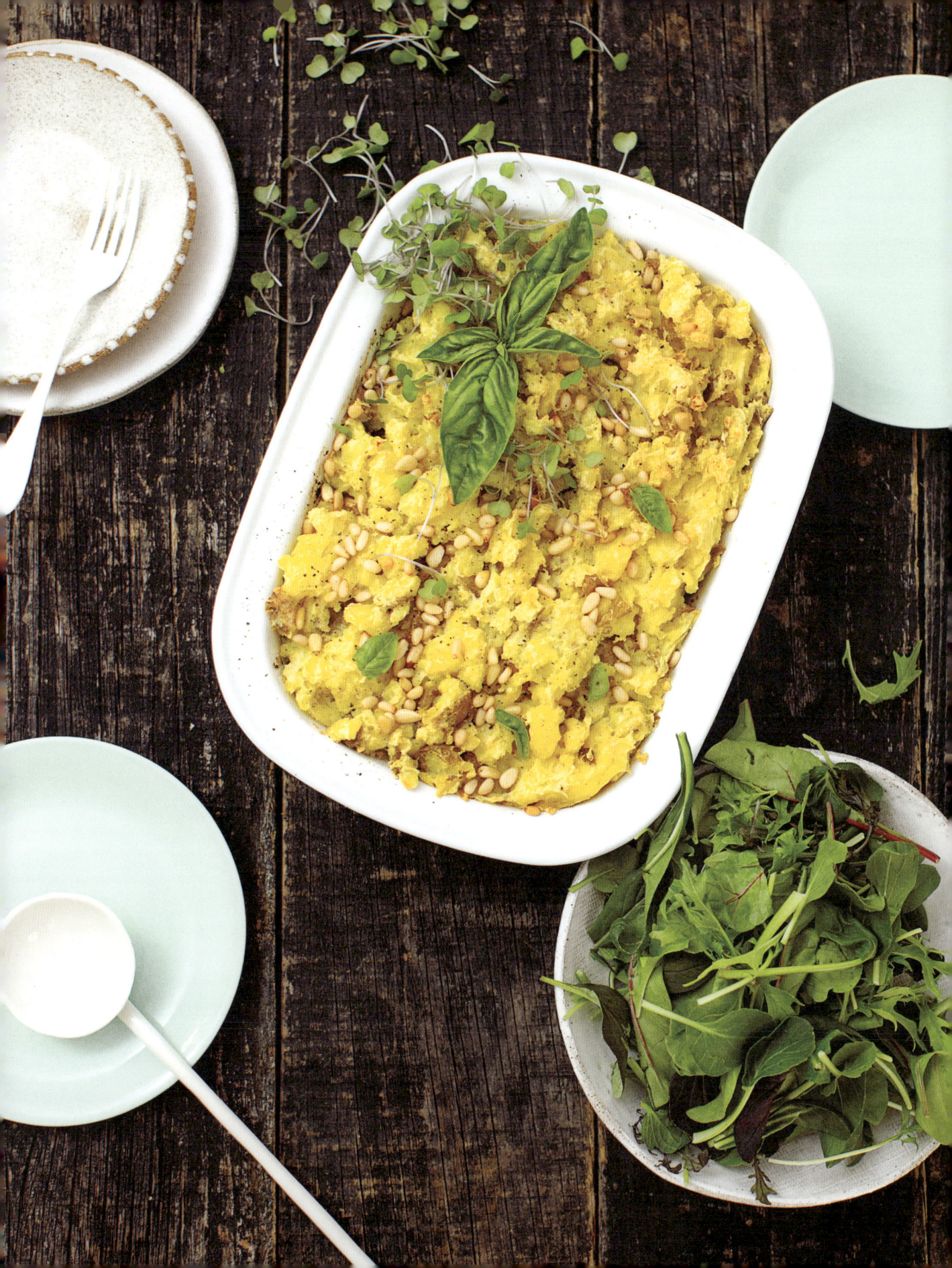

CREAMY SUNFLOWER AND VEGETABLE TART

SERVES 4–6

Buckwheat and Chia Pastry (see page 293), chilled

Tart filling
1 cup peeled and sliced carrots
1 cup peeled and cubed kūmara
2 cups peeled and cubed pumpkin
1 tablespoon olive, avocado or coconut oil (optional)
1 red onion, diced
3 cloves garlic, diced
2 cups mushrooms, sliced
3 packed cups baby spinach leaves
3 tablespoons sunflower seeds, plus extra for topping
1 tablespoon mixed herbs
1 teaspoon caraway seeds
2 cups Cashew Cheese Sauce (see page 279)

To serve (optional)
fresh leafy greens (spinach, mesclun or rocket leaves)

On my travels through Western Australia last year, I found a little organic health food store that served a vegan and gluten-free tart. It was so good I had to try to recreate it. This creamy tart will not disappoint, made with gluten-free Buckwheat and Chia Pastry (see page 293), and the tastiest Cashew Cheese Sauce (see page 279). I find it to be a great pie to bake when I have a little more time, like on a Sunday afternoon. Serve with a nutritious side of fresh garden greens.

Preheat the oven to 180°C (350°F) fan bake. Grease a 20 cm (8 in) round dish with olive oil.

Prepare the Buckwheat and Chia Pastry for the base according to the recipe instructions (see page 293). Chill in the fridge until needed.

For the tart filling, bring a saucepan of water to a boil. Place the carrots, kūmara and pumpkin in a colander over the water, cover, and steam for 15 minutes, or until just tender.

Heat the oil in a large frying pan over medium-high heat. Add the onion, garlic and mushrooms and cook, stirring frequently, for 5–7 minutes, until soft and fragrant. Add the spinach leaves, sunflower seeds, mixed herbs and caraway seeds and cook for an additional 2–3 minutes, until the spinach is wilted.

Remove from the heat and add the kūmara, pumpkin, carrots and cheese sauce to the pan. Gently mix to combine all the ingredients.

Remove the prepared pie dish from the fridge. Tip in the filling and spread out evenly around the pie dish. Scatter over a few sunflower seeds. Bake for 40–45 minutes, until golden brown.

Allow to cool for 5–7 minutes before slicing. This is an important step as it allows the tart the time it needs to set.

Serve with a side of fresh garden greens, if desired.

NOTE: For faster preparation, simply pre-make the pastry and store in the fridge or freezer until you're ready to use it.

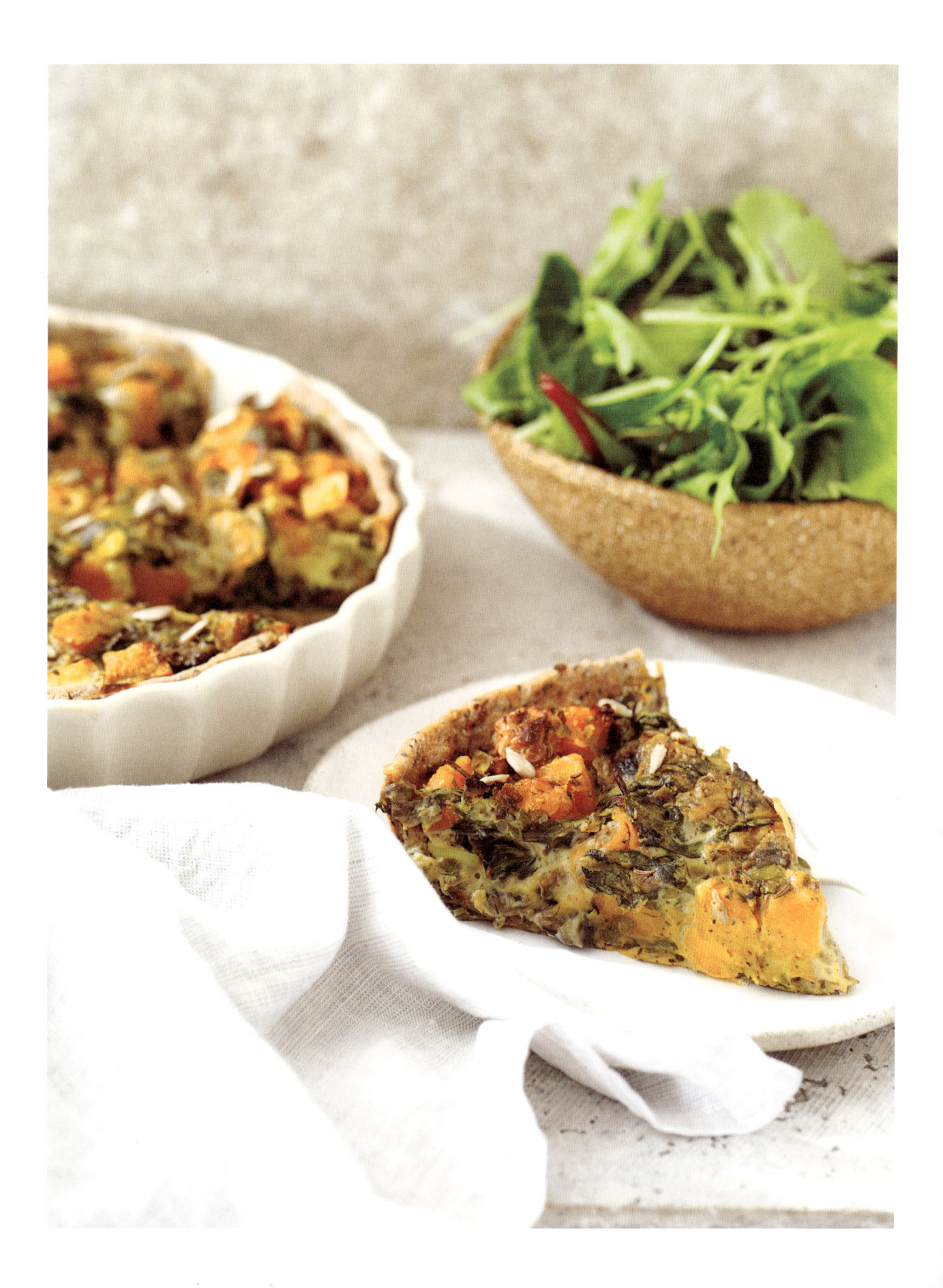

BLACK BEAN MEXICAN BOWLS with KŪMARA and VEGAN SOUR CREAM

SERVES 4–6

2 large orange kūmara, cut into small cubes

sea salt and cracked pepper, to taste

1 teaspoon olive, avocado or coconut oil (optional)

2 corn cobs, husks and silks removed

400 g (14 oz) can black beans, drained and rinsed (or 1½ cups cooked black beans)

1 cup cherry tomatoes, cut into quarters

¾ cup chopped coriander

½ small red onion, finely diced

1 small red capsicum, finely diced

½ cup black pitted olives, sliced

1 tablespoon lime zest

¼ cup lime juice

2 cloves garlic, crushed

1 teaspoon cumin seeds

1 teaspoon sweet paprika

½ teaspoon ground cinnamon

½ teaspoon ground chipotle (omit for children)

2 large avocados, stoned and diced into cubes

½ cup Vegan Sour Cream (see page 279) or coconut yoghurt

To serve (optional)
fresh coriander or basil, chopped
chilli flakes
sliced jalapeños
lime wedges
brown rice

I absolutely love Mexican food, and I especially love the raw, juicy flavours of this meal. I was originally going to create a warm chilli for this book, but I am so pleased that I decided on a mildly raw chilli instead; topped with many of my favourite things—kūmara, avocado, Vegan Sour Cream, fresh coriander and lots of zesty lime juice. These bowls make such an easy and nutritiously fun meal that the whole family will enjoy.

Preheat the oven to 180°C (350°F) fan bake. Line a large baking tray with baking paper.

Place the kūmara on the baking tray and spread out into a single layer. Drizzle over a dash of olive oil, if desired, and season to taste. Bake for 30–35 minutes, or until tender and golden.

Heat the oil in a large frying pan over medium heat. Add the corn cobs and cook, turning occasionally, for 8–10 minutes, until the corn is charred. Remove from the heat and set aside to cool.

Place the black beans, tomatoes, coriander, onion, capsicum, olives, lime zest and juice, garlic, cumin, paprika, cinnamon and chipotle in a large bowl. Slice the corn kernels from the cobs and add to the bowl. Season and toss to combine all the ingredients.

To serve, place the raw chilli bean mix in serving bowls. Divide the kūmara among the bowls, and scatter over the avocado followed by a dollop of sour cream. Finish each bowl with a sprinkle of coriander or basil, chilli flakes, jalapeños and a wedge of lime, and serve with brown rice, if desired.

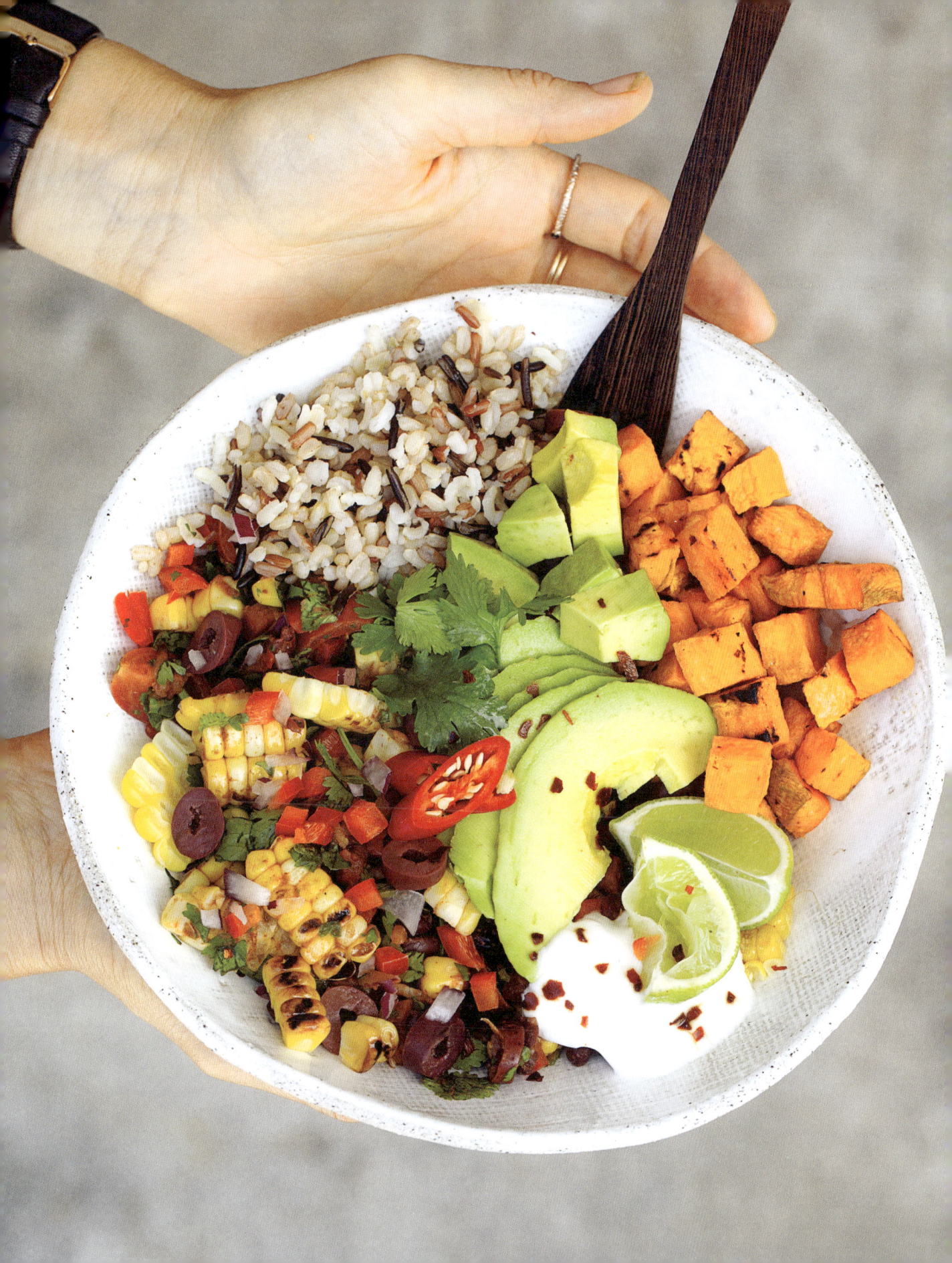

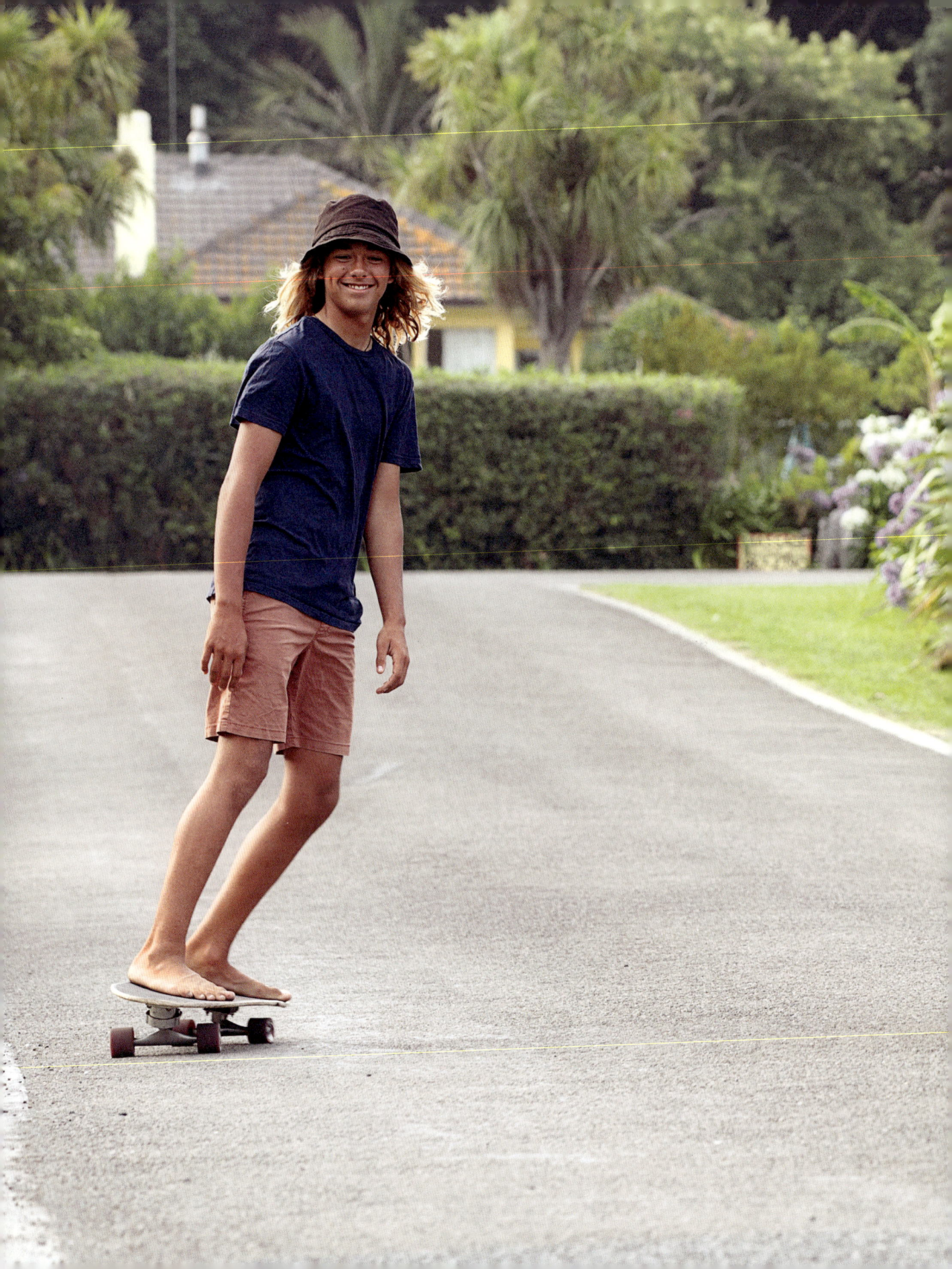

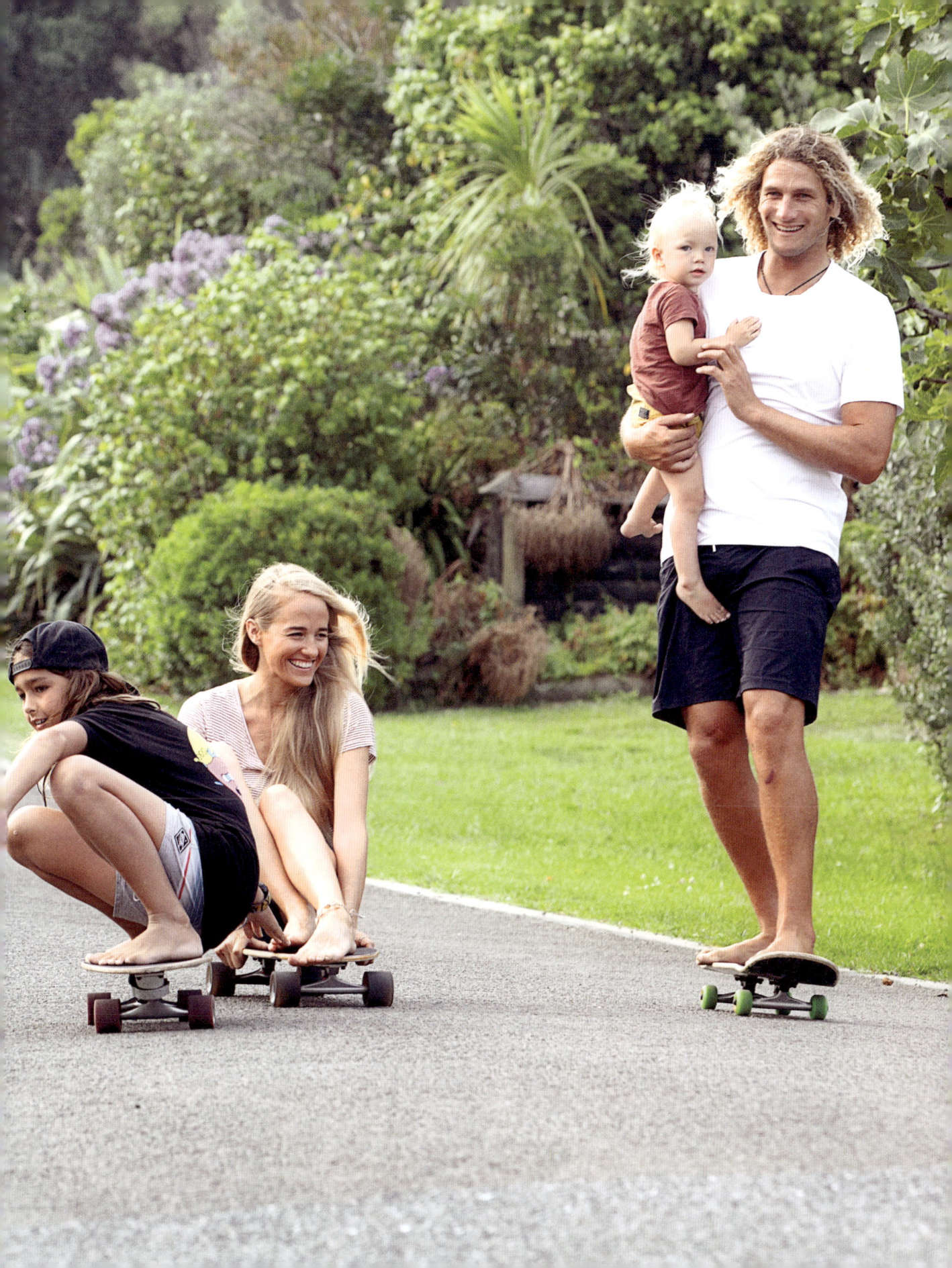

SESAME PEANUTTY PUMPKIN with SWEET MISO ASIAN SLAW

SERVES 4

Pumpkin
1 large clove garlic, minced
2 tablespoons sesame oil
2 tablespoons smooth peanut butter (or almond butter)
1½ tablespoons tamari
1½ tablespoons pure maple syrup
1 tablespoon black or white sesame seeds
pinch of chilli flakes (omit for children)
1 kg (2 lb 4 oz) pumpkin, deseeded and cut into 3 cm (1¼ in) wedges

Sweet miso dressing
3 tablespoons sesame oil
2 tablespoons tamari
2 teaspoons pure maple syrup
2 teaspoons miso paste
2 tablespoons water

Asian slaw
1 Chinese cabbage, finely shredded (approx. 5 cups)
2 cups mung bean sprouts
3 spring onions, sliced
large handful coriander, roughly chopped
2 tablespoons diced chives
3 tablespoons raw crushed peanuts, plus extra to serve
2 tablespoons black sesame seeds, plus extra to serve

To serve (optional)
2 avocados
brown rice noodles or quinoa or rice

These Asian-inspired Buddha bowls are such an easy and highly nutritious bowlful of goodness. I love the peanutty sesame-infused pumpkin, especially paired with the fresh and crunchy slaw. With a sweet and sour tang, this beautiful slaw is another tasty way to eat an abundance of raw cabbage, boosting your vitamin C, vitamin K and folate intake, and it only takes 10 minutes to make. For a larger meal, these bowls are amazing served with your favourite gluten-free grain or noodles, and, if you like, finished with a sliced avocado.

Preheat the oven to 180°C (350°F) fan bake. Line a baking tray with baking paper.

For the pumpkin, place the garlic, sesame oil, peanut butter, tamari, maple and sesame seeds into a small bowl and whisk to combine. Tip the dressing into a large shallow bowl. Coat each piece of pumpkin in the marinade and place onto the prepared tray. Drizzle over any remaining marinade and lightly sprinkle with chilli flakes and extra sesame seeds. Bake for 40–45 minutes.

For the dressing, place all the ingredients in a bowl and whisk together.

For the slaw, place all the ingredients in a large bowl. Add the dressing and toss to combine.

To serve, divide the pumpkin wedges evenly among 4 shallow bowls. Add a large serving of the Asian slaw to each bowl along with half a sliced avocado. Choose your favourite extra additions such as brown rice, noodles, sprouts or broccolini. Garnish with a sprinkle of crushed peanuts, sesame seeds and lime wedges.

NOTE: Store any leftover salad in the fridge for up to 3 days.

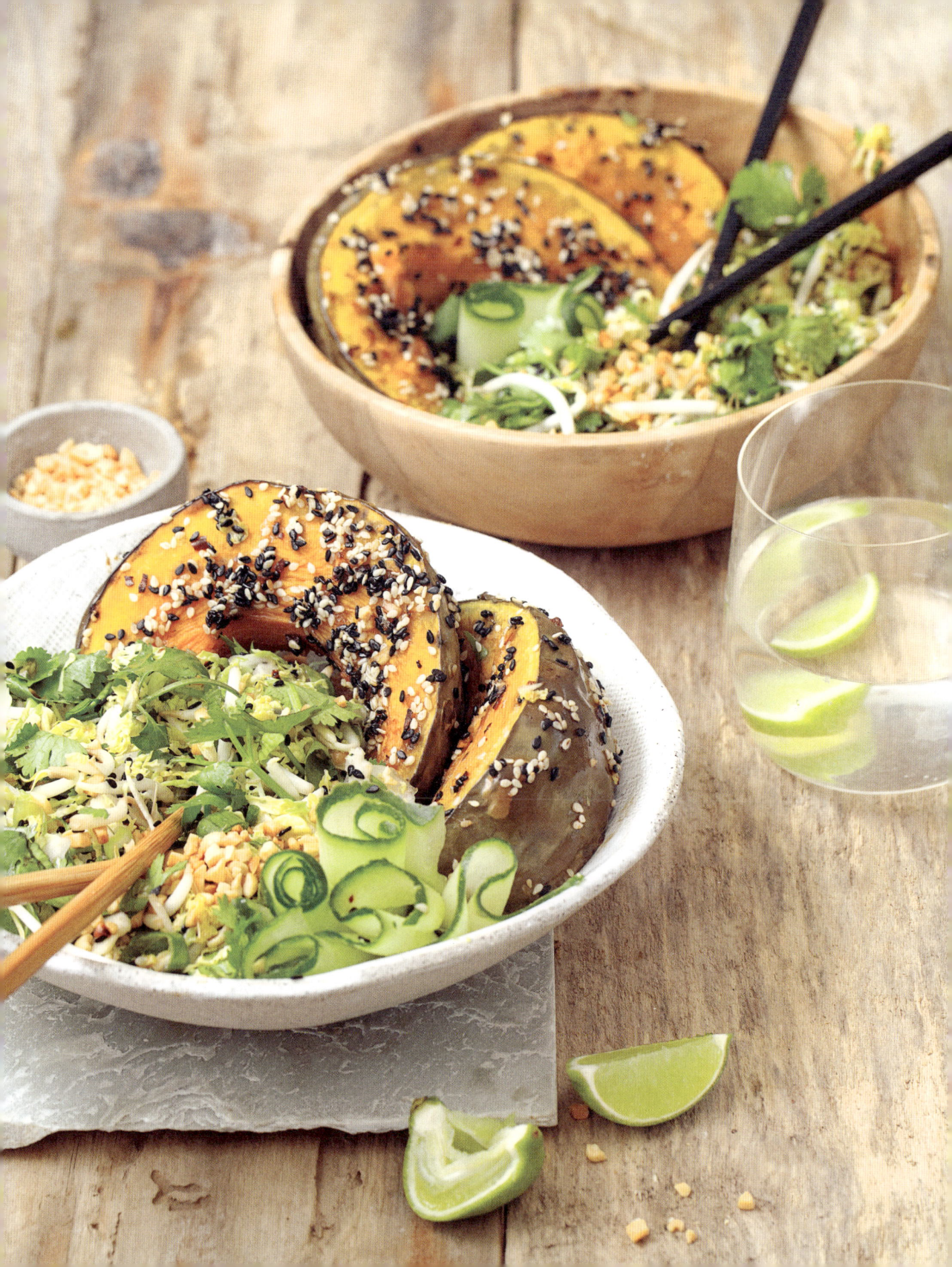

DUKKHA-BAKED KŪMARA, RAW BROCCOLI and PINE NUT SALAD with SUMAC TAHINI DRIZZLE

SERVES 4

Dukkha-baked kūmara
4 medium kūmara, sliced in half lengthways
1 teaspoon olive, avocado or coconut oil (optional)
¼ cup Dukkha (see page 282) or store-bought dukkha

Salad
¾ cup pine nuts
2 small heads broccoli (approx. 500 g / 1 lb 2 oz), trimmed and broken into large florets
¾ cup pitted dates, finely chopped
2 tablespoons sesame seeds
handful coriander, chopped
¼ cup finely diced red onion
¼ teaspoon chilli flakes (omit for children)
½ cup baby snow pea shoots, diced
juice of 1 medium lemon

To serve
½ cup Sumac Tahini Drizzle (see page 134)
fresh coriander leaves
pinch of ground sumac
2 tablespoons Dukkha (see page 282) or store-bought dukkha
lemon wedges

This beautiful plate is me to a tee. It's jam-packed with many of my favourite things: warming Egyptian-flavour-infused kūmara, a raw broccoli rice salad with toasted pine nuts and sweet chewy dates, and finished off with a drizzle of creamy sumac tahini. Kūmara is an incredibly versatile, hearty and highly nutritious root vegetable that is an absolute staple in my life. I enjoy it almost every evening, either baked or steamed, alongside a variety of raw salads and dressings. Always leave the skins on, as both kūmara and potatoes are more alkalising in the body when cooked and eaten with their skin. This salad is a great way to enjoy raw broccoli and makes a beautiful lunch idea.

Preheat the oven to 180°C (350°F) fan bake. Line a baking tray with baking paper.

Place the kūmara, flesh side up, on the prepared baking tray with the oil, if using, and evenly sprinkle over the dukkha. Bake for about 40 minutes, or until fork tender and the kūmara begins to caramelise.

Heat a small frying pan over medium heat. Add the pine nuts and cook, tossing constantly, for about 2 minutes, or until lightly browned and fragrant.

Place the broccoli in a food processor and pulse for about 5 seconds, until the broccoli resembles rice.

Place the pine nuts, broccoli and remaining salad ingredients in a bowl and toss to combine.

To serve, place two kūmara halves on each plate and top with broccoli salad. Drizzle over the sumac tahini, and sprinkle over the fresh coriander leaves, ground sumac and dukkha. Garnish with a lemon wedge.

NOTE: Store any leftover salad in the fridge for up to 3 days.

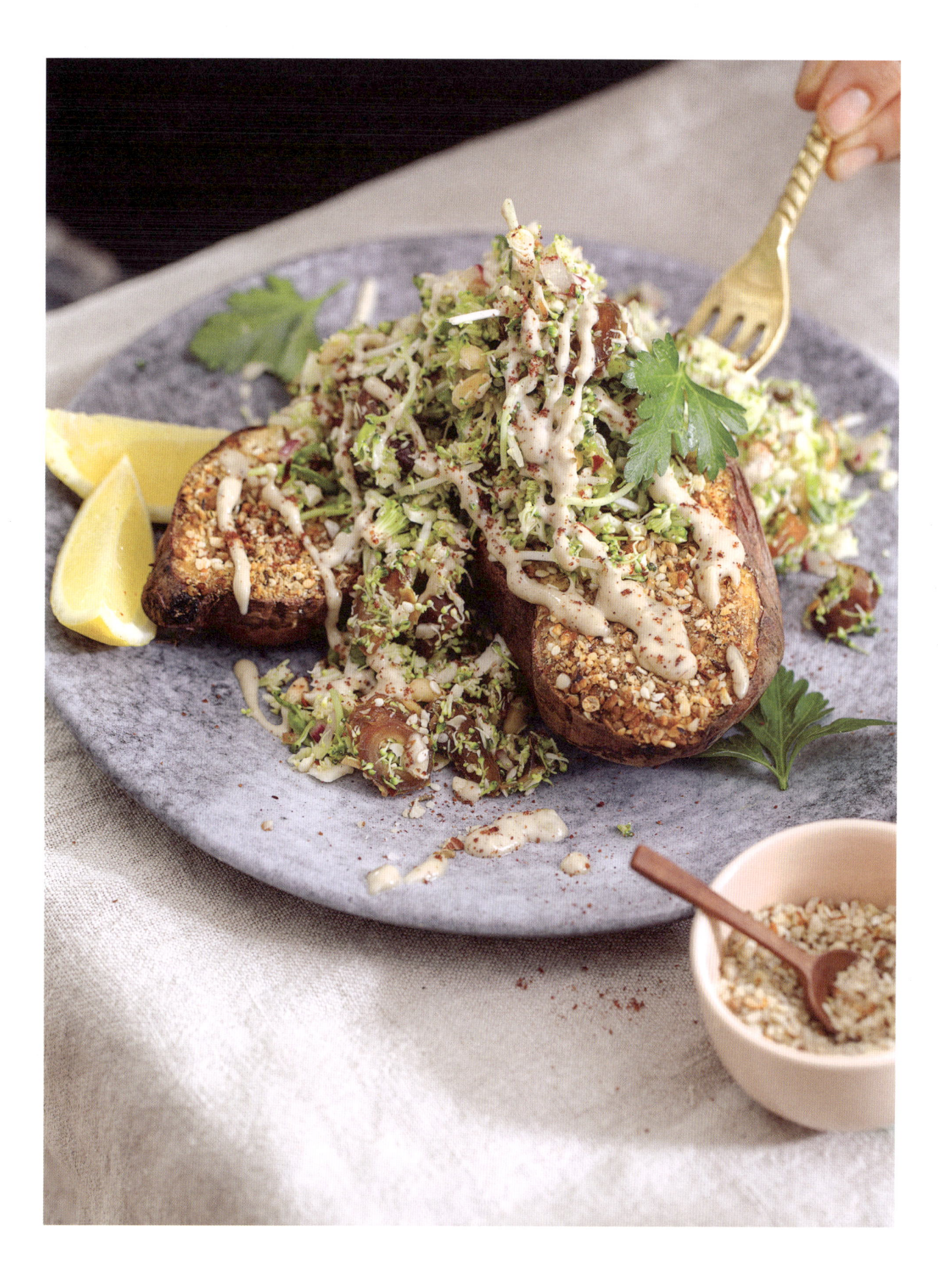

GREEK BLACK RICE STUFFED CAPSICUMS with CAPER and PARSLEY YOGHURT

SERVES 4

1 cup black rice (or wild rice mix)
2 cups water
4 large capsicums, halved lengthways and deseeded
1 teaspoon olive, avocado or coconut oil (optional)
5 spring onions, sliced
½ red onion, finely diced
3 cloves garlic, diced
½ cup raw pistachio nuts
¼ cup raw mixed seeds (pumpkin, sunflower, sesame)
½ cup green olives, sliced
large handful fresh parsley, finely chopped
3 tablespoons balsamic vinegar
3 tablespoons nutritional yeast flakes

Caper and parsley yoghurt
⅔ packed cup fresh parsley
⅔ cup coconut yoghurt
1½ teaspoons capers
2 teaspoons lemon juice
1 teaspoon apple cider vinegar
1 clove garlic, diced
¼ teaspoon sea salt

To serve
fresh leafy greens

If you're looking for a crowd-pleasing main, try this effortlessly stylish and tasty dish. The juicy capsicums are a true match with the Greek black rice mix, and to top it all off the dressing is incredible. My brother, a vegetarian his entire life, was the person who originally inspired me to get creative with stuffed capsicums, and I became hooked from the beginning. Try filling them with Mexican beans and guacamole or Moroccan chickpeas and hummus for other scrumptious meal ideas.

For the Caper and Parsley Yoghurt, place all the ingredients in a blender and blend for 20–30 seconds, until smooth. Transfer to a bowl and place in the fridge for 30 minutes to set.

Preheat the oven to 180°C (350°F) fan bake. Line a baking tray with baking paper.

Place the rice and water in a saucepan, cover and bring to a boil. Once boiling, reduce the heat to low and simmer for about 25 minutes, until the water has been absorbed and the rice is soft.

Place the capsicums on the prepared baking tray and bake for 15–20 minutes, until soft and juicy.

Meanwhile, heat the oil in a small frying pan over medium-high heat. Add the spring onion, red onion and garlic and cook, stirring frequently, for 5–7 minutes, until soft and fragrant. Add the pistachios and seeds and cook, stirring occasionally, for another 3 minutes.

Remove and transfer to a large bowl. Add the rice, olives, parsley, balsamic vinegar and nutritional yeast, and mix to combine all the ingredients.

Remove the capsicums from the oven and divide the filling evenly among the capsicum halves.

To serve, top with a dollop of the Caper and Parsley Yoghurt and serve with a side of fresh leafy greens.

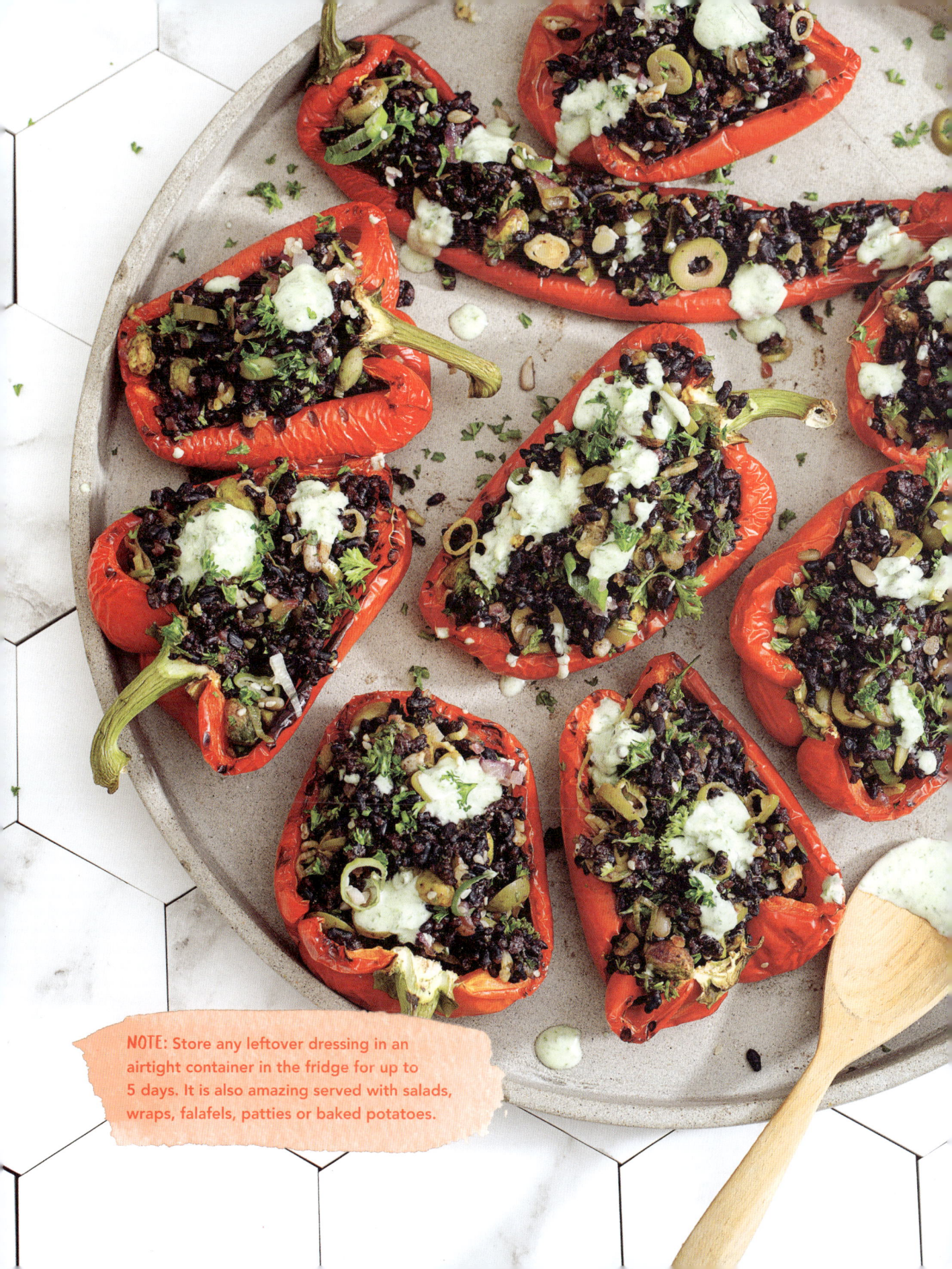

NOTE: Store any leftover dressing in an airtight container in the fridge for up to 5 days. It is also amazing served with salads, wraps, falafels, patties or baked potatoes.

CHEESY KALE, PESTO and PINE NUT PIZZA

SERVES 2–4

Pizza base

¼ head cauliflower (approx. 2 packed cups)
2 tablespoons dried oregano
1 teaspoon sea salt
1 tablespoon onion powder
1 tablespoon garlic powder
¾ cup buckwheat flour
1 tablespoon olive oil

Kale chips

2 cups cavolo nero or curly kale, stems removed and roughly chopped
1 teaspoon olive oil
1 tablespoon nutritional yeast flakes
sea salt and cracked pepper, to taste

Pizza toppings

½ cup Hemp, Spinach and Basil Pesto (see page 222) or store-bought pesto
½ cup mushrooms, thinly sliced
½ small red onion, thinly sliced
¾ cup cherry tomatoes, sliced
¼ cup pine nuts
¼ cup olives, sliced

Crispy 'cheesy' kale chips over a delish home-made pizza base with pesto, mushrooms, pine nuts and olives—so good. This pizza base has been a long-time staple in our home; it's an easy, gluten-free base that goes perfectly with all of your favourite pizza toppings. Eli and Milo love these kale chips; they also make for a great snack idea or lunch-box filler, with a crunchy, cheesy flavour from the nutritional yeast flakes.

Preheat the oven to 180°C (350°F) fan bake. Line a baking tray with baking paper.

For the pizza base, place the cauliflower, oregano, salt, onion powder and garlic powder in a food processor and blend for about 7 seconds, until the cauliflower resembles fine breadcrumbs. It is important not to over-blend, as the cauliflower will then become too moist and mushy.

Remove and add to a large bowl with the buckwheat flour and olive oil. Mix to combine then, using your hands, begin to knead the dough for about a minute, until it forms into a compact ball. If it feels too sticky, add a little more flour.

Place the dough on the prepared baking tray and gently roll it out into a round pizza base, about 5 mm (¼ in) thick. Bake for 15 minutes.

For the kale chips, place the kale and oil in a bowl. Using your hands, massage the oil into the leaves for 1–2 minutes, until they begin to soften. Add the nutritional yeast, season and mix through the leaves until evenly coated.

Remove the base from the oven and layer with the toppings, beginning with the pesto and finishing with the kale.

Return to the oven and bake for another 15–20 minutes. Slice and serve.

NOTE: Make extra cheesy kale chips to serve on the side or as a snack for later. Simply follow the kale step, then place on a lined tray and bake for 15 minutes, or until crispy.

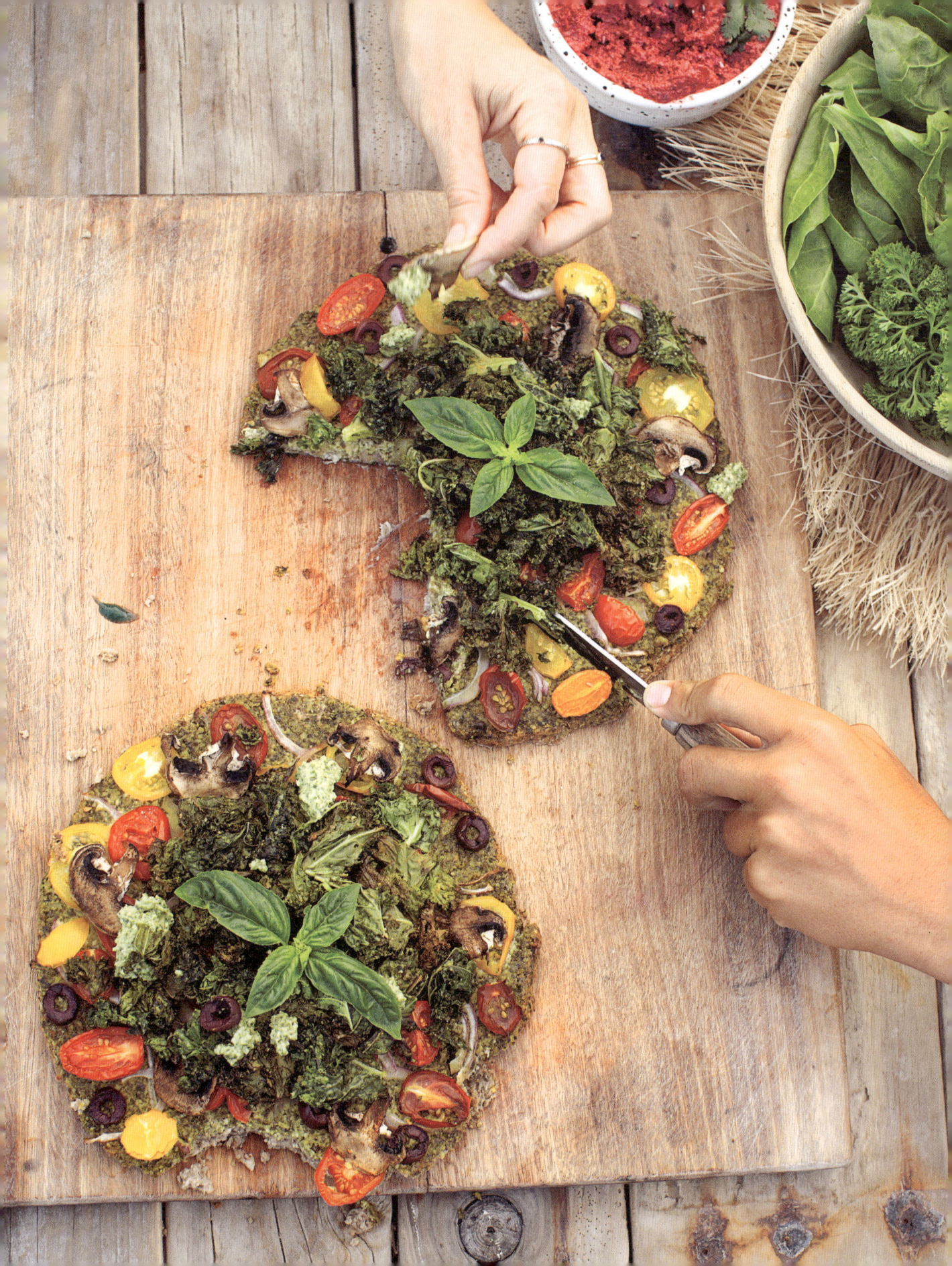

BALSAMIC CAJUN JACKFRUIT TACOS with APPLE SLAW

SERVES 4–6

Balsamic Cajun jackfruit
1 tablespoon paprika
1 teaspoon smoked paprika
2 teaspoons garlic powder
1 teaspoon onion powder
1 tablespoon dried oregano
½ teaspoon dried thyme
pinch of cayenne pepper (optional)
1 teaspoon olive, avocado or coconut oil (optional)
1 red onion, sliced
2 x 400 g (14 oz) cans young jackfruit, drained and broken into smaller pieces if necessary
1½ tablespoons tomato paste
2 tablespoons balsamic vinegar
3 tablespoons coconut sugar

Apple slaw
2 cups thinly shredded purple cabbage
2 carrots, peeled and julienned
1 apple, peeled and julienned
¼ cup fresh parsley, roughly chopped
⅓ cup coconut yoghurt
2 teaspoons apple cider vinegar

To serve
12 Easy Chickpea Tacos (see page 291) or store-bought tacos or 12 large lettuce leaves
1 large avocado, finely diced
½ cup Ranch Dressing (see page 278) or Aïoli (see page 276) (optional)

The first time I experienced jackfruit cooked this way was about four or five years ago, served in a mostly raw, plant-based café. And wow, what a flavour explosion. If you haven't tried marinated jackfruit before, then I highly recommend you do. In the vegan world it's often used as a light, juicy and super-tasty addition to burgers, tacos, nachos and curries. These tacos taste even better than they look. They're incredibly flavoursome and have fast become a family favourite in our home.

For the balsamic Cajun jackfruit, make a Cajun blend by mixing together the paprikas, garlic powder, onion powder, dried oregano, dried thyme and cayenne pepper, if using, in a small bowl. Set aside.

Heat the oil in a frying pan over medium-high heat. Add the onion and cook, stirring frequently, for 5–7 minutes, until soft and fragrant. Add the jackfruit, tomato paste, balsamic vinegar, coconut sugar and Cajun blend, and mix to combine. Reduce the heat to low and leave for 5–10 minutes, stirring occasionally, to allow the flavours to blend and the jackfruit to marinate.

For the apple slaw, place all the ingredients in a bowl and toss to combine.

To serve, layer each taco with the apple slaw, followed by the jackfruit and diced avocado. Finish with an optional drizzle of dressing and a squeeze of lime.

NOTES: Try this jackfruit in burgers, over nachos or added to a crisp cos lettuce salad.

My home-made Easy Chickpea Tacos (see page 291) are super-quick to make and contain no additives, unlike the majority of the store-bought ones. For a much quicker prep time, pre-make the tacos as they will store well in the fridge.

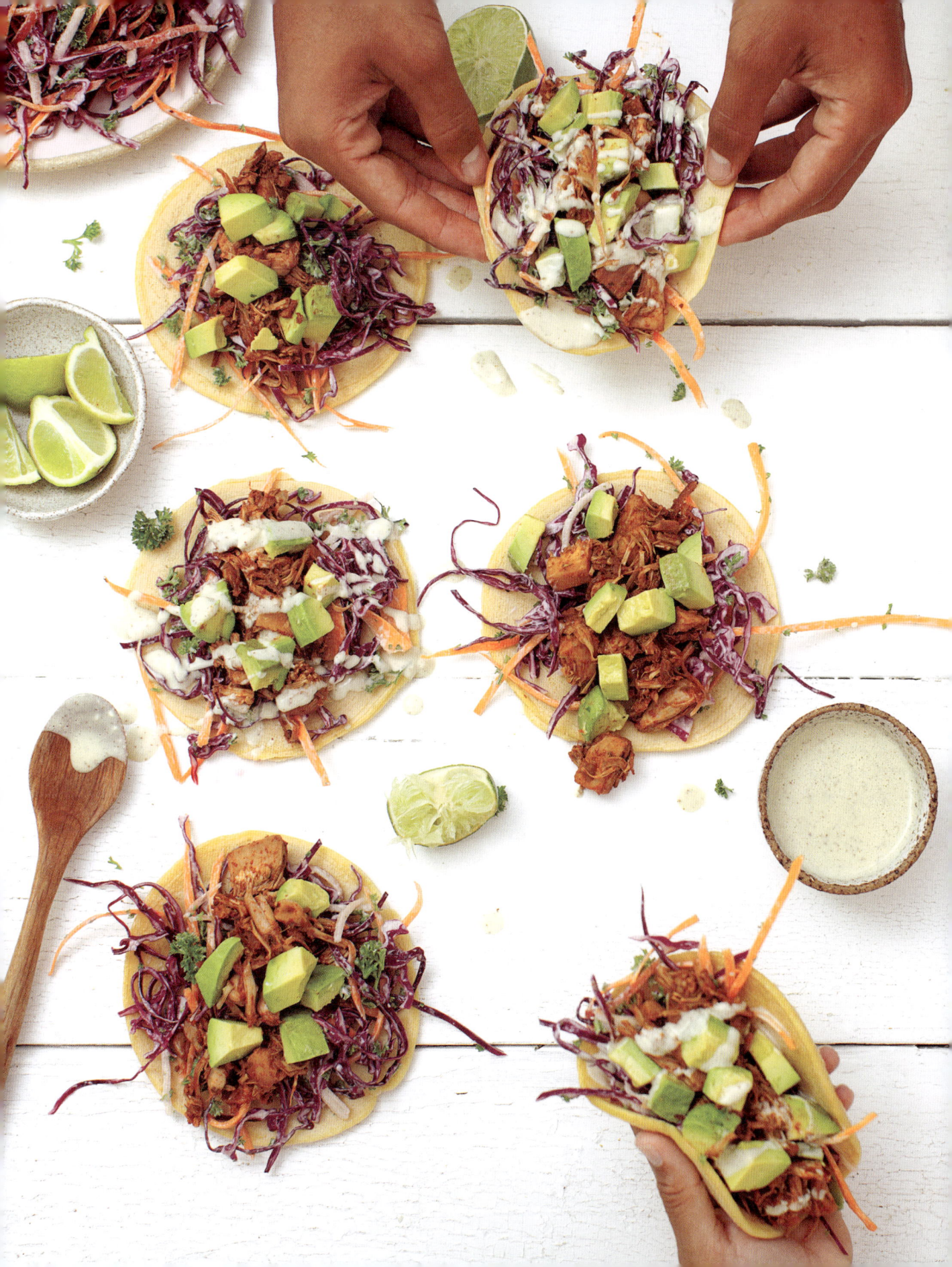

BEETROOT, ORANGE, WALNUT and QUINOA PATTIES, with LIME, DILL and YOGHURT DRESSING

MAKES 6 LARGE OR 8 SMALL PATTIES

Lime, dill and yoghurt dressing

½ cup coconut yoghurt
1 tablespoon roughly chopped fresh dill
1 teaspoon pure maple syrup
½ teaspoon garlic powder
zest and juice of 1 lime

Quinoa patties

½ cup quinoa, rinsed
1 cup water
1 teaspoon olive, avocado or coconut oil (optional)
1 red onion, thinly sliced
3 cloves garlic, diced
2 raw beetroot (approx. 500 g/ 1 lb 2 oz), peeled and grated
¾ cup buckwheat flour
small handful fresh dill, roughly chopped
small handful fresh mint, roughly chopped
2 tablespoons Dijon mustard
2 tablespoons orange zest
2 tablespoons orange juice
3 tablespoons crushed walnuts
1 teaspoon dried thyme
1 teaspoon fennel seeds
1½ teaspoons ground cumin
oil for cooking

To serve

leafy greens
cucumber, sliced into ribbons
avocado, sliced
gluten-free burger buns or lettuce leaves

Friday night takeout never looked better. These hearty patties would have to be another favourite of mine; bursting with fresh herby mint and dill flavours that are beautifully complemented by the hints of orange and fennel. Serve them alongside any salad, or create a gluten-free burger with a dollop of one of my favourite dressings in the book—Lime and Dill Yoghurt. This dressing also partners perfectly with raw vege sticks, Sesame Baked Falafel Bites (see page 224) or Quick 'n' Easy Carrot Fritters (see page 102).

For the Lime, Dill and Yoghurt Dressing, place all the ingredients in a bowl and mix to combine. Place in the fridge for about 30 minutes, to allow the dressing to set.

For the quinoa patties, place the quinoa and water in a saucepan, cover, and bring to a boil. Once boiling, reduce the heat to low and simmer for 12–15 minutes, until the water has been absorbed and the quinoa is soft and fluffy.

Heat the oil in a frying pan over medium-high heat. Once hot, add the onion and garlic and cook, stirring frequently, for 5–7 minutes, until soft and fragrant.

Remove and place in a large bowl with the quinoa, beetroot, flour, dill, mint, mustard, orange zest and juice, walnuts, thyme, fennel seeds and cumin. Mix until all the ingredients are combined.

Using your hands, mould the mixture into 6 large patties or 8 small patties.

Heat a dash of olive oil in a large non-stick frying pan over medium-high heat. Once the pan is hot, reduce heat to medium-low.

Place 3 patties in the pan and cook for 6–7 minutes, until golden brown. Flip and cook the other side for another 6–7 minutes. Remove and place on a paper towel to absorb any excess oil. You could then place in a warmed oven if you wish to keep the patties warm. Repeat with the remaining patties.

Serve with a side of fresh greens, cucumber and avocado, topped with a dollop of yoghurt dressing, or create a burger with a gluten-free bun or lettuce leaves.

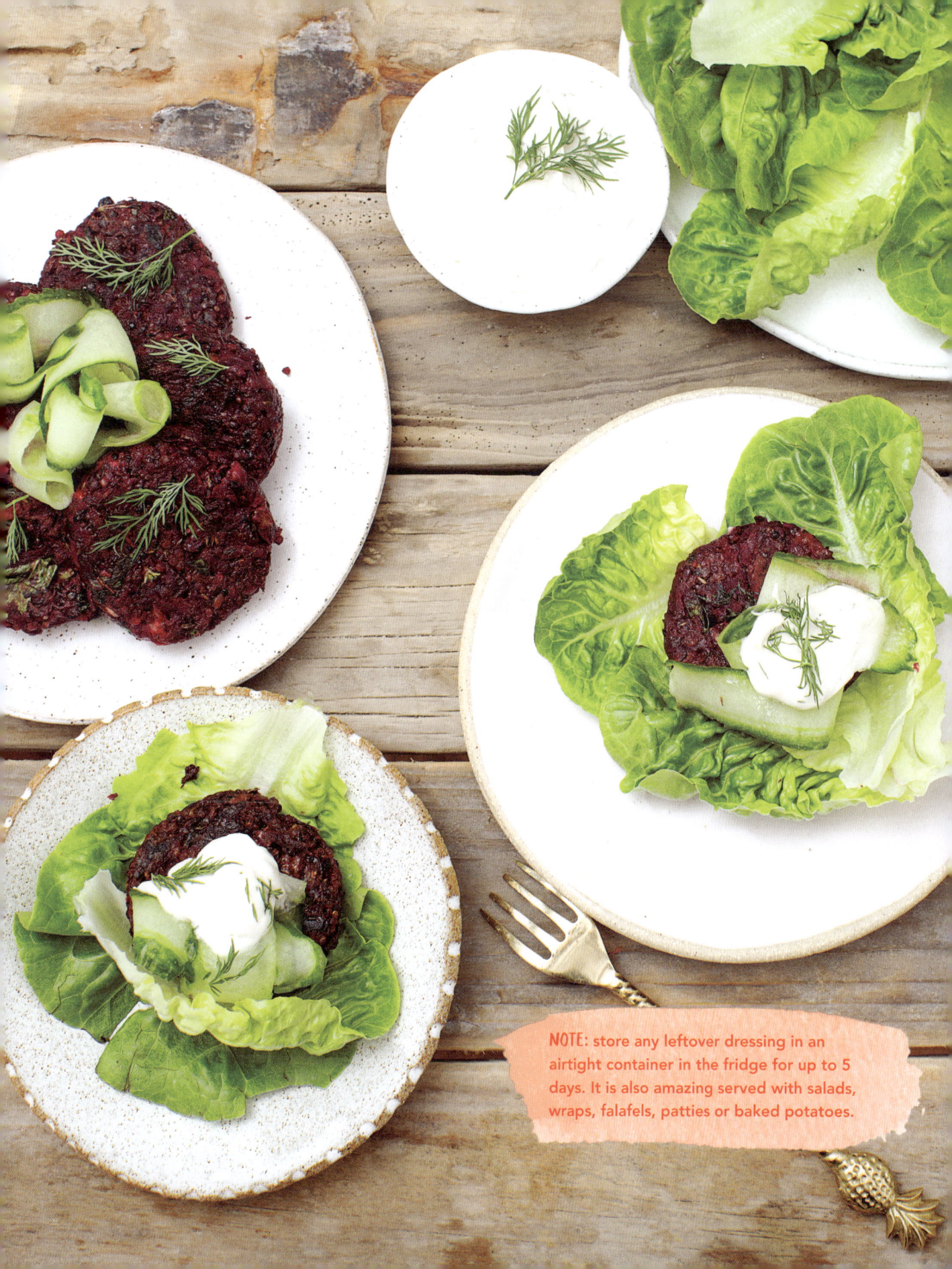

NOTE: store any leftover dressing in an airtight container in the fridge for up to 5 days. It is also amazing served with salads, wraps, falafels, patties or baked potatoes.

CARAWAY POTATO and CHICKPEA MINGLE with GARDEN GREENS and RANCH DRESSING

SERVES 4

Caraway potatoes
6 large potatoes (agria, russet, red, etc., approx. 1 kg / 2 lb 4 oz), cut into bite-sized cubes
2 tablespoons caraway seeds
olive oil, for cooking (optional)
sea salt and cracked pepper, to taste

Chickpea mingle
2 x 400 g (14 oz) cans chickpeas, drained and rinsed (or 3 cups cooked chickpeas)
1 large red onion, thinly sliced
½ red capsicum, finely diced
2 tablespoons apple cider vinegar
1 tablespoon buckwheat flour
1 teaspoon caraway seeds
1 tablespoon fennel seeds
1 tablespoon dried rosemary
1 tablespoon pure maple syrup

To serve
4 cups baby spinach or mesclun leaves
1 cup Ranch Dressing (see page 278)
finely chopped fresh parsley

This simply tasteful mingle is another one of my favourites. I don't eat many beans and legumes, but there is definitely something about this mingle that wins me over every time. The crunchy chickpeas with hints of rosemary and fennel mingled with caraway-roasted potatoes make for the perfect lunch or dinner, served over fresh greens and finished with a drizzle of my creamy Ranch Dressing (see page 278).

Preheat the oven to 180°C (350°F) fan bake. Line a large baking tray with baking paper.

Bring a saucepan of water to a boil. Place the potatoes in a colander over the water, cover, and steam for about 15–20 minutes, until the potatoes are just tender.

Place all of the Chickpea Mingle ingredients in a bowl and mix to combine, ensuring all of the chickpeas are well coated in the mixture.

Drain the potatoes and tip onto the prepared baking tray. Evenly sprinkle over the caraway seeds and a drizzle of olive oil, if using. Lightly season. Add the chickpea mix to the tray and gently mix through the potatoes to combine. Bake for 25–30 minutes until the potatoes are golden brown.

To serve, place the mingle on a bed of leaves and drizzle over the Ranch Dressing. Garnish with a light sprinkle of parsley.

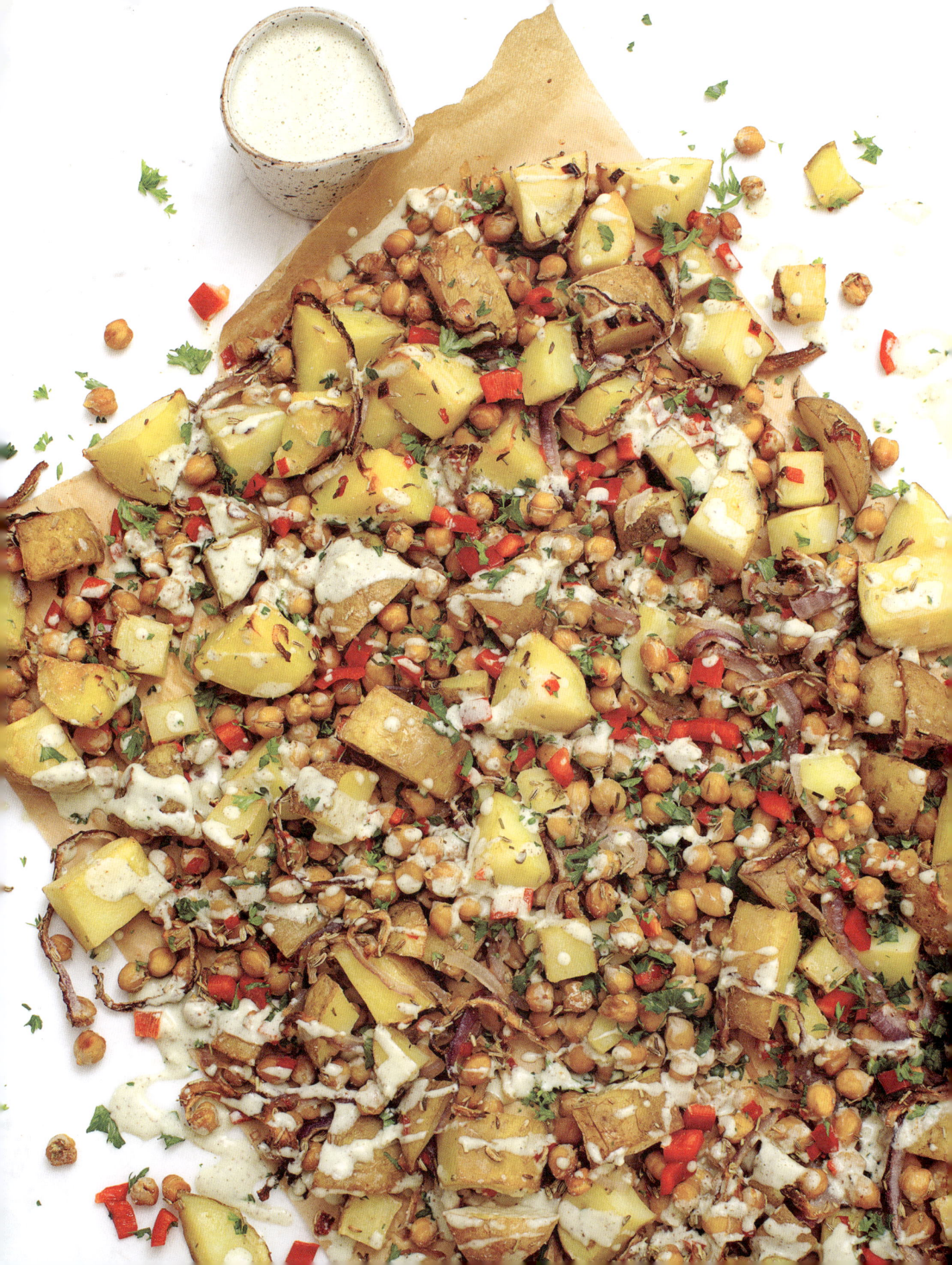

CAULIFLOWER KOFTA BALLS with MINT AÏOLI

SERVES 4 (MAKES APPROX. 14 BALLS)

- 2 medium agria potatoes, cut into bite-sized pieces (approx. 3 cups)
- ⅓ head cauliflower, cut into small florets (approx. 3 cups)
- 1 teaspoon olive, avocado or coconut oil (optional)
- 1 onion, diced
- 3 cloves garlic, diced
- 2 carrots, peeled and finely grated (approx. ¾ cup)
- 1 cup roughly chopped coriander
- 1 teaspoon garam masala
- ½ teaspoon curry powder
- ½ teaspoon ground turmeric
- 2 tablespoons nutritional yeast
- 1 teaspoon ground ginger
- ¾ cup chickpea flour
- ½ teaspoon sea salt
- ⅛ teaspoon white pepper

To serve
- 1 cup Mint Aïoli (see page 276)
- leafy greens
- Raw Cleansing Beetroot, Carrot and Walnut Salad (optional, see page 116)

When I first created these beautifully spiced kofta balls I almost ate half the batch in one sitting. They're super soft and fluffy with warming aromatic Indian flavours and partner really well with my Raw Cleansing Beetroot, Carrot and Walnut Salad (see page 116) and a drizzle of Mint Aïoli (see page 276). Any leftovers make an excellent ready-to-go snack to store in the fridge, or throw them in a bowl with fresh raw greens, grated beetroot and a drizzle of my creamy Ranch Dressing (see page 278).

Preheat the oven to 180°C (350°F) fan bake. Line a baking tray with baking paper.

Bring a large saucepan of water to a boil. Place the potatoes in a colander over the water, cover, and steam for 18–20 minutes, or until tender. Add the cauliflower for the last 5–7 minutes of cooking time.

Heat the oil in a frying pan over medium-high heat. Add the onion and garlic and cook, stirring frequently, for 5–7 minutes, until soft and fragrant.

Transfer to a bowl along with the potatoes, cauliflower and carrots. Mash until mostly smooth, leaving a few small chunks. Add the coriander, garam masala, curry powder, turmeric, nutritional yeast, ginger, flour, salt and pepper. Mix to combine.

Using your hands, roll about 3 tablespoons (or more for larger koftas) of the mixture into a ball, and place on the prepared tray. Repeat with the remaining mixture.

Bake for 30 minutes, or until golden brown.

Serve over fresh leafy greens with a drizzle of Mint Aïoli or with a side of my Raw Cleansing Beetroot, Carrot and Walnut salad.

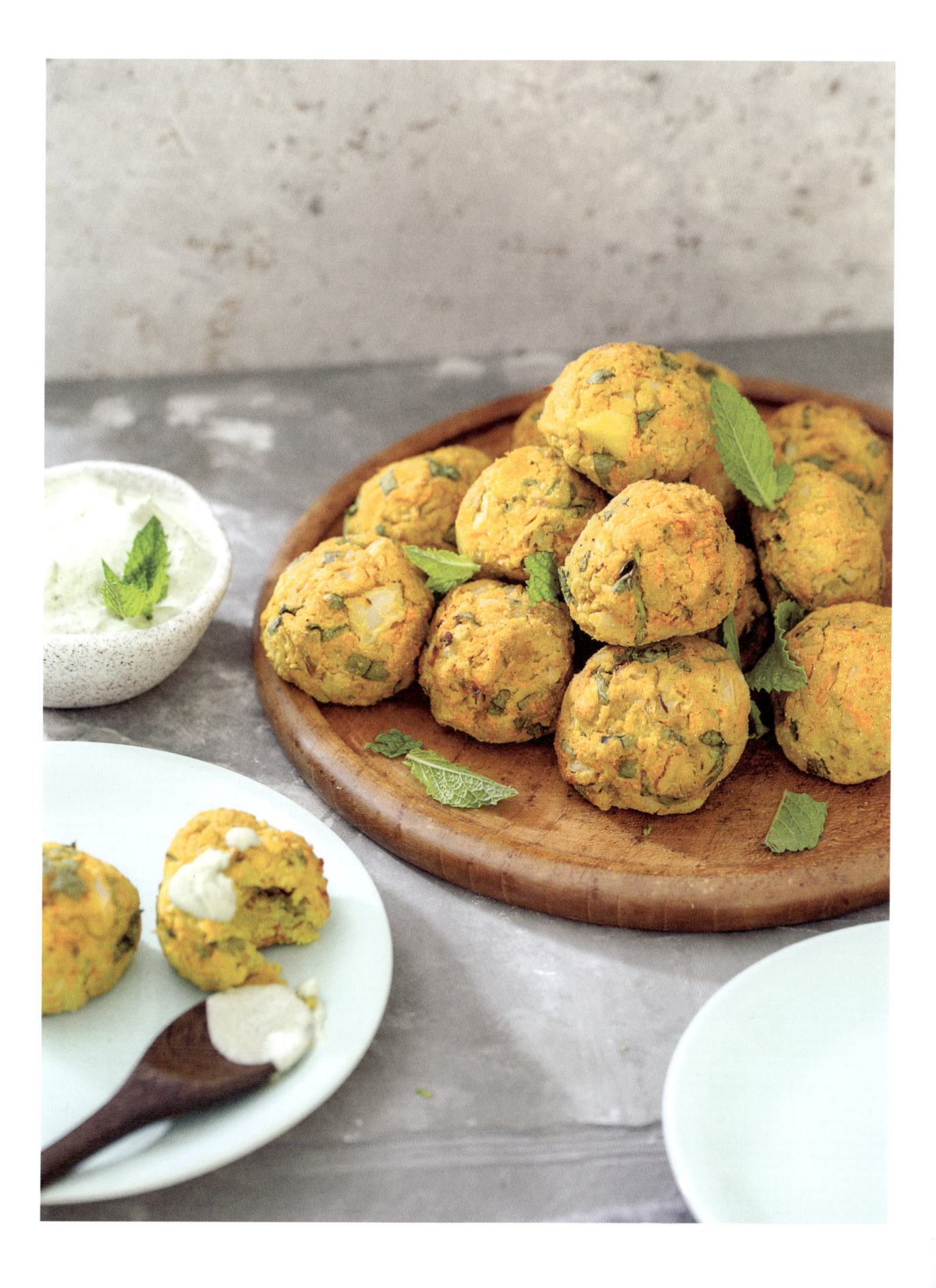

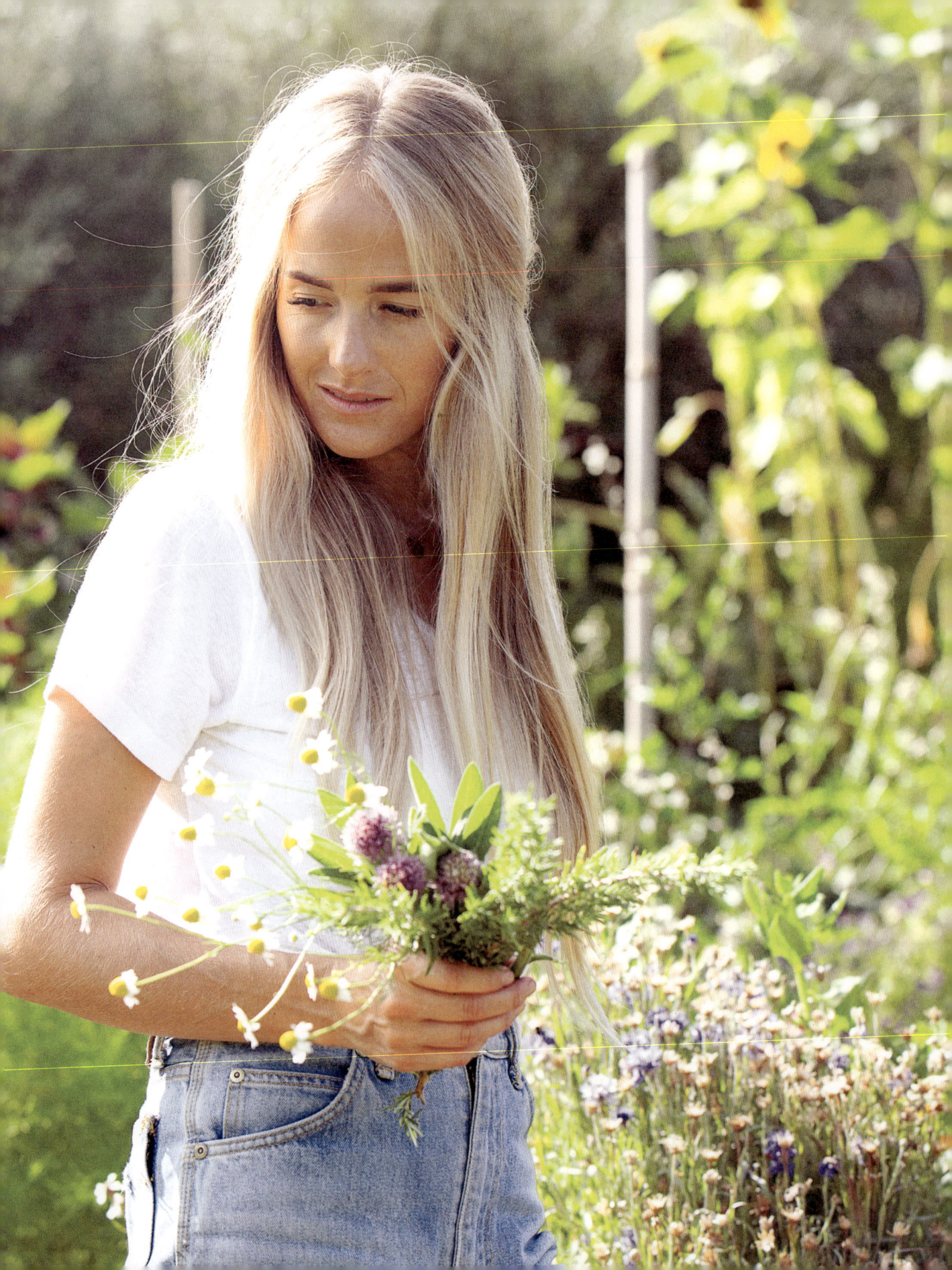

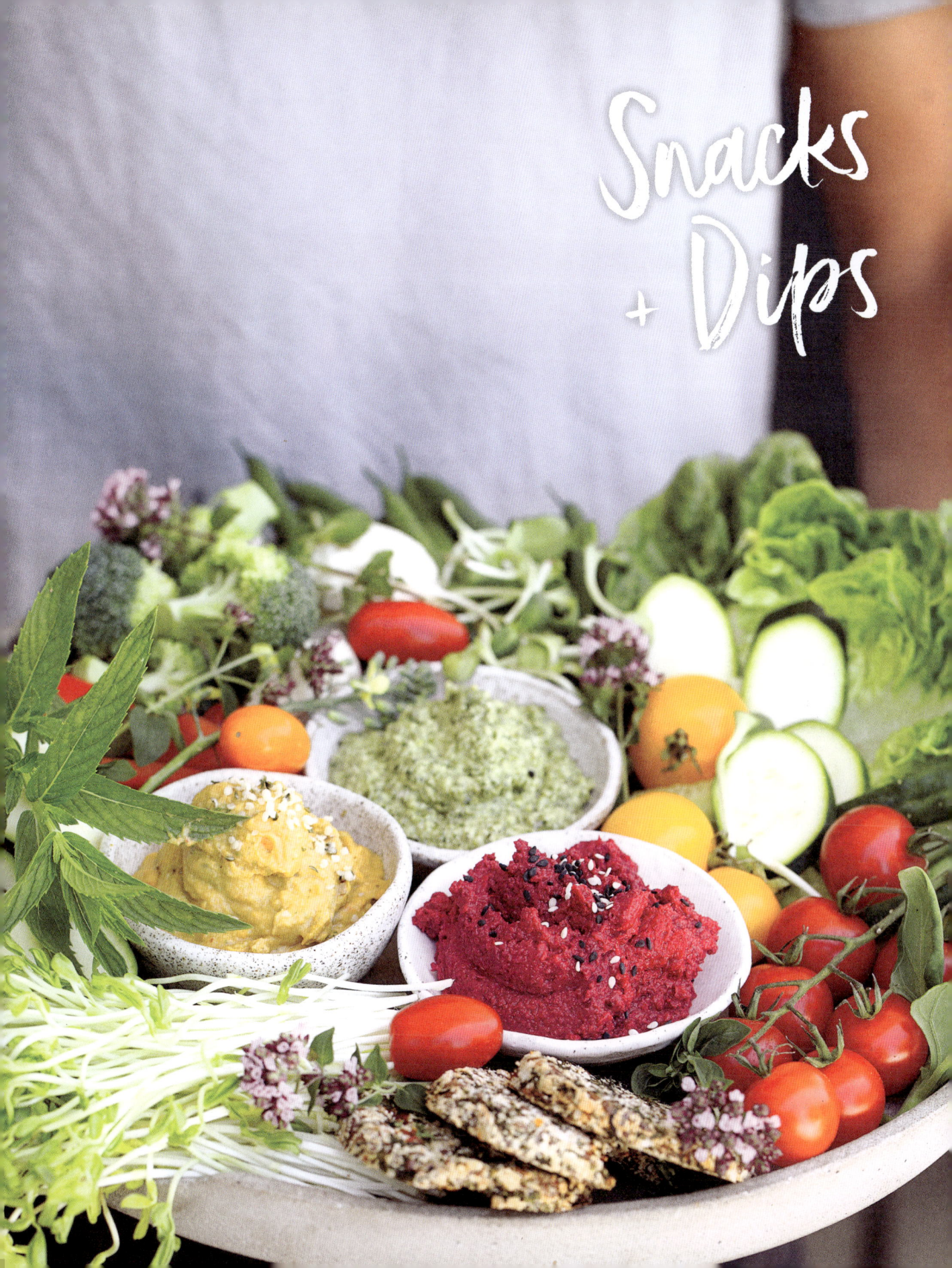

Snacks + Dips

Snacks + Dips

Creating a healthy snacking habit is essential to living a wholesome lifestyle. When we need a quick fix, we tend to reach for processed foods, but these foods are dead foods that are stripped of nutrients. Not only are they detrimental to our health and addictive, but they also completely deplete us of what we were needing in the first place—energy.

The best, most simple snacks are the ready-to-go foods that Nature so perfectly designed for us. Fruit, veges, nuts and seeds provide nutrient-dense, energising and perfectly balanced food, jam-packed with the many vitamins and minerals we need to feel refreshed, energised and ready to go again. And the best part—they require no preparation.

I personally choose to eat mostly raw, live foods throughout the day (fruit, in particular, in abundance) and I feel absolutely amazing for it. Here are some of my favourite everyday snacks, which are all simple wholefoods that contribute to a healthy lifestyle.

- Mono meals of fresh seasonal fruit or fruit platters
- Smoothies (see pages 52–54)
- Smoothie bowls (see pages 56–60)
- Fruity Whips (nice cream) (see pages 64–66)
- Fresh fruit and vegetable juices (see page 70)
- Nuts and seeds
- Frozen pitted medjool dates (a must-try; when frozen they become extra chewy and taste like chewy caramel sweets)
- Dried fruit—especially figs, dates, apricots, goji berries and raisins (100 per cent natural, with no sulphates, colours or preservatives)
- Raw bliss balls—the recipes are endless (see pages 236–238)
- Raw vege sticks, such as carrots, celery or cucumber, with home-made dips such as guacamole
- Dehydrated crackers or brown rice crackers with almond butter, tomato, avocado and sprouts, or fresh dips such as hummus
- Spinach or lettuce wraps with fresh veges and dips
- Sun-dried tomatoes (natural, oil- and salt-free) with a dollop of natural peanut or almond butter (it's a great combination)

My family and I are BIG on smoothies, juices and fruity whips (nice cream). They create a super nutritious, refreshing and alkalising glass of goodness that works wonders in increasing your fruit and vege intake, making them the perfect light meal for any time of the day. For more snacking recipes and smoothie tips, refer to the Smoothies and Juices chapter of this book (see page 50).

QUICK TIPS FOR WHOLESOME SNACKING

» **REMOVE UNHEALTHY TEMPTATIONS FROM YOUR HOME:** Get rid of *all* the highly processed food that is wreaking absolute havoc in your body. This way you will create a healthful environment and avoid reaching for artificial food choices when in desperate need of a quick fix.

» **BE PREPARED:** Have a variety of wholesome snacks on hand, such as fresh fruit, smoothie ingredients, avocados, hummus, vege sticks, dried fruit, nuts, seeds and bliss balls. I quite often pre-cut fresh fruit, such as melons, oranges or pineapple, into bite-sized pieces and store them in containers in the fridge. That way you can simply grab a fork and enjoy a mono meal of fresh fruit on the go. You can also do the same with vege sticks. Ensure you eat these nutritious options *before* reaching for anything else. This way you'll feel full, energised and satisfied without the need for unhealthy food—when you eat more of the good, it leaves less room for the bad.

» **THINK AHEAD:** Stop and think about how an unhealthy food choice will make you feel *after* you've consumed it. When I used to consume highly processed, unhealthy snacks, it only ever left me feeling absolutely terrible and often sent me straight to the couch. One of the things that helped me to overcome these bad choices was to remind myself of this feeling *before* diving into the packet of chocolate biscuits.

» **DRINK PLENTY OF WATER:** I try to drink at least 2–3 litres (70–100 fl oz) of water per day. When you're feeling dehydrated, it's easy to mistake the feeling for hunger.

» **GIVE YOUR TREATS A MAKEOVER:** Use wholefoods to recreate a healthier version of your favourite daily snack/treat. There is often a way to replicate a wholesome version of it, and by doing this, you don't feel like you're missing out on your favourite things. I personally like to experiment with smoothies and dips.

» **SET A TARGET:** Challenge yourself (and your family) to a one- or two-week 'plant over processed' trial. This would involve cutting out all highly processed and artificial packet foods and reaching for healthy wholefoods instead. The first few days might seem impossible, but as you continue, your taste buds (and sugar cravings) will adapt and you'll be surprised by how good you feel. It's now been five years without highly processed food in my diet, and it has made the world of difference to both my physical and my mental well-being.

» Alongside the list of my favourite everyday snacks, this chapter provides you with a handful of snacking ideas that make for fantastic lunch-box fillers, as well as heavenly dips to accompany raw vege sticks, wholesome crackers or Buddha bowls. Enjoy.

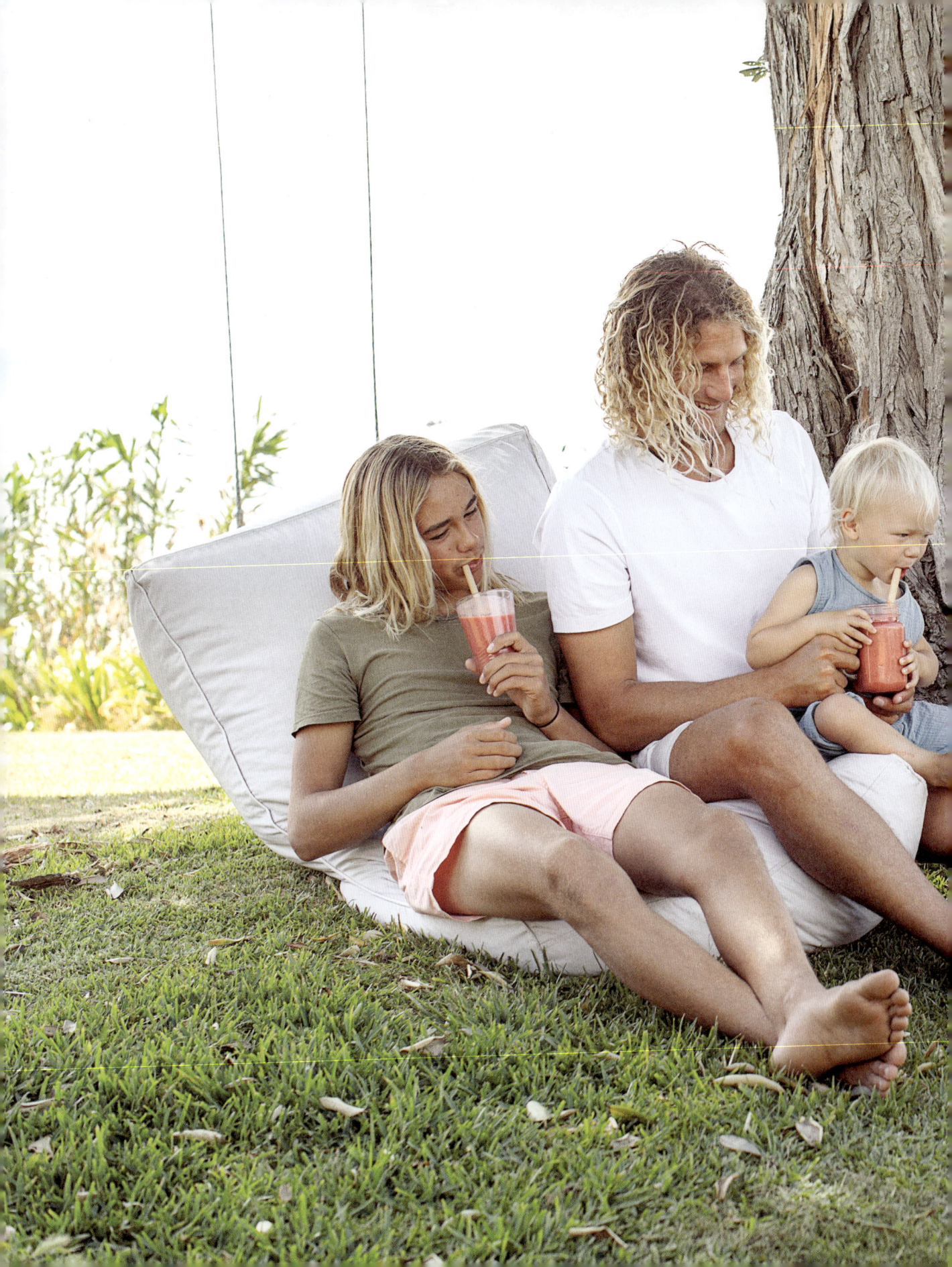

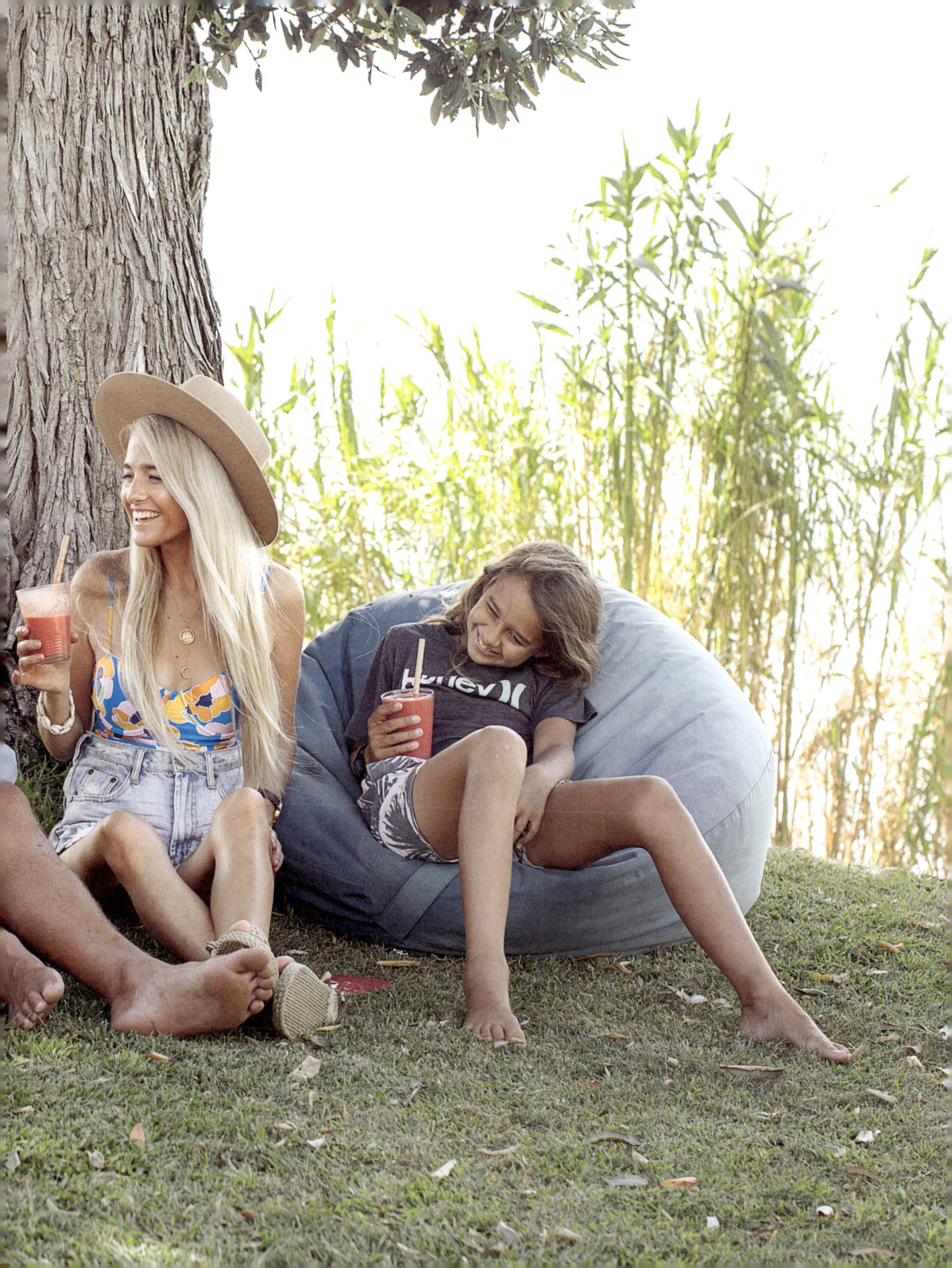

RAINBOW WRAPS AND CUCUMBER ROLLS with THAI LIME AND COCONUT DIPPING SAUCE

SERVES 3–4

Cucumber rolls (makes 10)
1 large cucumber
1 small yellow capsicum, thinly sliced lengthways
1 small red capsicum, thinly sliced lengthways
100 g (3½ oz) baby snow pea shoots, halved
1 tablespoon white sesame seeds
1 tablespoon black sesame seeds

Rainbow wraps (makes 8)
8 sheets rice paper
8–12 lettuce leaves, washed
2 cups thinly sliced red cabbage
2 carrots, julienned
large bunch coriander, trimmed
1 large avocado, stoned, quartered and thickly sliced

Thai lime and coconut dipping sauce (makes 1½ cups)
⅔ cup coconut milk (from a can)
½ cup peanut butter
2 tablespoons red Thai curry paste (vegan)
3 tablespoons coconut sugar
1 teaspoon grated fresh ginger
¼ cup lime juice
coriander leaves, to garnish

This beautiful snacking platter filled with raw vibrant veges offers heaps of flavour and nutrients. The cucumber rolls are super cute, light and fresh, and make a quick snack to whip up or are perfect as a wholesome party plate idea. I became obsessed with these rainbow wraps (rice paper rolls) when I was pregnant with Jai. They are a great way to pack in a variety of raw herbs and veges and pair so beautifully with this utterly delicious Thai dipping sauce.

For the Cucumber Rolls, use a vegetable peeler to peel the cucumber into thin strips, discarding the first few strips of skin. You should get about 10–12 before reaching the seeds. Save the rest of the cucumber for another dish.

Arrange a few slices of capsicum and a small handful of snow pea shoots on one end of a cucumber strip. Sprinkle with sesame seeds then roll firmly. Trim the ends if you want to serve the rolls standing. Repeat with the remaining cucumber strips and filling.

For the Rainbow Wraps, place one sheet of rice paper on a flat plate of warm–hot water, for 20 seconds, or until just softening. Remove and gently place on a clean, flat service. Lay the lettuce on the centre of the sheet, followed by a little cabbage, carrot, coriander and avocado. Fold in both sides, then the end closest to you and firmly continue to roll. Slice in half (optional) and place on a platter. Repeat with the remaining rice paper sheets and filling.

For the dipping sauce, place all the ingredients except the coriander garnish in a blender and blend until smooth. Pour into a serving bowl and garnish with the fresh coriander leaves. Store any leftover dip in an airtight container in the fridge for up to 5 days.

NOTE: Rice paper wraps can be tricky to get the hang of, so don't give up after your first try.

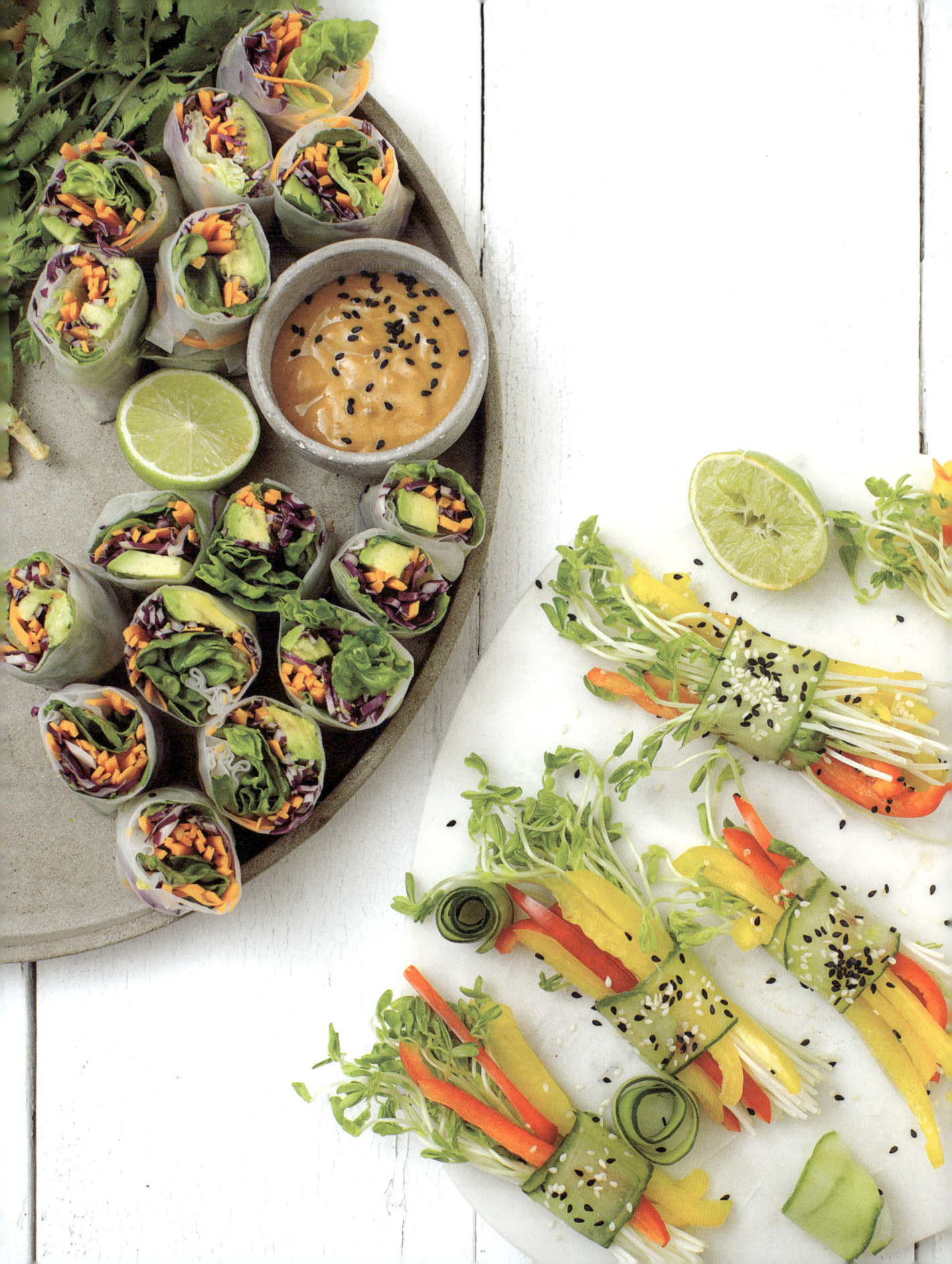

PUMPKIN, KŪMARA and CAPSICUM DIP

MAKES ABOUT 2 CUPS

250 g (9 oz) butternut pumpkin (about ¼ small butternut), peeled and cut into small cubes (2 cups)

250 g (9 oz) kūmara (1 medium), peeled and cut into small cubes

1 red capsicum, halved, trimmed and deseeded

⅓ cup hulled tahini

⅓ cup chopped parsley

1 tablespoon cumin seeds

2 cloves garlic

1 teaspoon dried thyme

1 tablespoon apple cider vinegar

1 teaspoon pure maple syrup

1 tablespoon olive oil

½ teaspoon sea salt

¼ teaspoon white pepper

¼ cup water

To serve (optional)
fresh parsley
Dukkha (see page 282)

This heavenly dip would have to be one of my favourite recipes in the entire book. I know that's a big call, but the flavours just blend so perfectly together, creating a totally moreish taste experience. It's a creamy, hearty blend and a true staple, making the perfect addition to sandwiches, burgers, salads, crackers and fresh vege sticks—or you could just eat it by the spoonful like I do.

Preheat the oven to 180°C (350°F) fan bake. Line a large baking tray with baking paper.

Place the pumpkin and kūmara on the tray and spread them out into a single layer. Bake for 25–30 minutes, until tender.

Remove the pumpkin and kūmara from the oven and place in a food processor. Add the remaining ingredients and blend for 20–30 seconds, until smooth, stopping to scrape down the sides of the blender if necessary.

To serve, place in a serving bowl and garnish with fresh parsley and a sprinkle of Dukkha, if desired.

Store in a sealed jar or container in the fridge for up to 5 days.

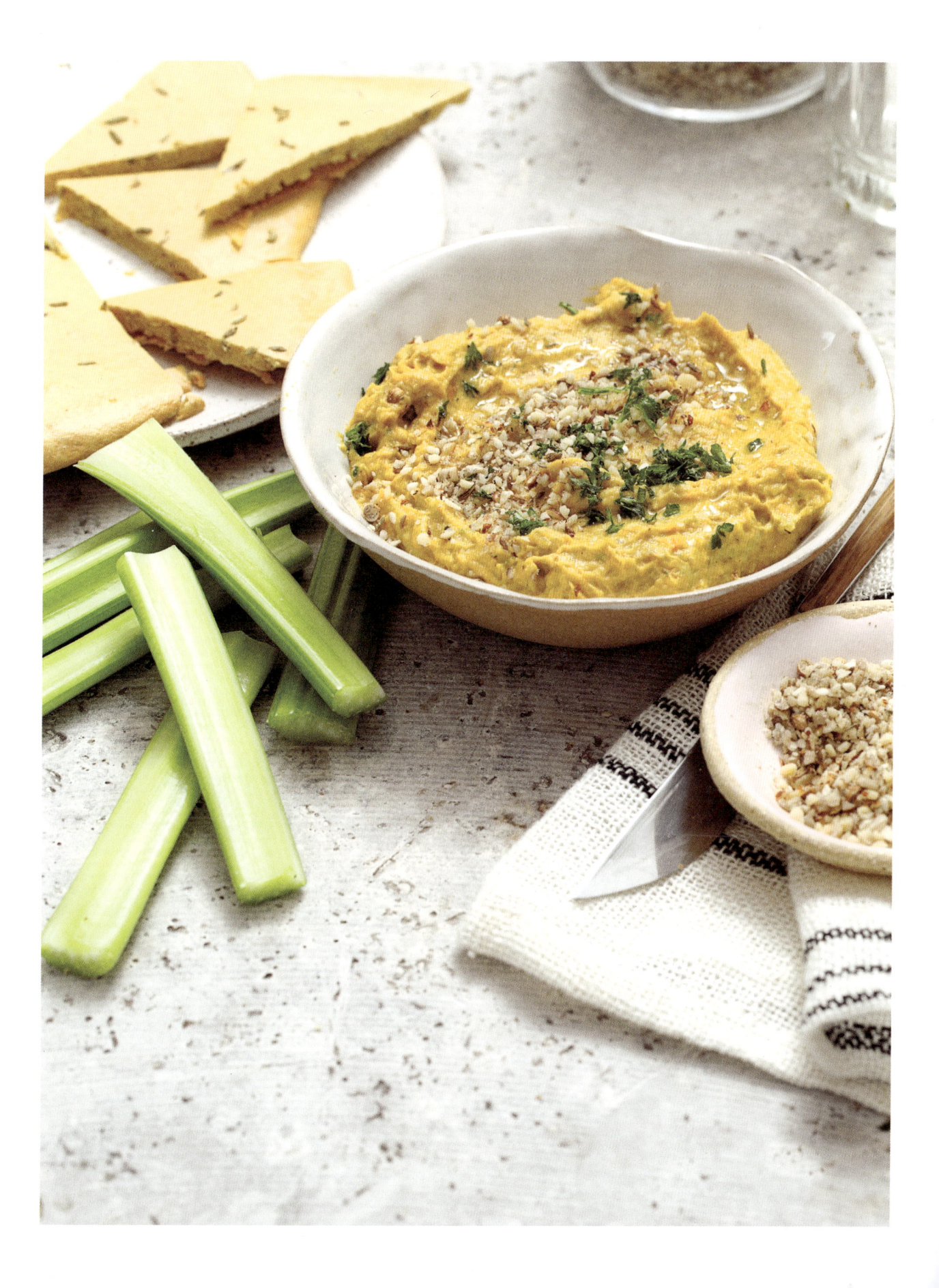

EGGPLANT, CORIANDER and BALSAMIC DIP

MAKES 1½ CUPS

1 large eggplant (500 g/ 1 lb 2 oz), halved lengthways
½ cup hulled tahini
⅓ cup chopped coriander
2 cloves garlic
¼ cup lemon juice
2 teaspoons balsamic vinegar
1½ tablespoons pure maple syrup
1 tablespoon olive oil
1 teaspoon ground cumin
½ teaspoon sea salt
¼ teaspoon chilli flakes

To serve (optional)
fresh coriander
chilli flakes or sliced fresh chilli
lemon or lime wedge

This version of baba ganoush is another totally divine dip. It has hints of tangy balsamic, cumin, chilli and coriander blended through baked eggplant flesh. I love adding this dip to roasted vegetables, Buddha bowls and salads, or try a dollop on cucumber slices to create a scrumptious snack.

Preheat the oven to 180°C (350°F) fan bake. Line a large baking tray with baking paper.

Place the eggplant halves on the tray, flesh side up. Bake for 25–30 minutes, until tender. Let cool for 5 minutes, and once cool enough to handle, gently peel off the skin.

Place the eggplant flesh in a food processor with the remaining ingredients. Blend for 20–30 seconds, until smooth, stopping to scrape down the sides of the blender if necessary.

To serve, place in a serving bowl and garnish with fresh coriander, a light sprinkle of chilli flakes or fresh chilli, and a wedge of lemon or lime, if desired.

Store in a sealed jar or container in the fridge for up to 5 days.

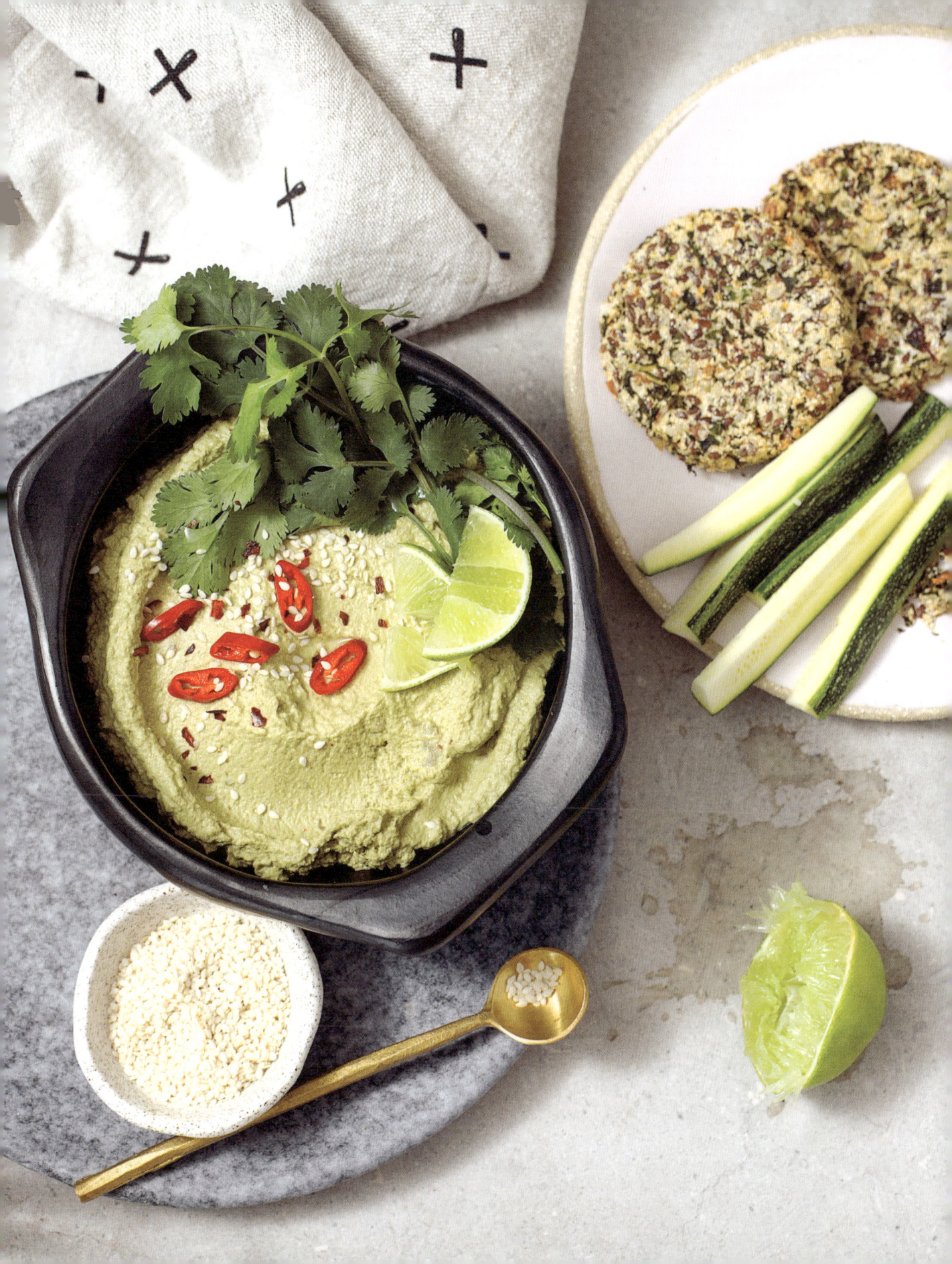

HERBY SUNFLOWER SEED HUMMUS

MAKES 2 CUPS

1 cup sunflower seeds, presoaked (see Recipe Notes page 47)
1 cup water
3 tablespoons dried Italian herbs (or fresh herbs)
1 teaspoon cumin seeds
2 cloves garlic
3 tablespoons orange juice
2 tablespoons apple cider vinegar
1 teaspoon pure maple syrup
¼ teaspoon chilli flakes
½ teaspoon sea salt

To serve
macro greens
sunflower seeds

I love this sunflower hummus, with its hints of chilli and herbs; it adds a wholesome dollop of goodness to any meal. Sunflower seeds, boasting calcium, iron, manganese and zinc, have a mild flavour and a creamy texture, making them a great substitute for cashews in dips and dressings. If you're making this for children, you might like to use less chilli flakes or omit altogether.

Place all the ingredients in a food processor. Blend for 20–30 seconds, until smooth, stopping to scrape down the sides of the blender if necessary.

Transfer to a serving bowl and scatter with the macro greens and sunflower seeds.

REVITALISING RAW BEETROOT HUMMUS

MAKES ABOUT 2 CUPS

400 g (14 oz) can chickpeas, drained and rinsed (or 1½ cups cooked chickpeas)
1 medium-large beetroot, peeled and diced
⅓ cup hulled tahini
¼ cup lemon juice
1 teaspoon ground cumin
3 tablespoons olive oil
2 cloves garlic
½ teaspoon sea salt

To serve
fresh coriander, finely chopped
black and white sesame seeds

This hummus is light, earthy, slightly sweet and vibrant. It's easy to adapt the recipe to make traditional hummus, simply by leaving the beetroot out. It's fantastic served with my Garlic Chickpea Flatbread (see page 291).

Place all the ingredients in a food processor. Blend for 20–30 seconds, until smooth, stopping to scrape down the sides of the blender if necessary.

Serve in a bowl with a sprinkle of coriander and sesame seeds.

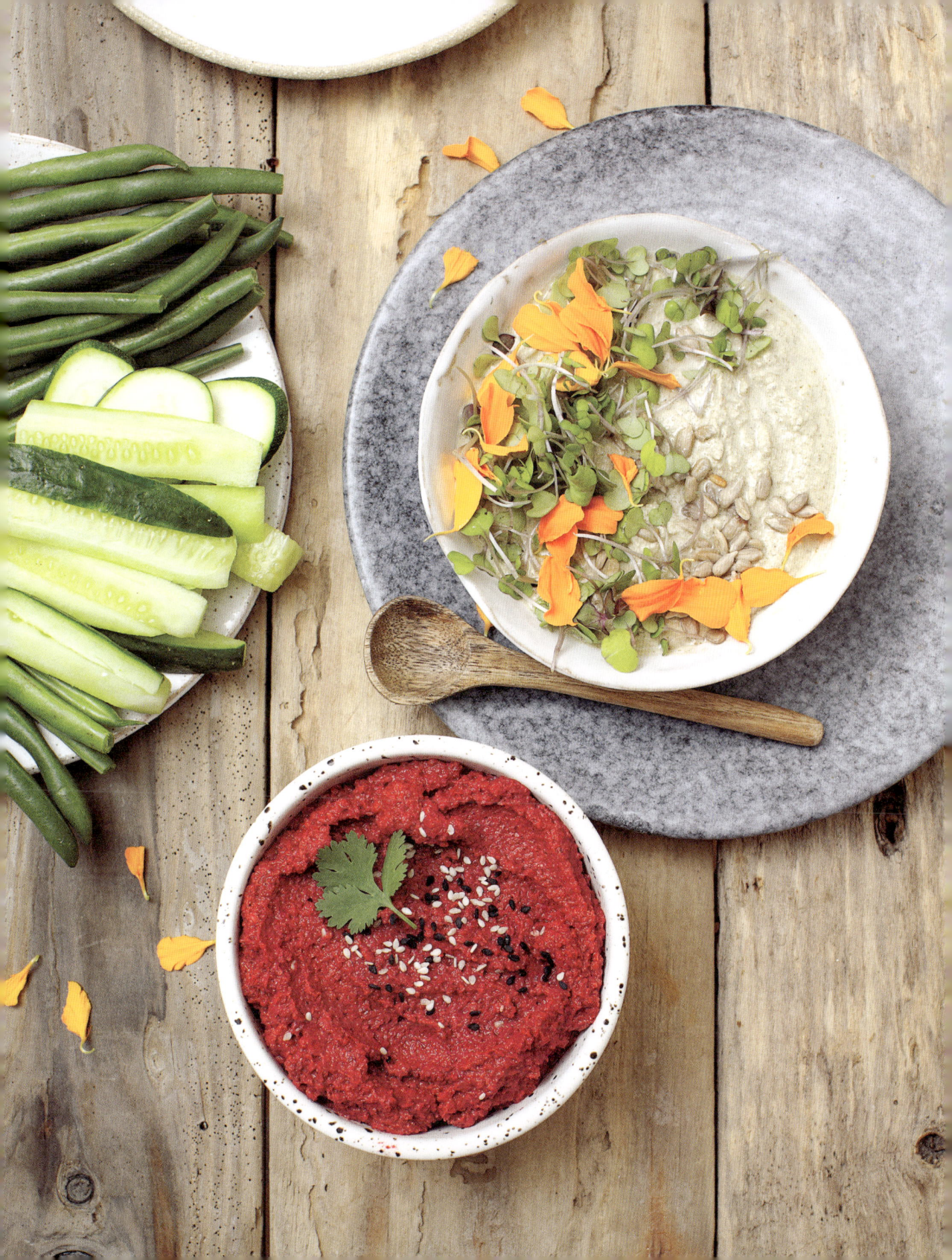

HEMP, SPINACH and BASIL PESTO

MAKES 2 CUPS

3 cups fresh basil
3 cups fresh spinach
¼ cup hempseeds
⅓ cup nutritional yeast
⅓ cup pine nuts
⅓ cup macadamias
2 cloves garlic
¼ cup lemon juice
¼ cup olive oil
¼ cup water
½ teaspoon salt (optional)

This has always been my go-to wholesome pesto. It's incredibly nutritious, packed with flavour and has become a versatile kitchen staple in my home. I use it to create many meals, including warm pastas, salads, with raw zucchini noodles, as a toast topper or sandwich filler for the boys, or as a dip for Buddha bowls and raw vege sticks. Try it in my Basil Pesto Potato Top Pie (see page 184) or Basil Pesto and Zucchini Pasta Salad (see page 146).

Place all the ingredients in a food processor and blend for 20–30 seconds, until mostly smooth.

Store in a sealed jar or container in the fridge for up to 5 days.

NOTE: To create a traditional basil pesto, simply replace the 3 cups of spinach leaves with fresh basil and omit the hempseeds.

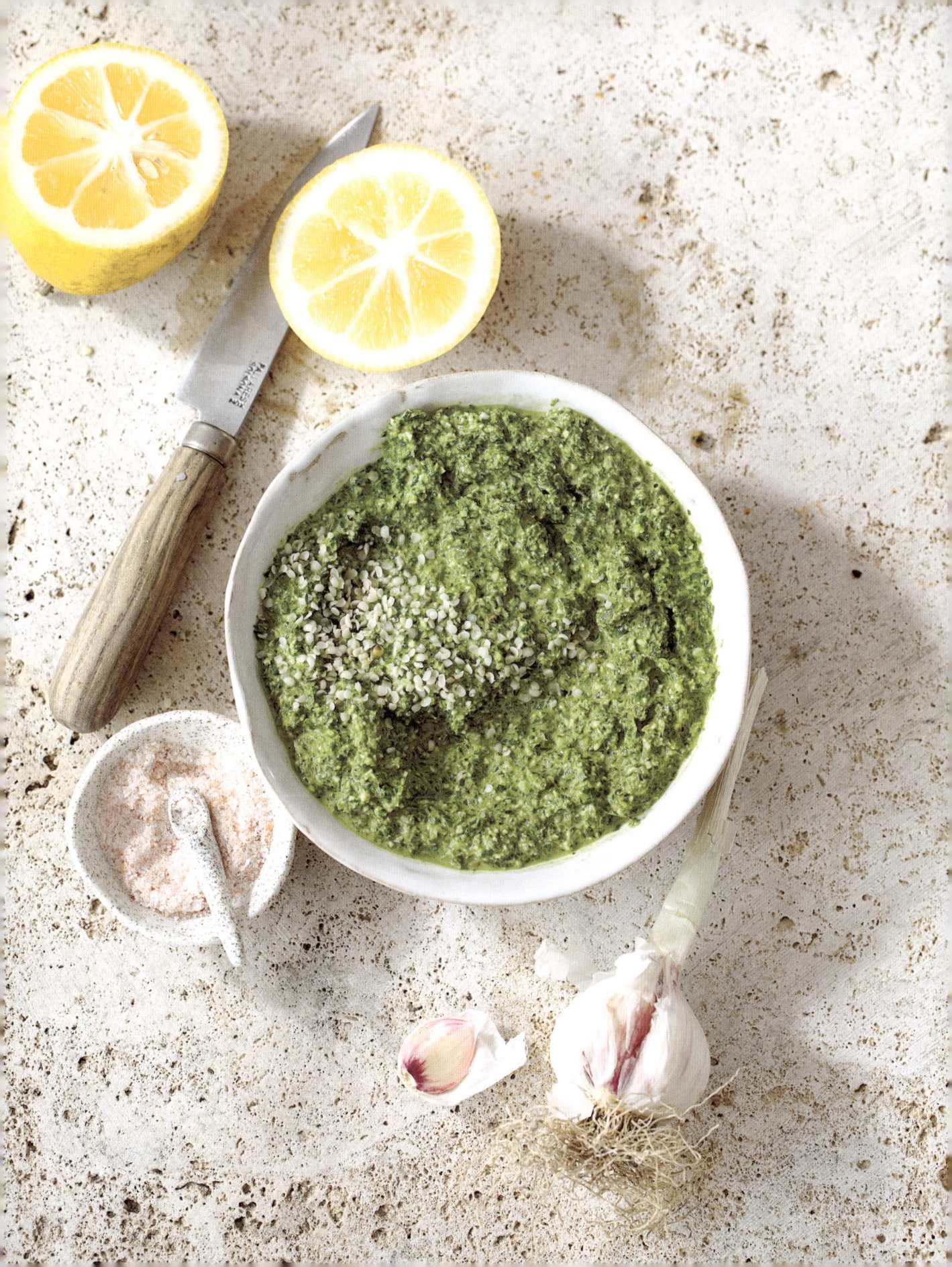

SESAME BAKED FALAFEL BITES with TZATZIKI DIP

MAKES 10 BITES

Sesame baked falafel bites
400 g (14 oz) can chickpeas, drained and rinsed (or 1½ cups cooked chickpeas)
2 cloves garlic, diced
2 spring onions, diced
2 tablespoons lemon juice
1 cup chopped fresh parsley
1 tablespoon ground cumin
1 tablespoon ground coriander
¼ red onion, diced
½ teaspoon sea salt
1 teaspoon baking powder
2½ tablespoons chickpea flour
¼ cup sesame seeds

Tzatziki dip (makes 1½ cups)
½ large cucumber
1 cup coconut yoghurt
2 cloves garlic, crushed
1 tablespoon finely chopped mint leaves
2 tablespoons finely chopped dill
2 tablespoon lemon juice
½ teaspoon sea salt
2 tablespoons finely diced cucumber

We all love a good falafel, and this winning combo definitely hits the spot. Falafel balls are a fantastic addition to salads, wraps, sandwiches and lunch boxes, as well as making a beautiful snack with various dips and dressings. Tzatziki is an incredibly refreshing Greek dip; the combination of fresh dill, mint and cucumber with zesty lemon, garlic and creamy coconut yoghurt will seriously make you want to eat it by the spoonful.

Preheat the oven to 180°C (350°F) fan bake. Line a baking tray with baking paper.

For the falafel bites, place all the ingredients except the sesame seeds in a food processor and blend for about 10 seconds, or until the mixture is mostly smooth with a few small chunks remaining.

Sprinkle the sesame seeds onto a large plate. Use your hands to roll 2 tablespoons of the mixture into a ball, then roll through the sesame seeds to lightly coat. Place on the prepared baking tray and repeat with the remaining mixture.

Bake for 25–30 minutes, until golden.

For the Tzatziki Dip, finely grate the cucumber and squeeze out as much liquid as you can. Place it in a small bowl with the yoghurt, garlic, mint, dill, lemon juice and salt. Mix to combine all the ingredients.

To serve, place the tzatziki in a small serving bowl, top with the diced cucumber and serve with the falafel bites.

Store any leftover dip in an airtight container in the fridge for up to 5 days. Store the falafel bites in the fridge for up to 4–5 days, or freeze for up to 1 month.

NOTE: This recipe can easily be doubled to make extra falafels.

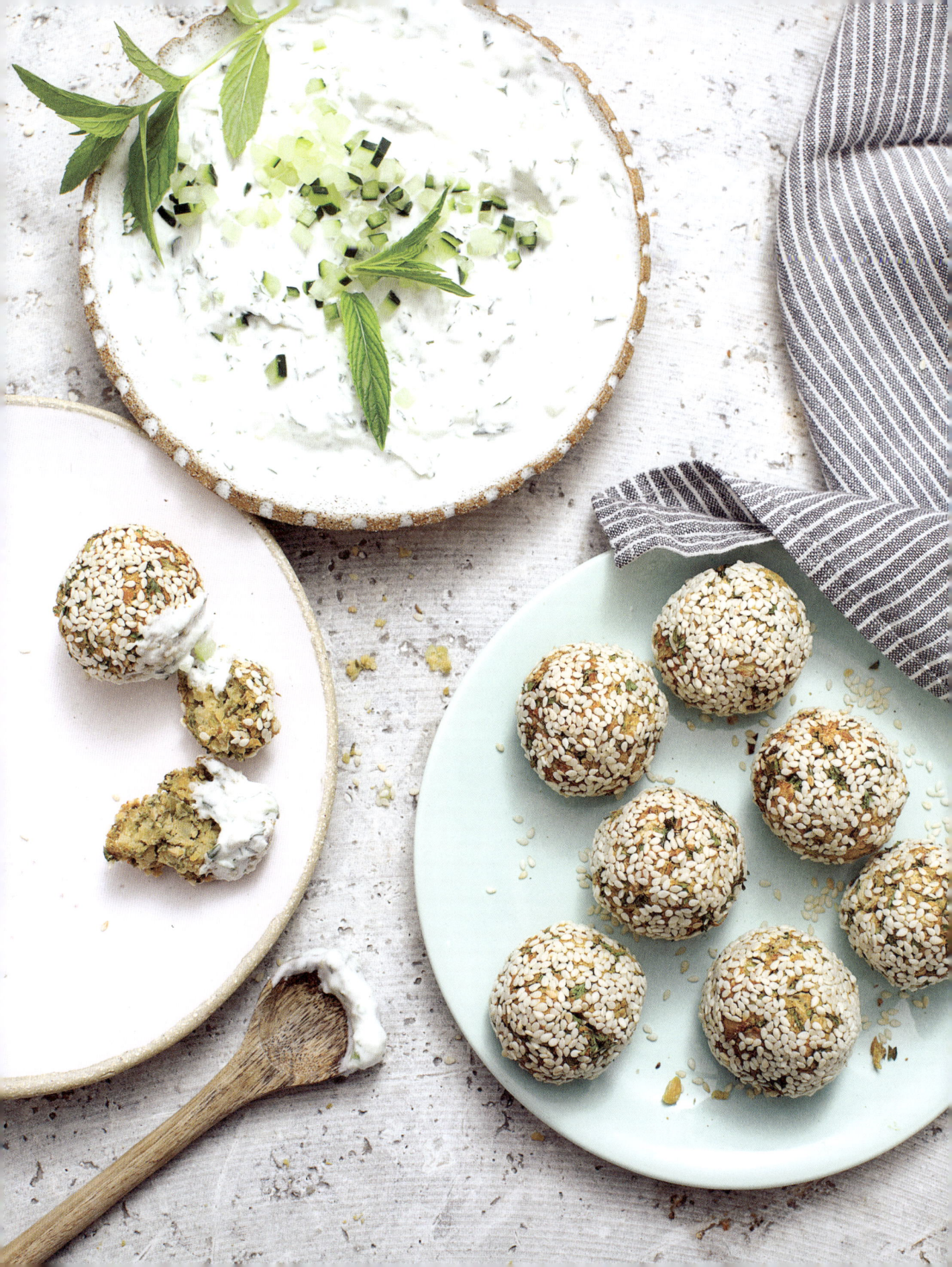

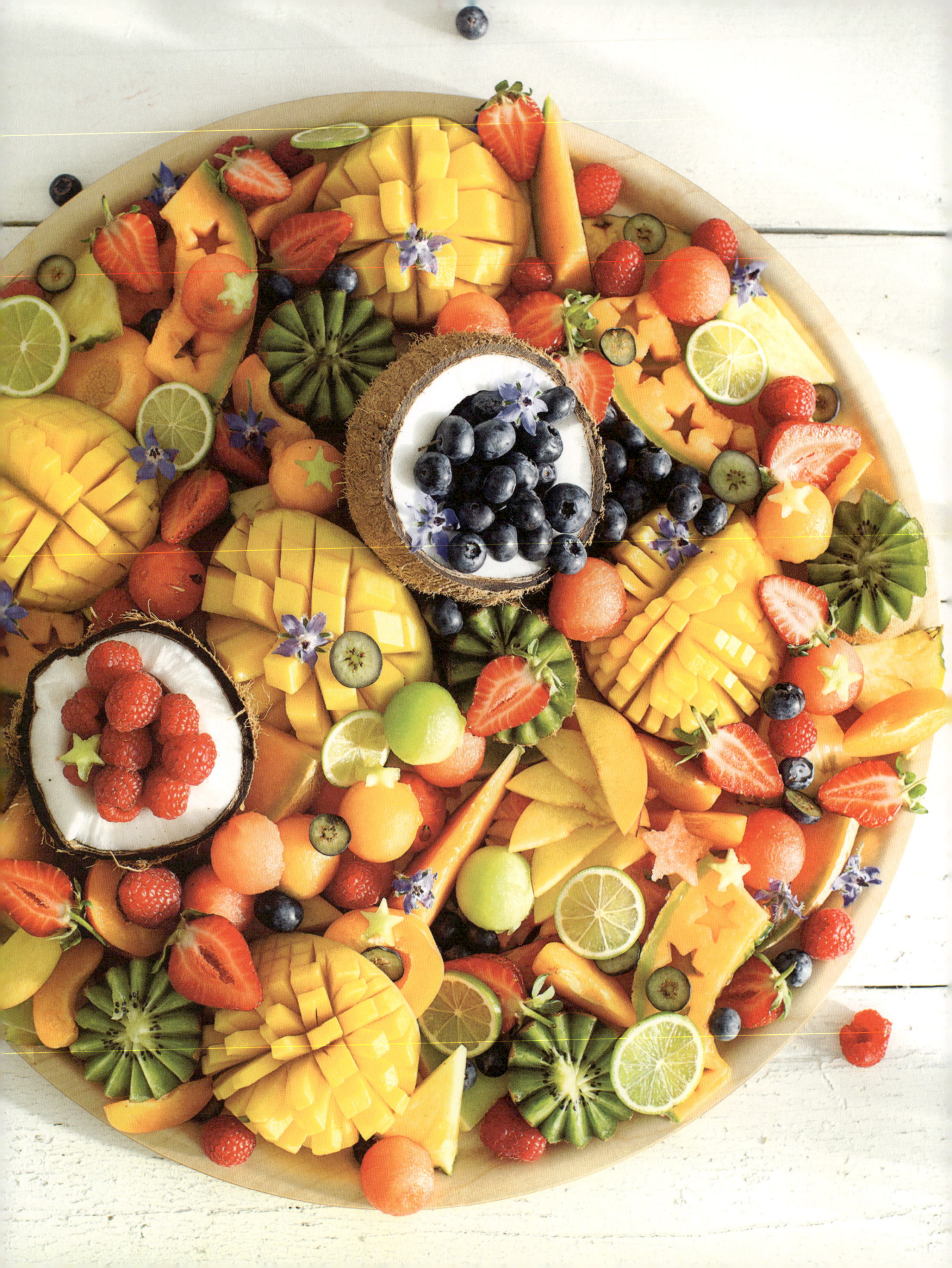

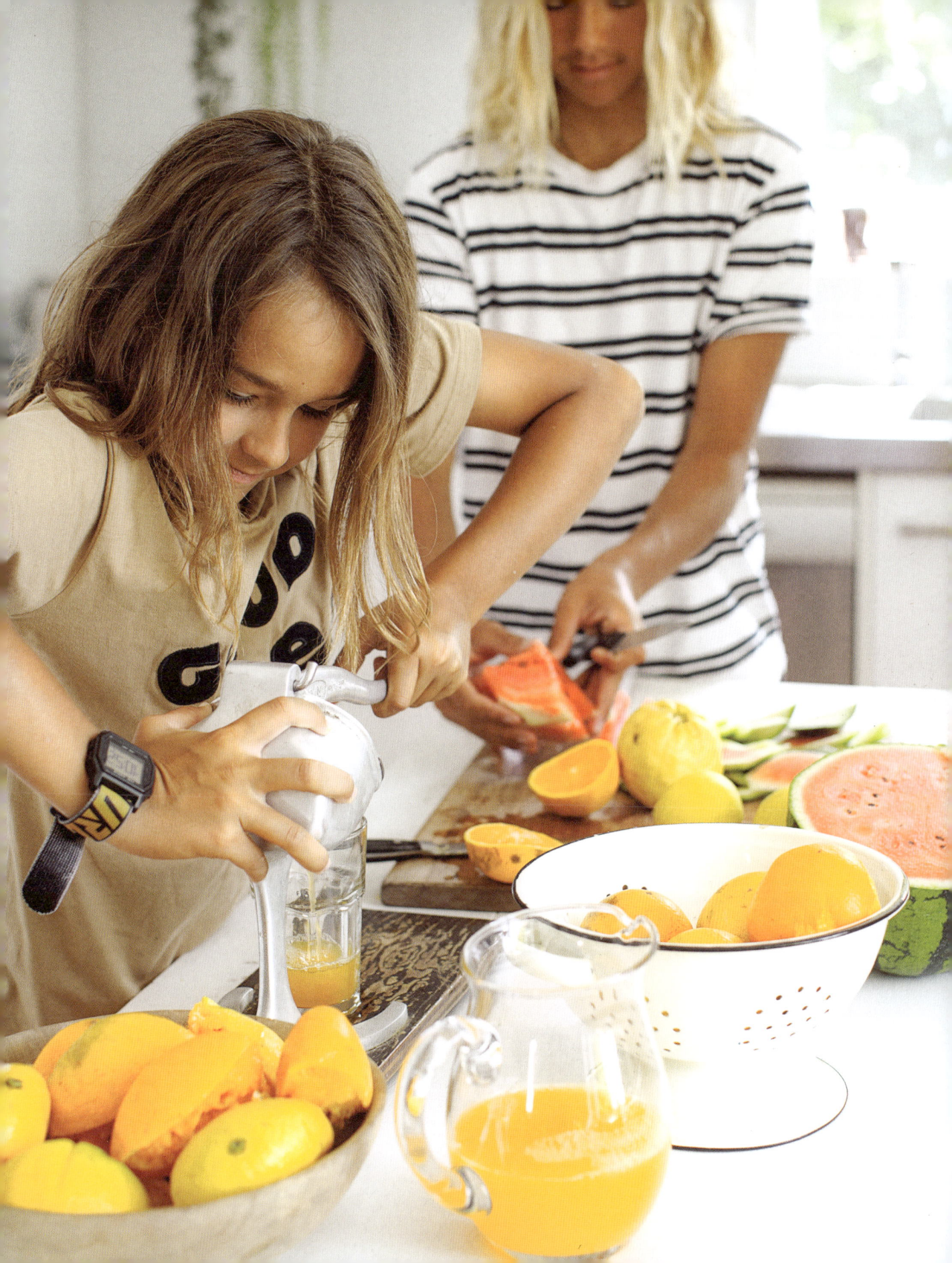

LIME, HERB and CHILLI CASHEWS

MAKES 2 CUPS

2 cups raw cashews
1 teaspoon olive oil
1½ tablespoons dried oregano
1 tablespoon garlic powder
1½ tablespoons coconut sugar
2 teaspoons lime zest
½ teaspoon sea salt
⅛ teaspoon cayenne pepper
2 tablespoons lime juice
1 tablespoon apple cider vinegar
3 tablespoons buckwheat flour

I'm a little obsessed with these chewy, crunchy, lime-infused cashews. And I'm not the only one—whenever I make a batch, they never seem to last very long. They are baked to perfection in a lightly coated batter, with slightly sweet, chilli, herby, garlicky and zesty flavours, and make the most delish snack or crunchy salad topper.

Preheat the oven to 180°C (350°F) fan bake. Line a baking tray with baking paper.

Place the cashews, oil, oregano, garlic powder, coconut sugar, lime zest, sea salt and cayenne pepper in a bowl and mix together.

In a separate small bowl, mix the lime juice, apple cider vinegar and buckwheat flour together until it forms a paste.

Add the paste to the cashews and mix everything together until all of the cashews are coated in the paste.

Tip the cashews onto the prepared baking tray and spread out into a single layer. Bake for 8–10 minutes, tossing halfway through, until golden brown. Watch closely for the last few minutes as they will burn quickly. Let cool for 5 minutes before serving.

Store in a sealed jar for up to 7 days.

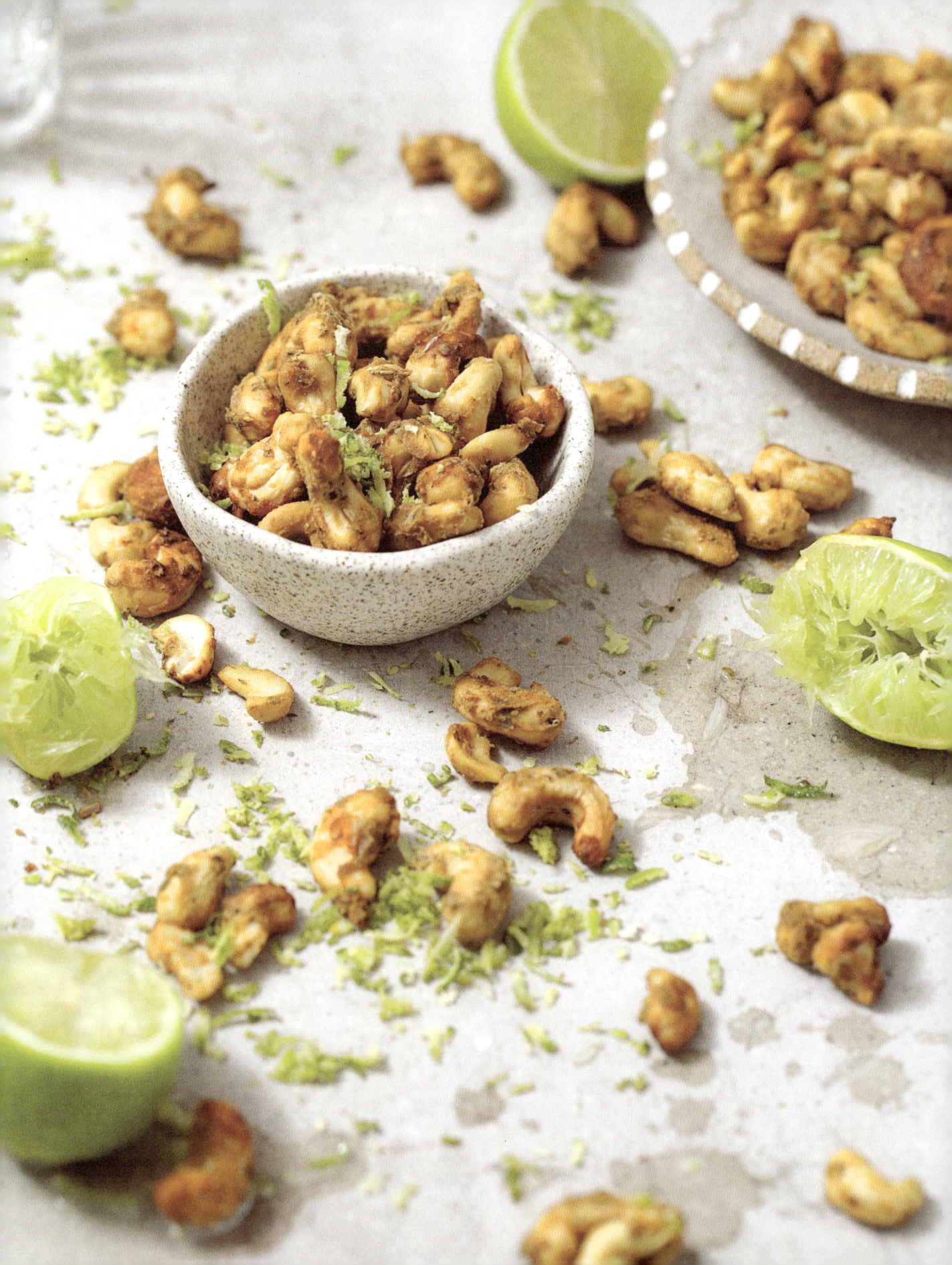

ITALIAN HERB CRACKER ROUNDS

MAKES 18 CRACKERS

1½ cups ground golden flaxseed (linseed)
1 cup water
1 bunch kale, stems removed (about 250 g/9 oz)
1 cup raw almonds
1 cup coconut flour or almond flour
½ cup oil-free sun-dried tomatoes, finely diced
2 tablespoons Italian dried herbs
⅓ cup nutritional yeast
sea salt to taste

These hearty protein-packed crackers are super-handy to have in the pantry as a wholesome snack. They're nutrient-dense with a cheesy, herby flavour, and are baked on a lower temp for a longer period of time so that they dehydrate. I absolutely love this tasty recipe, and often enjoy these crackers with a dollop of hummus.

Preheat the oven to 120°C (250°F). Line a large baking tray with baking paper.

Place the ground flaxseed and water in a bowl and mix to combine. Leave to sit for 10 minutes to allow the mixture to thicken.

Meanwhile, place the kale in a food processor and pulse for about 3 seconds, until finely chopped. Transfer to a large bowl. Add the almonds to the processor and blitz for about 3 seconds, until broken into small pieces. If you don't have a food processor, finely chop the kale and almonds. Add the almonds to the kale along with the flaxseed mixture and all the other ingredients.

Mix to combine into a thick dough. Using your hands, knead into a ball. The mixture should be quite moist, but if too sticky then add a sprinkle of flour. If too dry, add a splash more water.

Line a clean surface with a large sheet of baking paper. Roll out the dough to about 7 mm (¼ in) thickness. Use a small, round cookie cutter (or glass) to cut into circles. Gently peel off and place on the prepared baking tray. Gather up the excess dough, knead again, then repeat the rolling and cutting to get about 18 crackers in total.

Bake for 75–80 minutes, or until lightly golden and crunchy around the edges. Let cool for 10 minutes and enjoy with your favourite toppings.

Store in an airtight container for 5–7 days.

NOTE: It is important to use finely ground flaxseeds (linseeds) to ensure this recipe binds well.

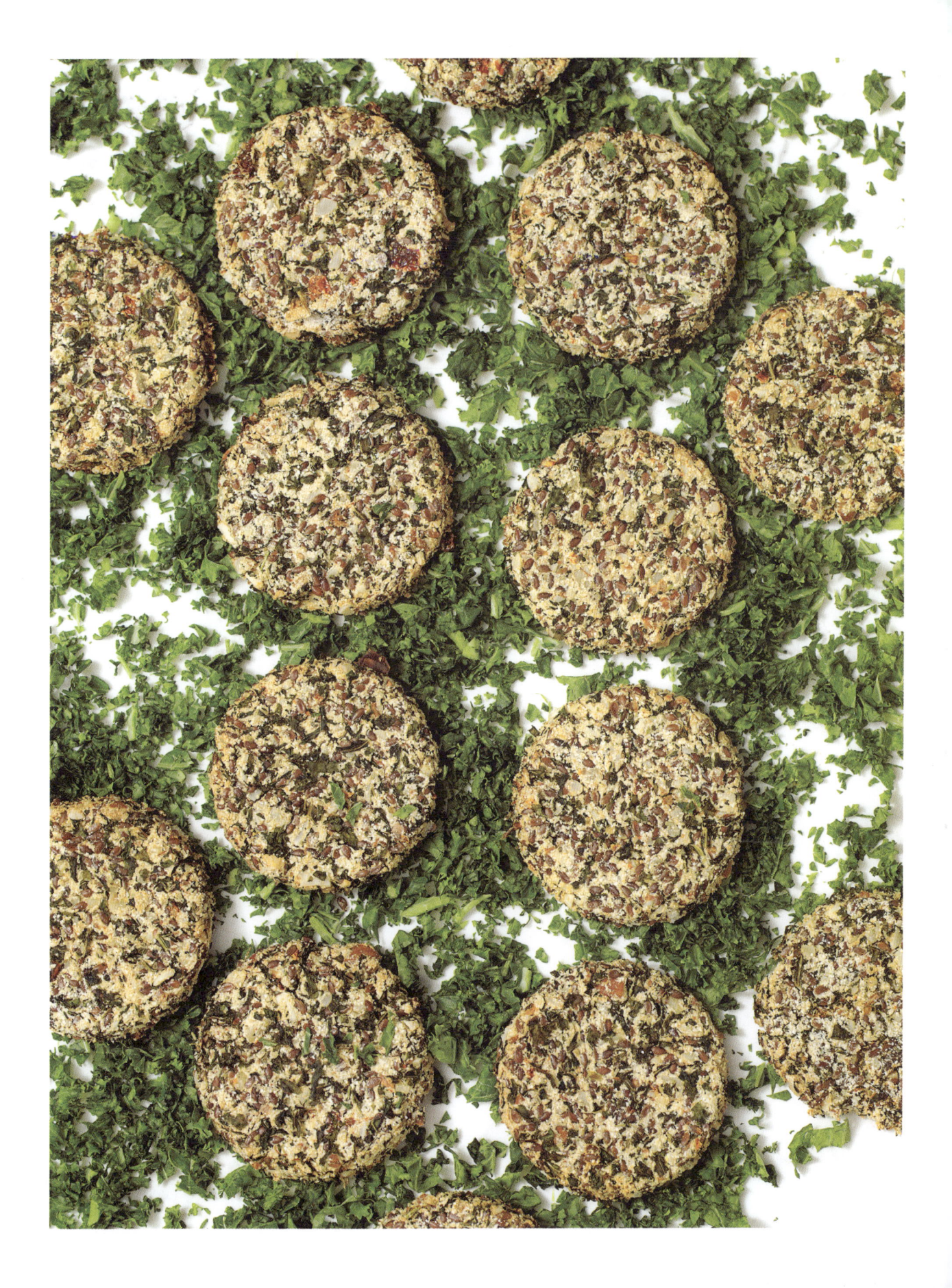

SUPERFOOD GRANOLA BARS

MAKES 12 BARS

1½ packed cups medjool dates (approx. 14–16 large dates), pitted
1 cup gluten-free rolled oats
1 cup roasted, unsalted almonds
2 tablespoons chia seeds
2 tablespoons hempseeds
1 tablespoon cacao nibs
¼ cup goji berries
¼ cup pure maple syrup
¼ cup almond butter

These gorgeous granola bars make for a perfectly healthy, balanced and super-tasty snack. The roasted almonds are a perfect match with the chewy goji berries and sweet medjool dates, creating an energising bite for any time of the day. I love that they require no baking. Medjool dates are a staple in our home; they're highly alkalising and are a fantastic natural sweetener, or perfect used as a base for bliss balls, snack bars, raw treats and in salads.

Line a 20 cm (8 in) square baking dish with baking paper.

Place the dates in a food processor and blend for 30 seconds, until smooth and the dates begin to form a large ball.

Transfer the dates to a large bowl and add the rolled oats, almonds, chia seeds, hempseeds, cacao nibs and goji berries. Mix together using a wooden spoon.

Place the maple syrup and almond butter in a saucepan over medium-high heat. Stir until the almond butter is completely melted and heated through.

Pour the maple syrup mixture into the date mixture and mix to combine.

Transfer the mixture to the prepared dish and spread out evenly. Using the back of a spoon, press down firmly over the mixture. Place in the freezer to set for 30 minutes.

Remove and slice into 12 bars.

Store in an airtight container in the fridge for up to 2 weeks.

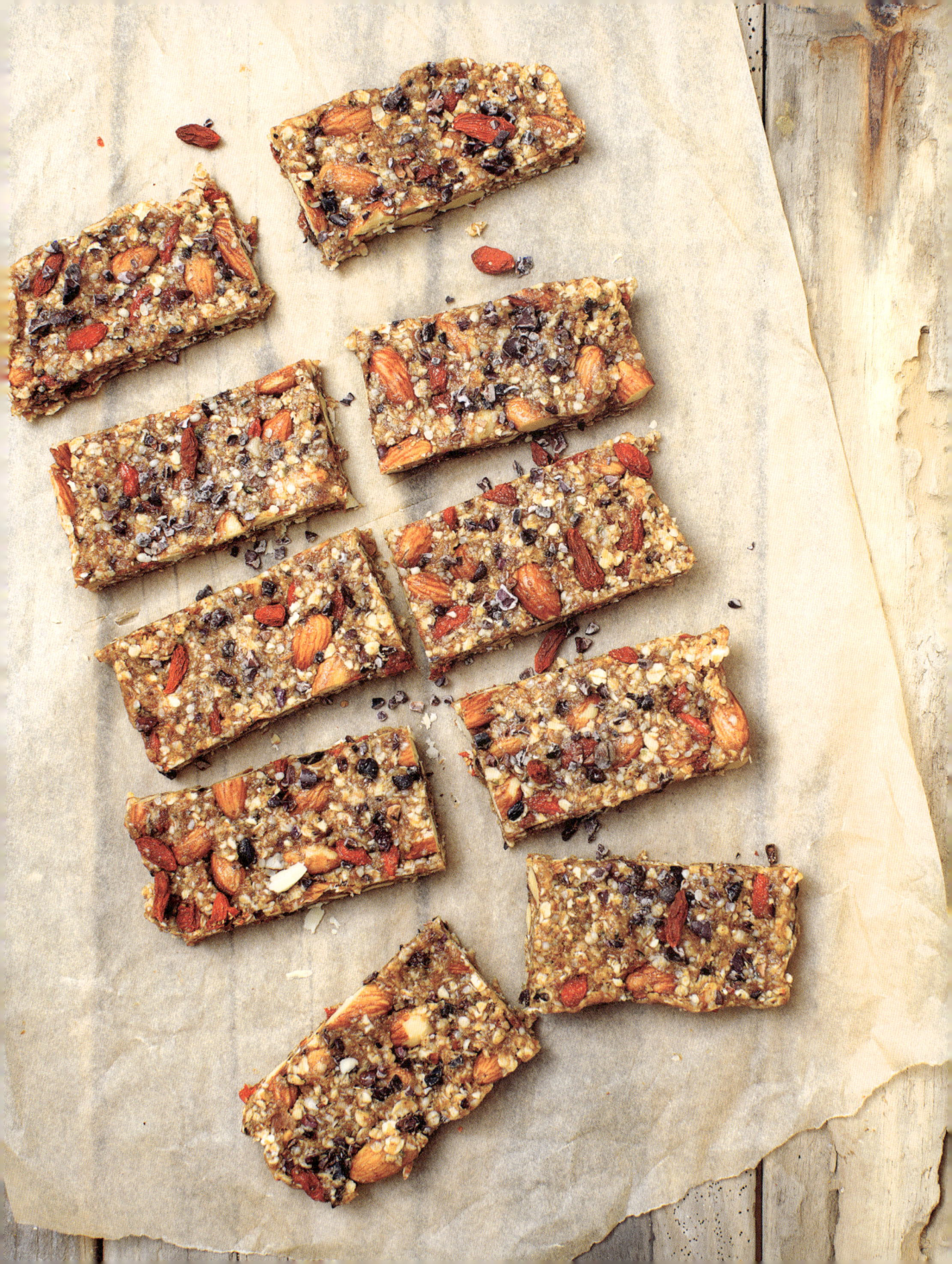

CHOC COCONUT QUINOA PUFF SNACK SQUARES

MAKES 12

1½ packed cups medjool dates (approx. 14–16 large dates), pitted
½ cup coconut milk (from a can)
½ cup desiccated coconut
¼ cup cacao powder
2 cups quinoa puffs

These epic chocolate treats are a nutritious take on the traditional rice puff bars, and the beauty of them is that they only require five ingredients. They're naturally sweetened by medjool dates with the perfect balance of cacao and coconut, combined with crunchy protein-packed quinoa puffs to create a blissful square of goodness.

Line a small square baking dish with baking paper.

Place the dates and coconut milk in a food processor and blend for about 30 seconds, until smooth. Add the desiccated coconut and cacao powder and blend for an additional 10 seconds, until fully combined.

Transfer to a large bowl and add the quinoa puffs. Mix to combine all the ingredients.

Transfer the mixture to the prepared dish and spread out evenly. Using the back of a spoon, press down firmly over the mixture. Place in the freezer to set for 30 minutes.

Remove and slice into 12 squares.

Store in an airtight container in the fridge for up to 1 week.

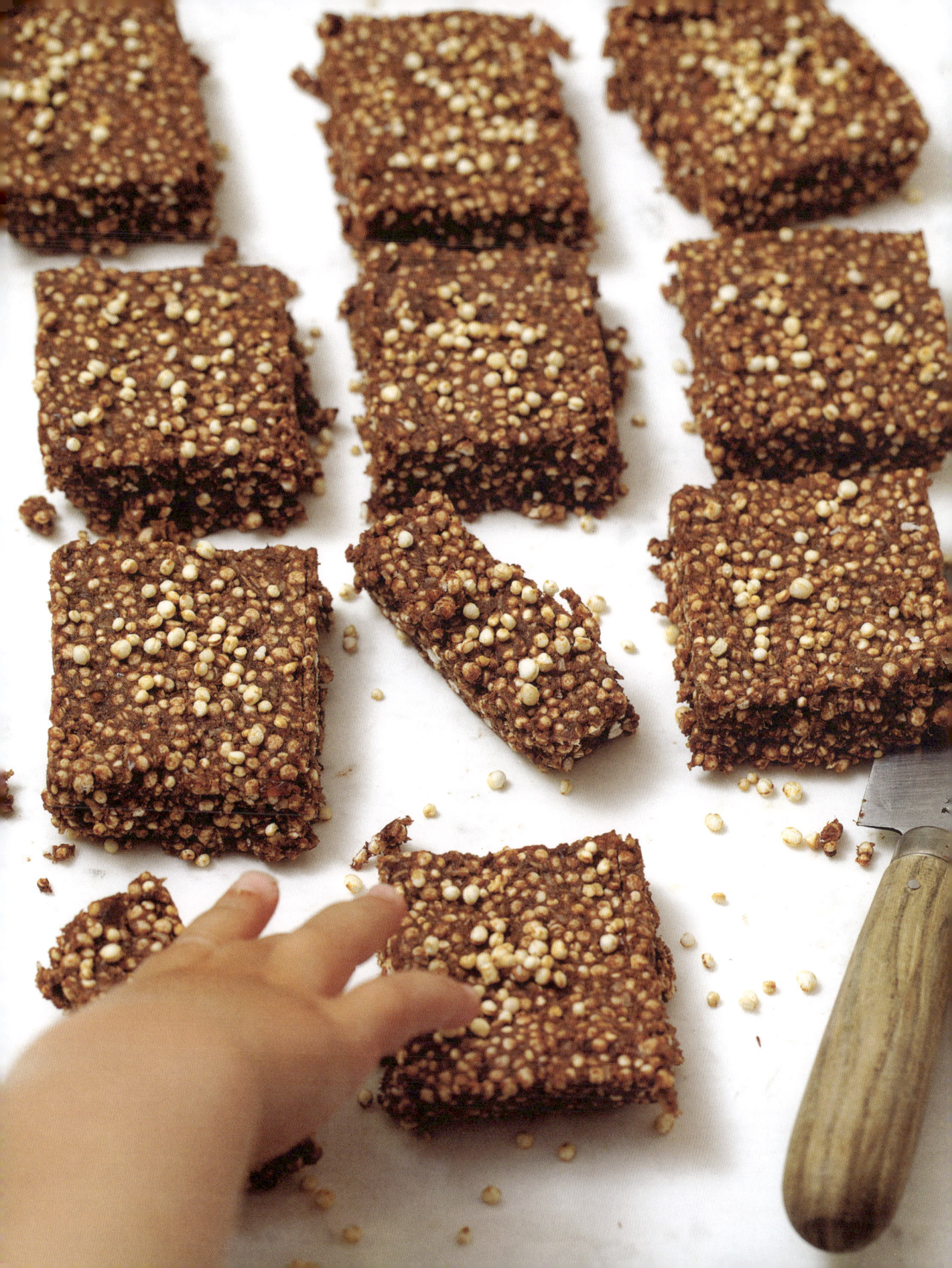

RAW BANANA BREAD BLISS BALLS

MAKES 10–12 BALLS

These simply delish balls taste just like banana bread. You can adapt the recipe and serve it as raw granola—simply skip the rolling step and store the crumbly mixture in an airtight jar.

1 cup dried dates
1 cup gluten-free oats (or almond meal)
2 medium ripe, spotty bananas, mashed
1 cup desiccated coconut
¼ cup coconut flour
1 teaspoon pure vanilla extract
1 teaspoon ground cinnamon

To coat
¼ cup desiccated coconut (optional)

MACADAMIA SALTED CARAMEL BLISS BALLS

MAKES 8–10 BALLS

These divine salted caramel balls have been a long-time family favourite; they're truly moreish.

1 cup dried dates
1 cup raw macadamias
½ cup melted coconut oil
½ cup pure maple syrup
¼ cup desiccated coconut
2 tablespoons tahini
2 teaspoons pure vanilla extract
½ teaspoon sea salt

To coat
¼ cup desiccated coconut, sesame seeds or crushed peanuts

LEMON AND POPPYSEED BLISS BALLS

MAKES 10–12 BALLS

Lemon and poppyseed is a popular combo used in many baked goods, and for good reason. These gorgeous bites have the most beautifully sweet and zesty flavours, making them one of my personal favourites.

1½ packed cups dried dates
1 cup raw cashews
1 cup almond meal
1 cup desiccated coconut
2 tablespoons poppyseeds
2 tablespoons lemon juice
1 tablespoon lemon zest
1 teaspoon pure vanilla extract (or paste)

To coat
¼ cup desiccated coconut

PEANUT, RAISIN AND CACAO BLISS BALLS

MAKES 10–12 BALLS

An energy-boosting fruit 'n' nut ball with a sweet and crunchy, slightly chocolatey vibe and only taking 2 seconds to whip up—simply blend, roll and eat.

1 cup medjool dates, pitted
1 cup raisins
1 cup desiccated coconut
1 tablespoon cacao powder
½ cup pumpkin seeds
½ cup raw crushed peanuts

METHOD OVERLEAF »

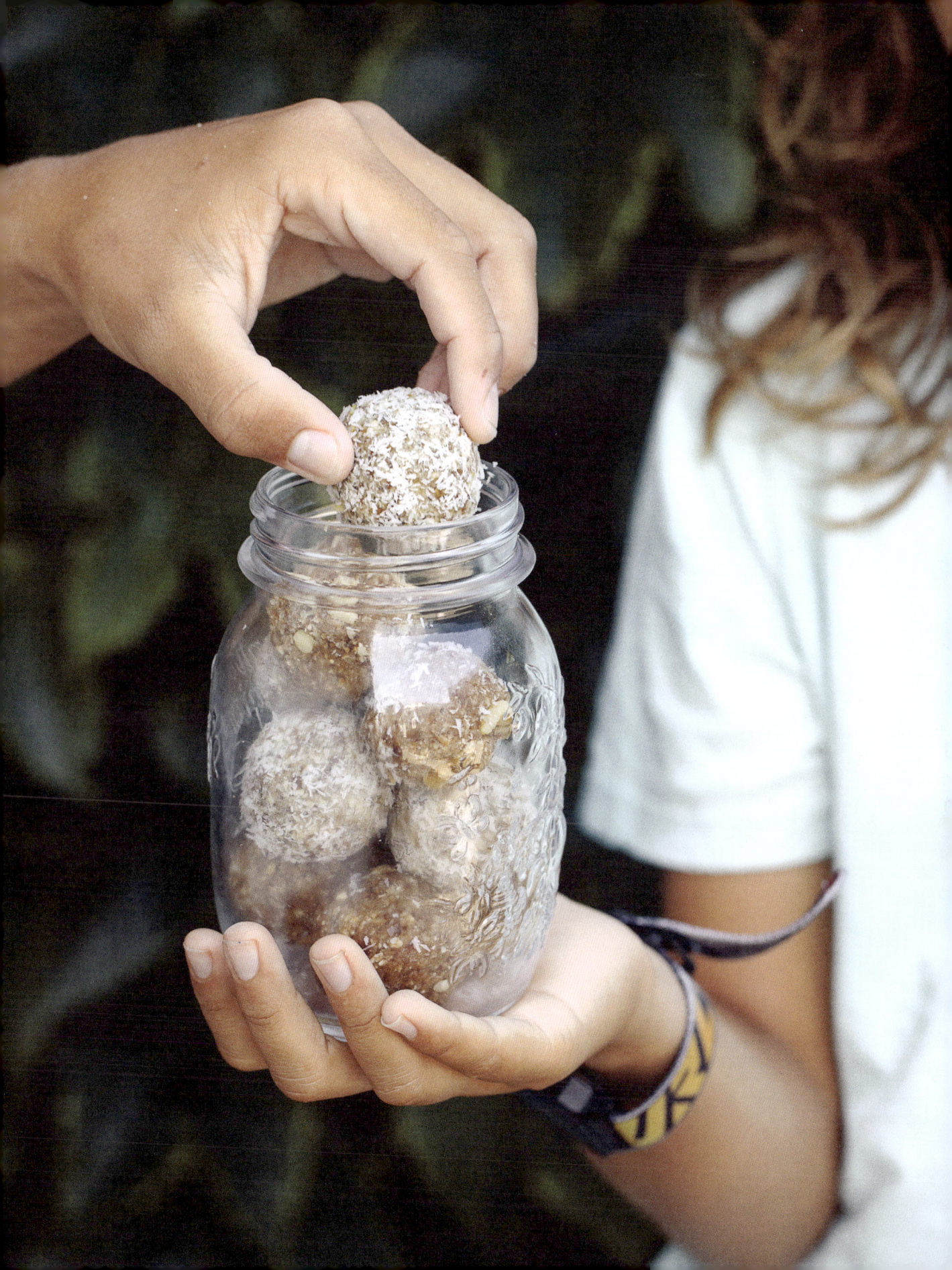

To make the bliss balls

Place the dates in a bowl and cover with warm-hot water (you will not need to soak medjool dates). Soak for 15 minutes, until they have softened. Drain and squeeze out any excess water.

Place all the ingredients, including the soaked dates, in a food processor. Blend for about 30 seconds, until smooth. You may need to stop the blender and scrape down the sides, then blend again.

For the macadamia salted caramel balls only, transfer to a bowl and place in the freezer for 30 minutes to set, or until firm enough to roll into balls.

Roll the bliss ball mixture into 10–12 balls.

Sprinkle the coating (coconut, sesame seeds or peanuts) onto a clean surface. Roll the bliss balls (except the peanut, raisin and cacao balls) through the coatings.

Store in an airtight container in the fridge for up to 2 weeks or in the freezer for up to 3 months—the Macadamia Salted Caramel Balls are best stored in the freezer.

NOTE: It's easy to get creative and experiment with bliss balls. Use equal amounts of dates and coconut as the base, then simply add in any other nuts, seeds, dried fruit and spices to create your own favourite combinations.

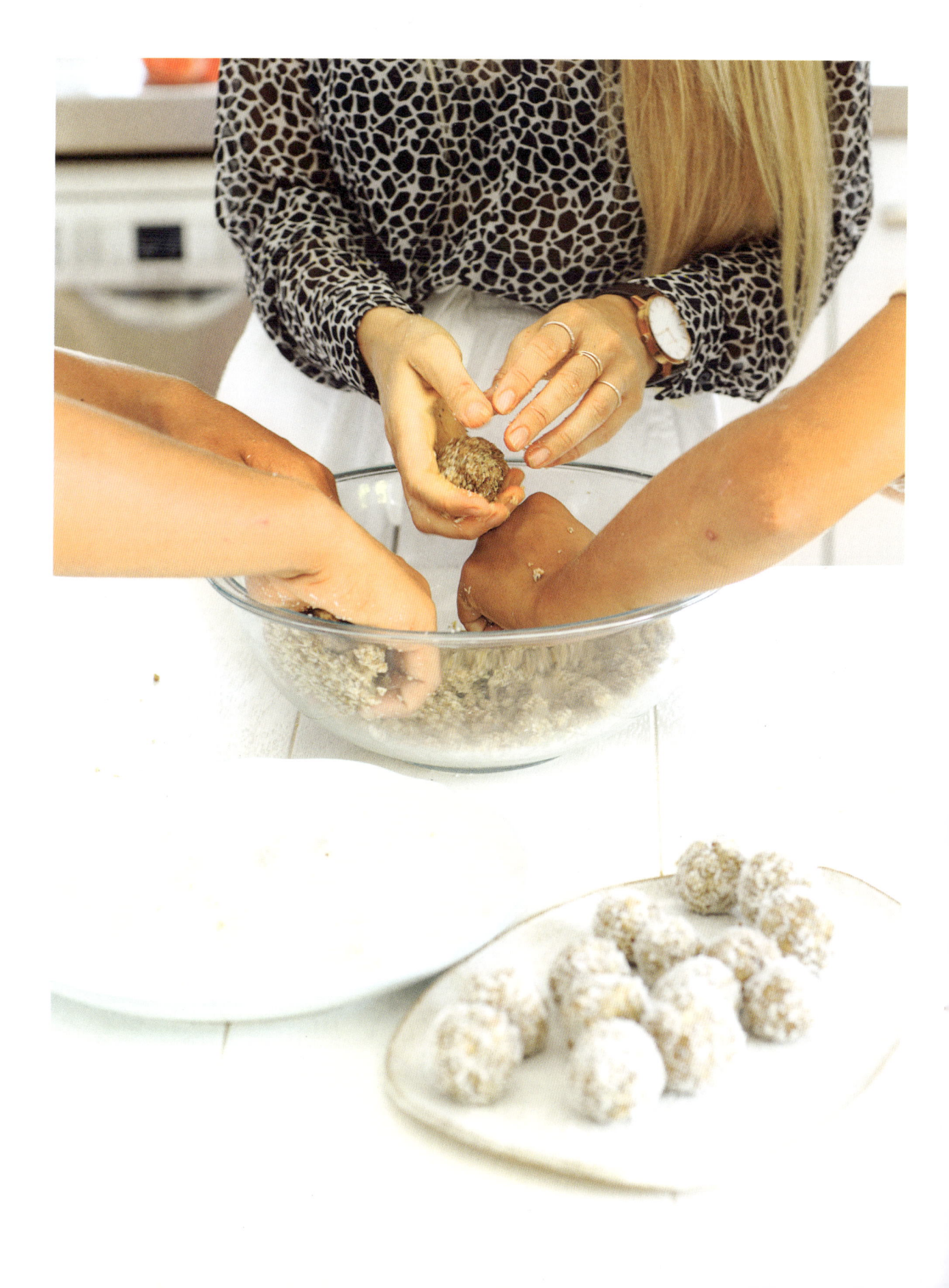

EASY TROPICANA COOKIES

MAKES 10 COOKIES

- ¾ cup fresh diced pineapple
- 1¾ cups gluten-free oats (or quinoa flakes)
- ½ cup raw cashews, roughly chopped
- ¼ cup orange juice
- 2 tablespoons orange zest
- ½ teaspoon ground cinnamon
- ½ cup shredded coconut
- ¼ cup pure maple syrup

These yummy tropical cookies are as easy as it gets—simply mix together and bake. They are inspired by a similar version we all fell in love with while in Europe and which happens to be one of Eli's favourites. The combination of pineapple, orange and coconut provides a sweet, tropical vibe and, with a hint of cinnamon, it makes these cookies a scrumptious snack that are also perfect as a lunch-box snack.

Preheat the oven to 180°C (350°F) fan bake. Line a baking tray with baking paper.

Place all of the ingredients in a bowl and mix to combine.

Roll the mixture into 10 balls and arrange on the prepared baking tray. Press down on each cookie with the back of a fork. Bake for 25–30 minutes, until golden. Remove and let cool for 5 minutes before serving.

Store in an airtight container for 3–5 days.

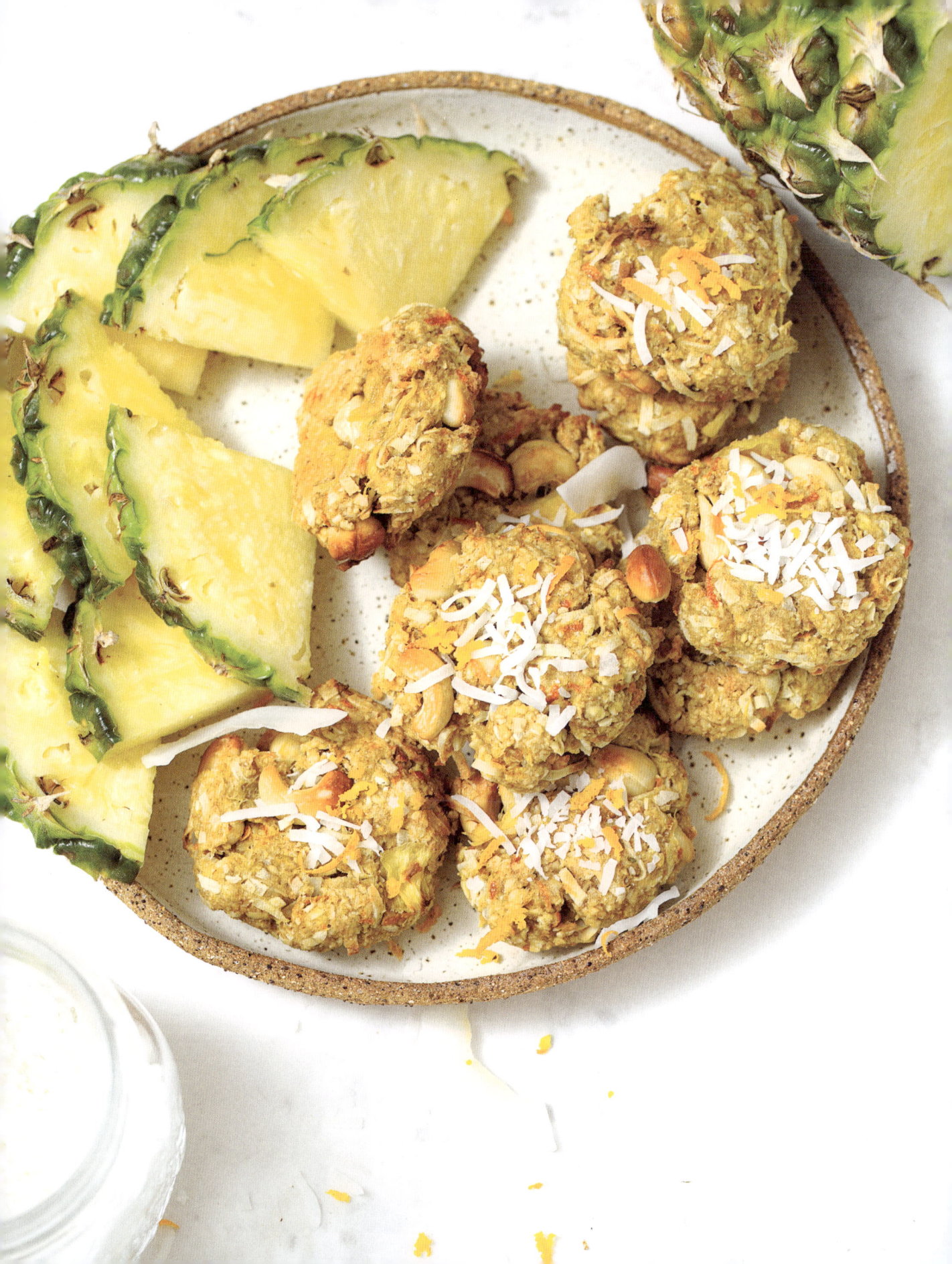

REFRESHING FRUITY SLUSHIES

There's nothing better than an icy cold, refreshing drink to cool you down on a hot summer's day. These healthy fruit-based slushies are our go-to after a long day at the beach; they're an awesome beverage to offer the boys and their mates when they come in from a surf. The flavour possibilities are endless, but these two are definitely our favourites.

PINEAPPLE, ORANGE AND PASSION FRUIT SLUSHIE

SERVES 2

2 cups diced frozen pineapple
1 orange, peeled
¼ cup passion fruit pulp
1 cup coconut water or water
1 tablespoon pure maple syrup
½ cup ice

This sweet tropical flavour would have to be one of my favourites; it will take you straight to the tropics while completely quenching your thirst.

Place all the ingredients in a blender and blend for about 10 seconds, until it resembles an icy slushie. Serve immediately.

RASPBERRY LEMONADE SLUSHIE

SERVES 2

2 cups frozen raspberries
¼ cup lemon juice
2 tablespoons pure maple syrup
1½ cups coconut water or water
½ cup ice

The classic raspberry lemonade is always a hit; it's naturally sweet from the raspberries with a refreshing zesty kick.

Place all the ingredients in a blender and blend for about 10 seconds, until it resembles an icy slushie. Serve immediately.

NOTE: These recipes also make great fruity ice blocks so pour any leftovers into ice block moulds and freeze.

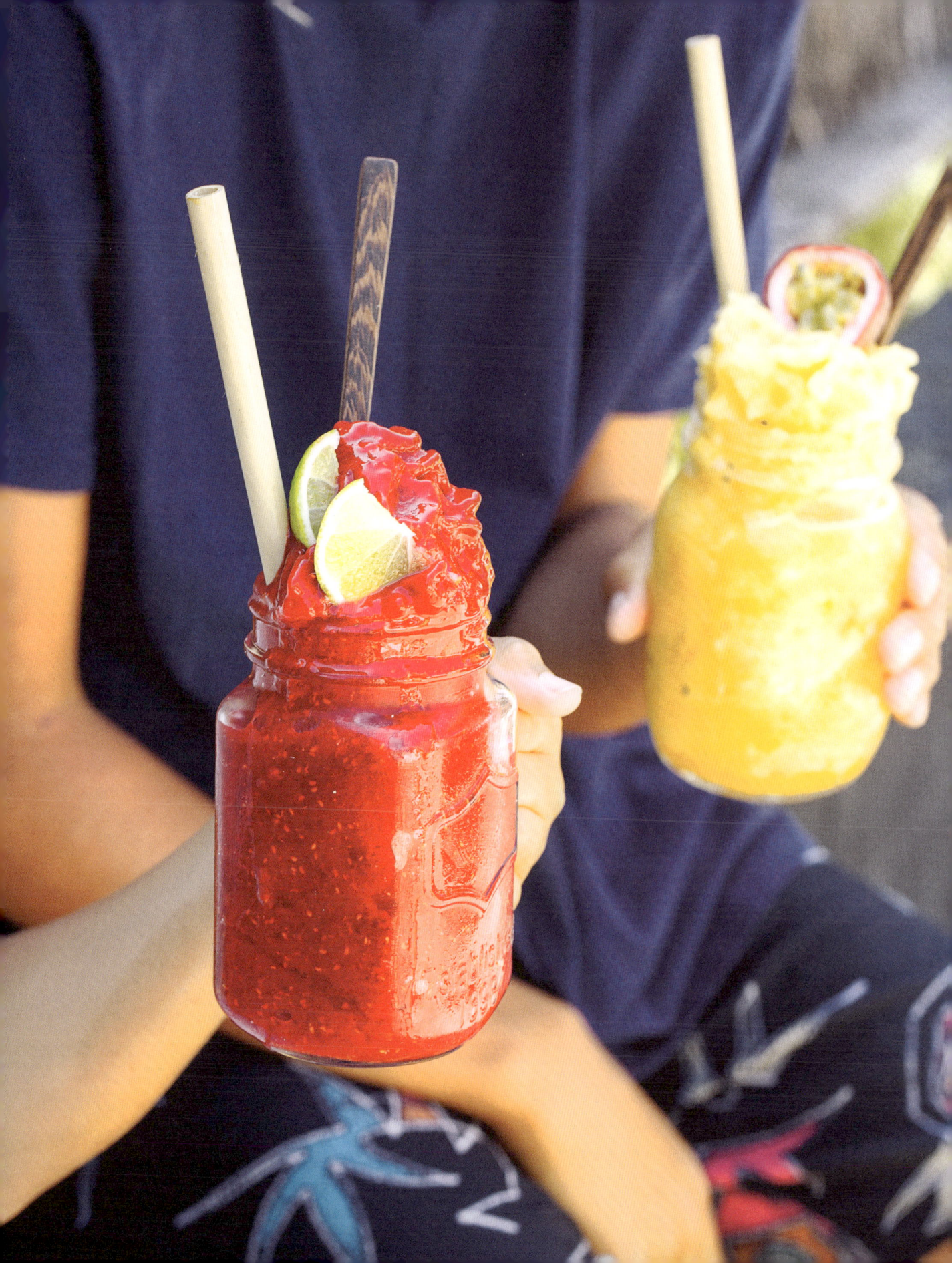

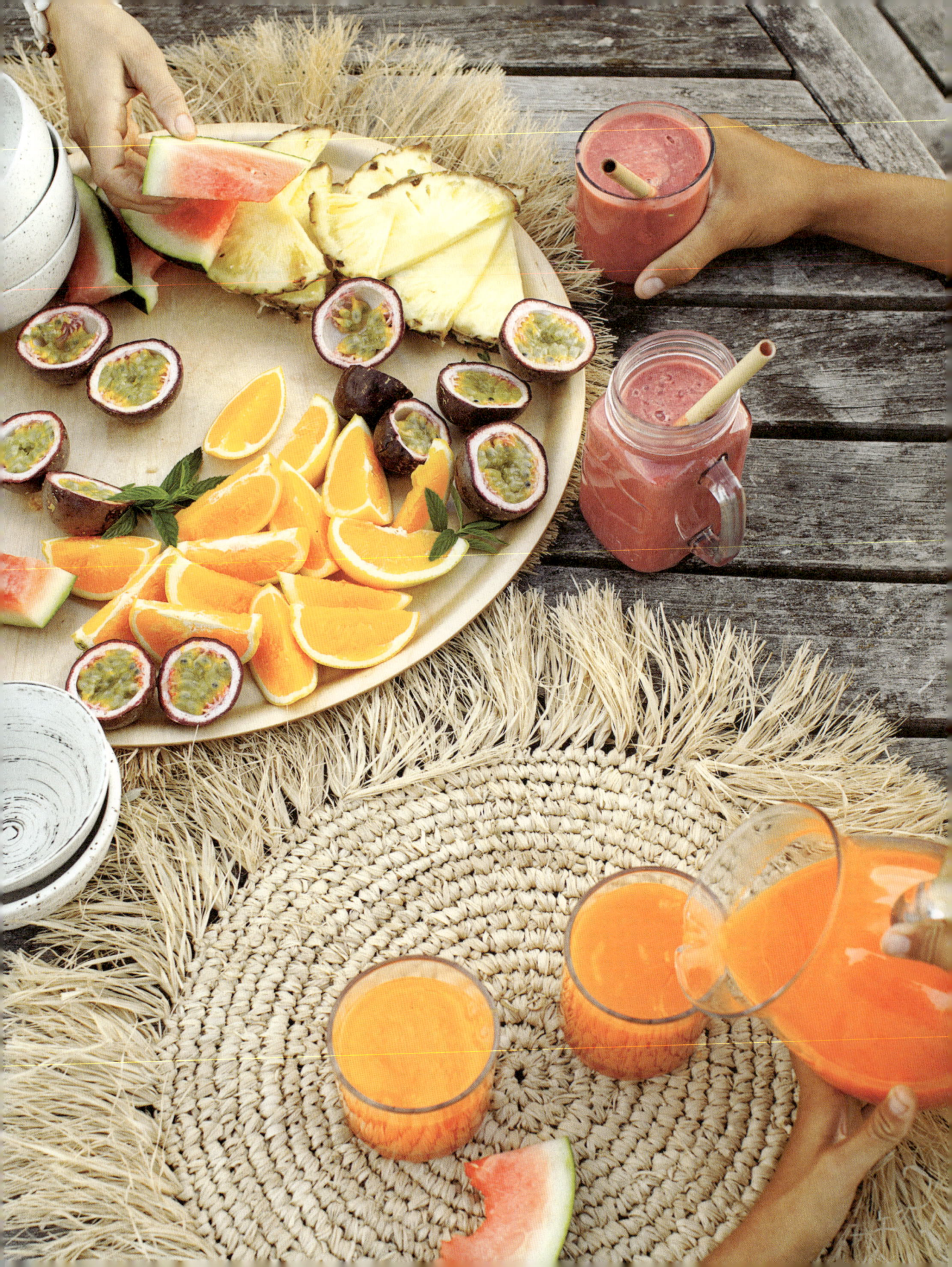

Raw Treats

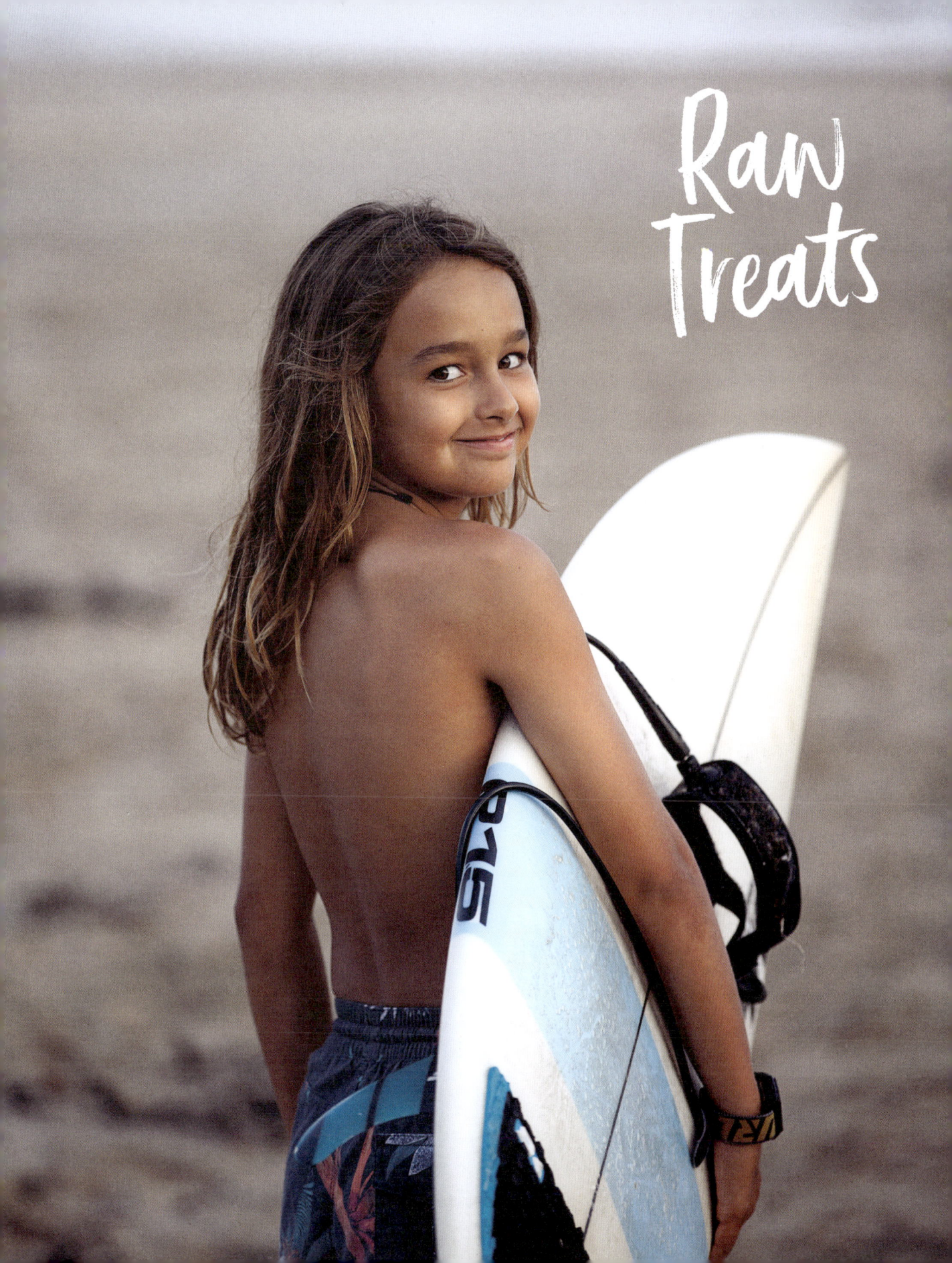

Raw Treats

Of course a piece of fruit is Nature's most nutritious candy, but we all love an indulgent treat from time to time. These fabulous recipes will fulfil your cravings while providing you with a handful of wonderful dessert ideas. Although these treats still contain unrefined sugars, overall they are more wholesome than traditional desserts as they use many more nutritious ingredients, such as nuts, seeds, coconut and dried and fresh fruit. To avoid softening or melting, they will need to be stored in either the fridge or the freezer. I store most of mine in the freezer—the beauty of this is that they last for longer and make the perfect welcoming treat for any unexpected guests.

Indulge a little and enjoy.

QUICK TIPS FOR RAW TREATS

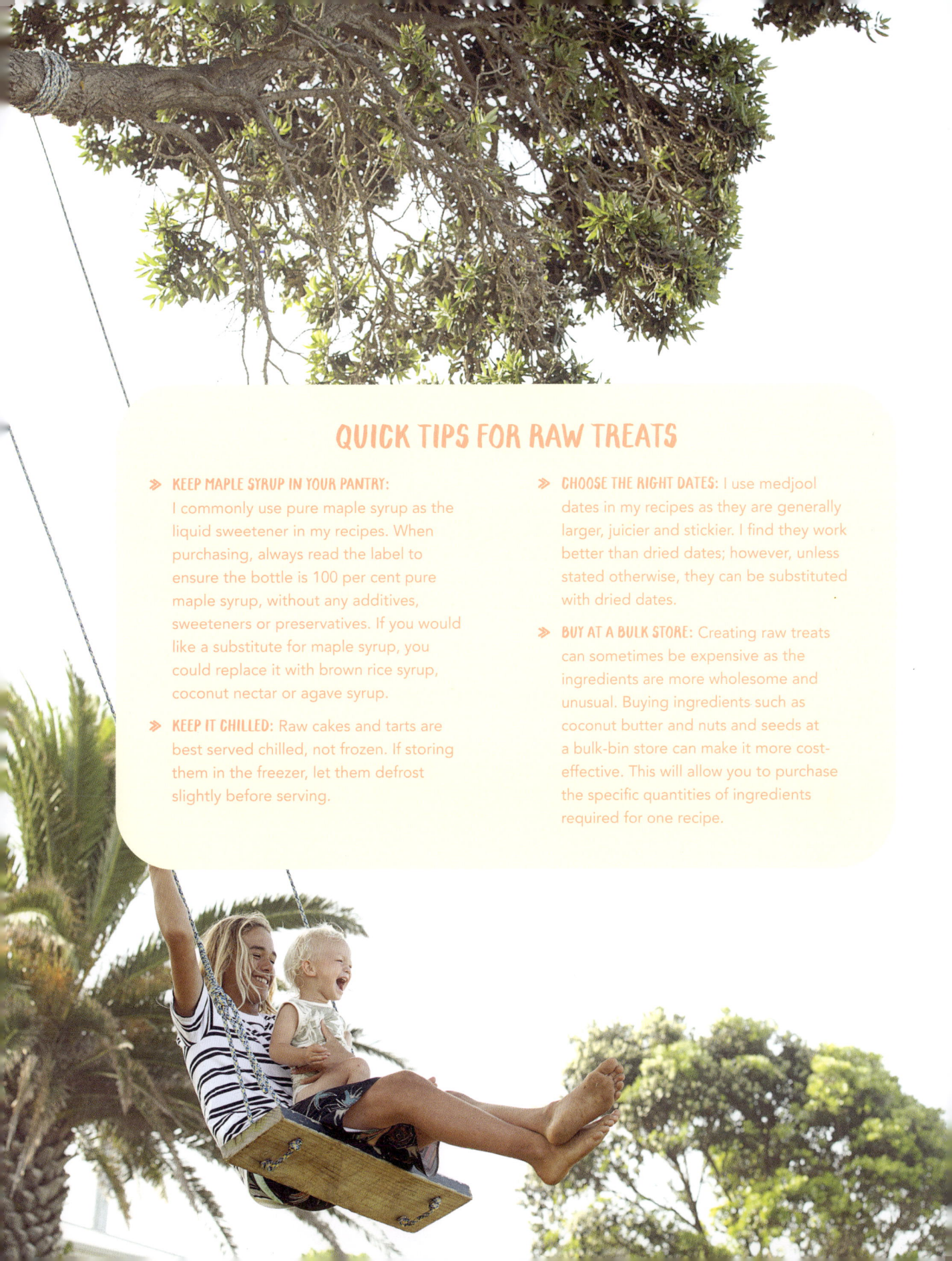

» **KEEP MAPLE SYRUP IN YOUR PANTRY:** I commonly use pure maple syrup as the liquid sweetener in my recipes. When purchasing, always read the label to ensure the bottle is 100 per cent pure maple syrup, without any additives, sweeteners or preservatives. If you would like a substitute for maple syrup, you could replace it with brown rice syrup, coconut nectar or agave syrup.

» **KEEP IT CHILLED:** Raw cakes and tarts are best served chilled, not frozen. If storing them in the freezer, let them defrost slightly before serving.

» **CHOOSE THE RIGHT DATES:** I use medjool dates in my recipes as they are generally larger, juicier and stickier. I find they work better than dried dates; however, unless stated otherwise, they can be substituted with dried dates.

» **BUY AT A BULK STORE:** Creating raw treats can sometimes be expensive as the ingredients are more wholesome and unusual. Buying ingredients such as coconut butter and nuts and seeds at a bulk-bin store can make it more cost-effective. This will allow you to purchase the specific quantities of ingredients required for one recipe.

RAW WHOLESOME CARROT CAKE with LEMON FROSTING

MAKES 1 CAKE

Cake
2 cups walnuts
2 cups medjool dates, pitted
1 cup desiccated coconut
3 cups grated carrot
¼ cup melted coconut oil
zest and juice of 1 lemon
¾ teaspoon ground ginger
2 teaspoons pure vanilla extract
1 teaspoon ground cinnamon
¼ teaspoon ground nutmeg
½ cup raisins

Frosting
1½ cups raw cashews, presoaked (see Recipe Notes page 47)
½ cup coconut cream (see Recipe Notes page 47)
¼ cup pure maple syrup
¼ cup lemon juice
2 tablespoons coconut oil
1 teaspoon pure vanilla extract
pinch of sea salt

Carrot cake has always been one of my favourite cakes. It was one of the indulgent treats I said goodbye to when I adapted a plant-based lifestyle—until I created this raw version. It's not only an incredibly moist and wholesome cake, but it's also super-speedy to make and I absolutely love the cashew-based lemony frosting.

Line the bottom of a 20 cm–24 cm (8 in–9½ in) springform cake tin with baking paper. Line the sides or lightly grease with coconut oil.

For the cake, place the walnuts and dates in a large food processor and blend until broken up into small pieces. Add the remaining ingredients except the raisins, and blend until the mixture sticks together and forms a semi-smooth mixture. It should be very moist and fairly smooth, but be careful not to over-blend as it will turn into mush. Remove the blade and stir through the raisins. Spoon the mixture into the prepared cake tin and press down evenly.

For the frosting, place all the ingredients in a blender and blend for about 20–30 seconds, until smooth.

Spoon the frosting onto the cake and spread evenly. Place in the freezer to set for at least 2–3 hours.

To serve, remove from the freezer and slice.

Store in the fridge for up to 1 week.

NOTES: This cake is best enjoyed chilled (not frozen).

Replace the raisins with crushed walnuts to add a crunchy, nutty texture.

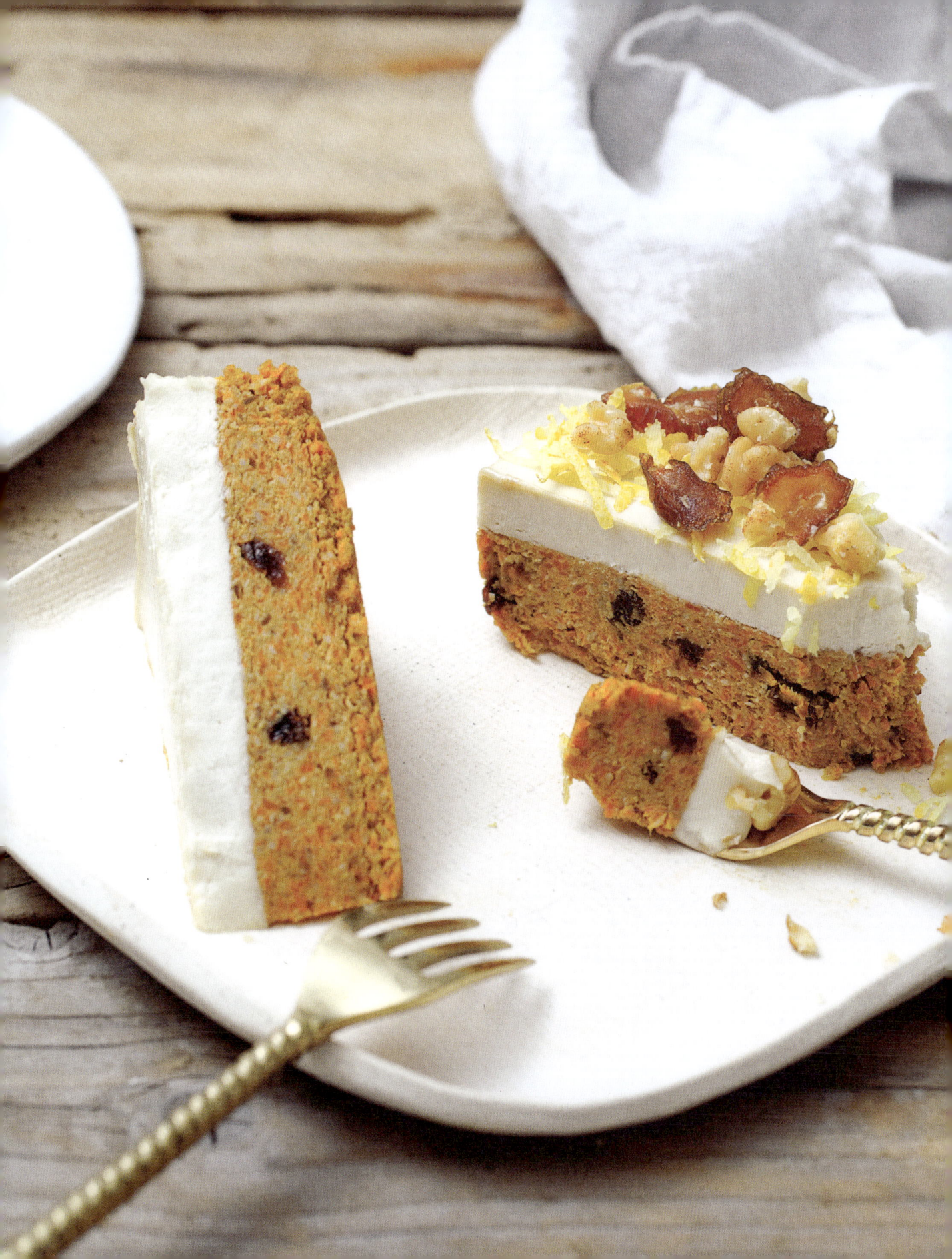

BANOFFEE FUDGE BITES

MAKES 12 BITES

½ cup cashew butter
¼ cup cacao butter
¼ cup coconut butter
¼ cup coconut cream (see Recipe Notes page 47)
¼ cup pure maple syrup
½ teaspoon pure vanilla extract
6 slices banana, halved
1 tablespoon chopped peanuts
1 tablespoon raw cacao nibs (optional)

These gorgeous melt-in-your-mouth bites make an absolutely divine dessert. I was excited with the idea of this recipe, but even more so when the outcome was more delicious than I had imagined. The slice of banana gives that beautiful banoffee touch. They are really sweet, so just one should hit the spot—with that said, it may also leave you craving more.

Heat a small saucepan over low-medium heat. Add the cashew butter, cacao butter and coconut butter, and stir until completely melted and well combined.

Remove from the heat and add the coconut cream, maple syrup and vanilla. Stir to combine.

Divide the mixture evenly among a mini 12-hole silicone mould. Poke a half-slice of banana halfway into the mixture and sprinkle with the chopped peanuts and cacao nibs, if using. Place in the freezer to set for 1½–2 hours.

Remove from the moulds and serve immediately.

Store in an airtight container in the freezer.

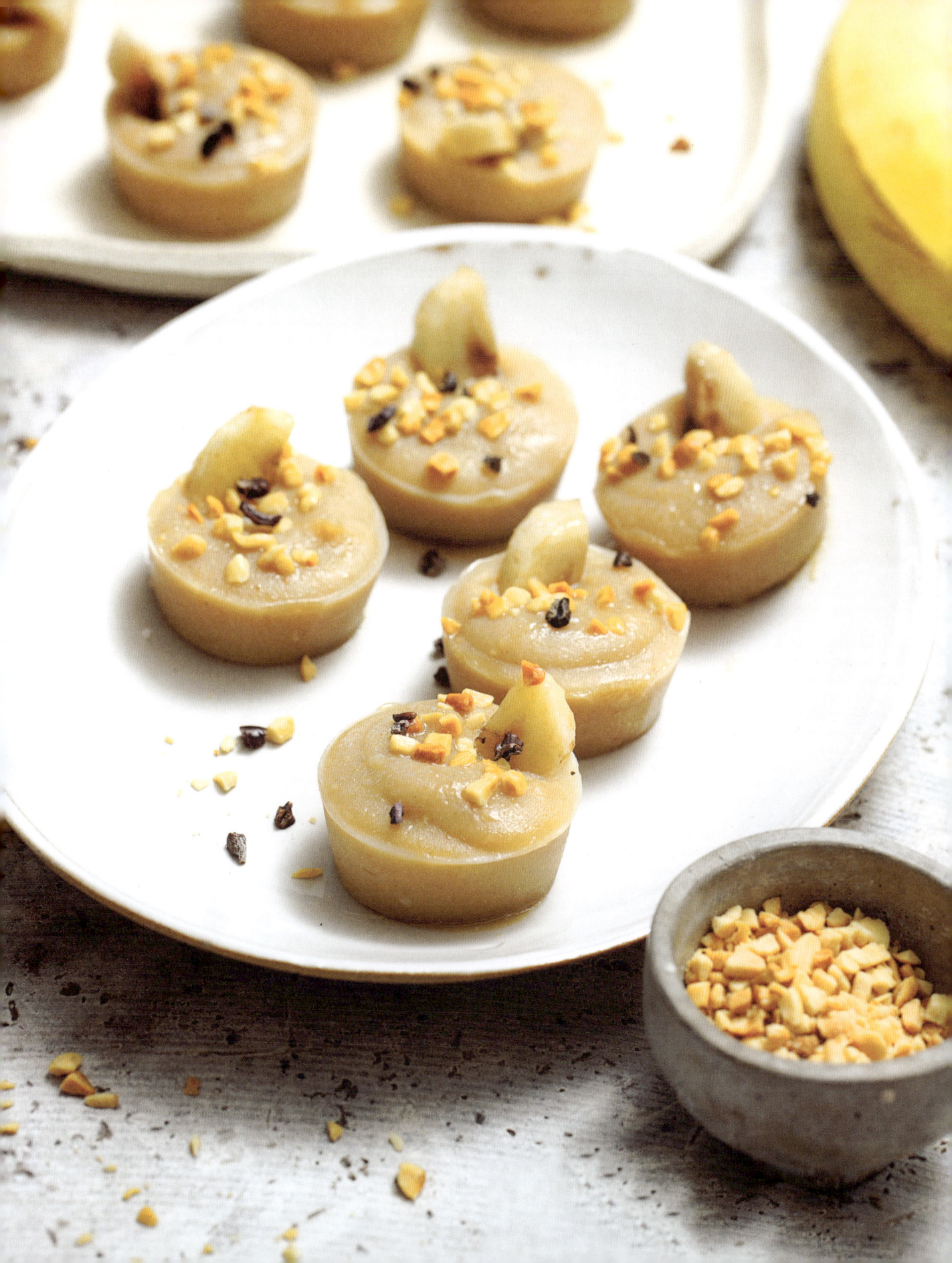

INDULGENT GINGER SLICE

MAKES 10 PIECES

Base
½ cup coconut flour
1 cup raw cashews
3 tablespoons melted coconut oil
¼ cup pure maple syrup
1 teaspoon pure vanilla extract

Ginger topping
¾ cup coconut butter, softened
½ cup pure maple syrup
2 tablespoons ground ginger
2 tablespoons water

This gorgeous slice truly is an indulgent treat, yet only requires minimal ingredients and effort. It tastes just like a classic New Zealand ginger crunch, without the overload of dairy, gluten or refined sugar. It melts in the mouth and is always a hit.

Line a small baking dish with baking paper.

For the base, place the ingredients in a large food processor and blend into a fine crumb-like texture. Tip the mixture into the baking dish and press down firmly to pack evenly. Place in freezer for 20 minutes to set.

For the ginger topping, place all the ingredients in a blender and blend into a smooth paste. Spoon onto the base and spread evenly— you will need to use a spatula for this. If the topping is too sticky to spread, add a little more water. Place in the freezer to set for 1 hour.

To serve, remove from the dish and slice into 10 pieces.

Store in a sealed container in the fridge.

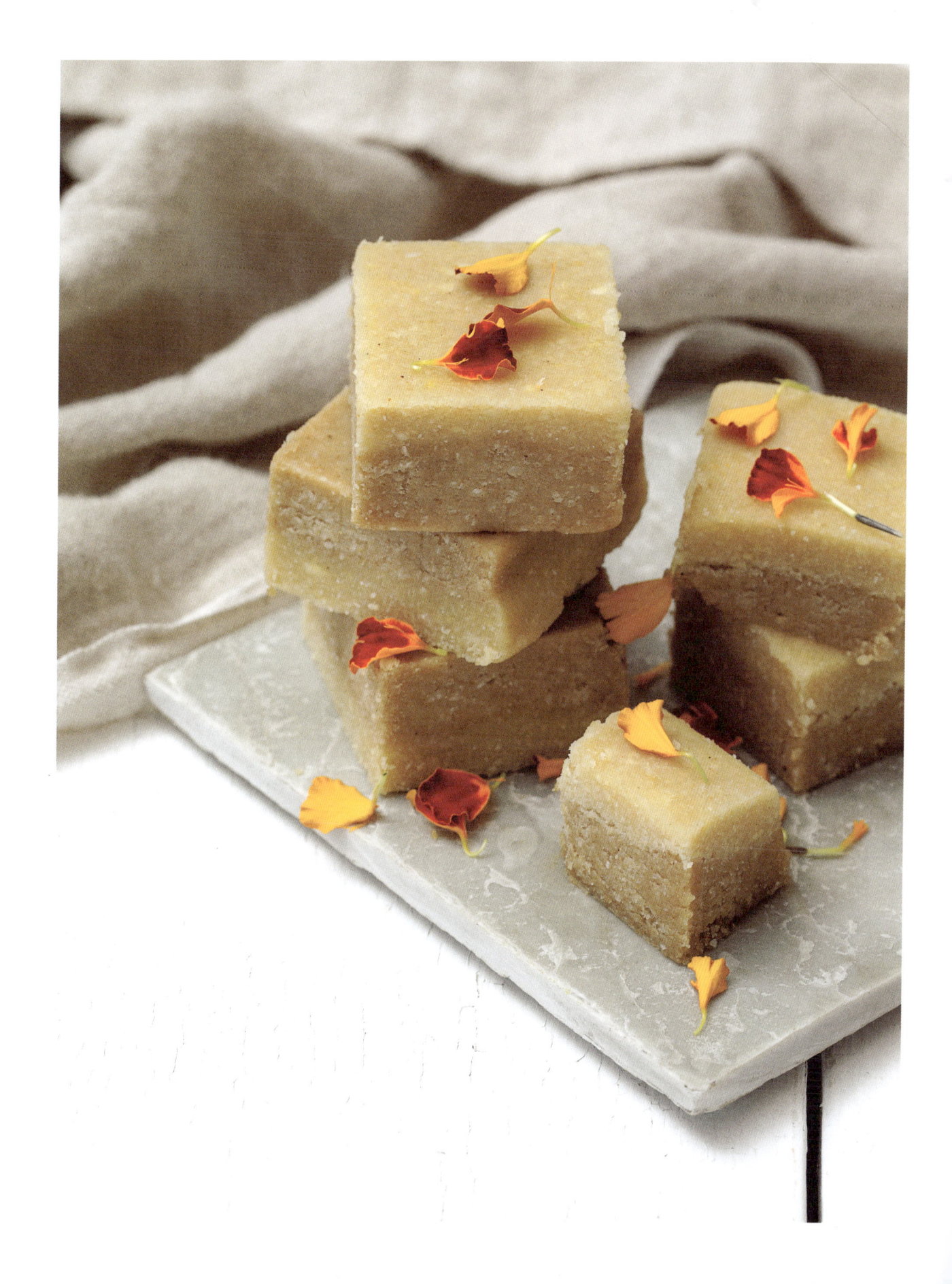

KEY LIME MOUSSE TART

MAKES 1 TART

Crust
1 cup pecans
1½ cups medjool dates, pitted
1 cup desiccated coconut
1 tablespoon lemon zest
1 teaspoon pure vanilla extract
pinch of sea salt

Mousse filling
1½ cups coconut yoghurt
¼ cup lime juice
1½ tablespoons lime zest
1 small–medium ripe avocado, stoned and peeled
⅔ cup cashews, presoaked (see Recipe Notes page 47)
3 tablespoons hempseeds (or use extra cashews)
3 tablespoons pure maple syrup
1 teaspoon pure vanilla extract
1 tablespoon melted coconut oil

Toppings (optional)
pistachios
lime zest and slices
hempseeds
kiwifruit
shredded coconut

This creamy tart makes a healthy dessert with a beautiful zesty flavour. The avocado and coconut yoghurt create a thick and creamy mousse, which also makes a beautiful dessert in its own right; simply top it with shredded coconut and fresh fruit before serving.

For the crust, place the ingredients in a large food processor and blend into a semi-fine texture. Tip the mixture into a 20 cm–25 cm (8 in–10 in) non-stick tart tin with a removeable base and press down firmly to pack evenly, using your hands to form an edge around the tin.

For the mousse filling, place the ingredients in a blender and blend until smooth and creamy. Spoon onto the base and spread evenly. Place in the freezer to set for at least 2–3 hours.

To serve, remove from the tart tin and garnish with your desired toppings. Slice and serve.

Store in an airtight container in the fridge for up to 1 week, or in the freezer for up to 1 month.

NOTE: This tart is best enjoyed chilled (not frozen). Take it out of the freezer 15 minutes before serving.

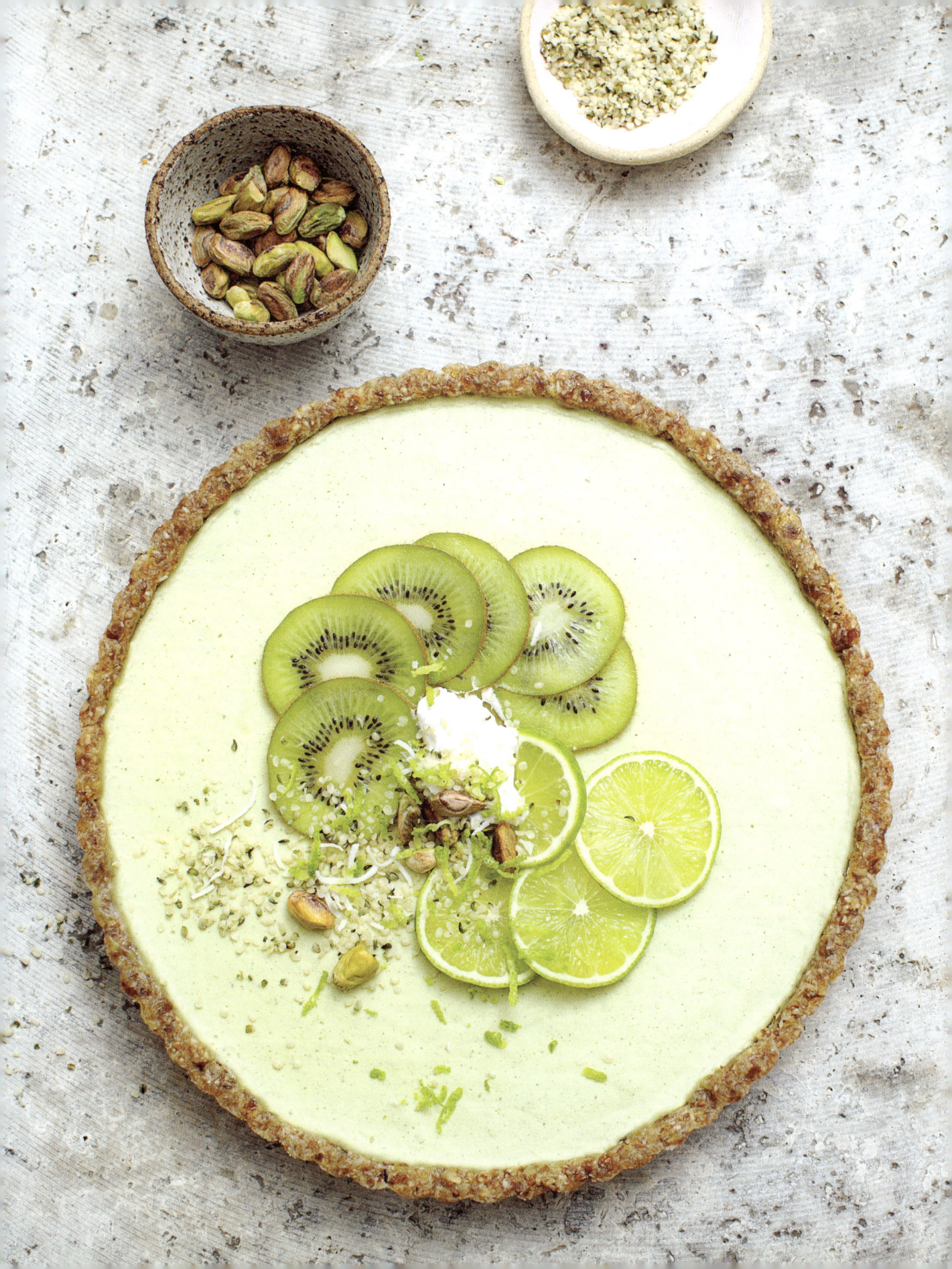

THE ULTIMATE SNICKERS SLICE

MAKES 12–15 PIECES

Base

⅔ cup almond meal
1 cup raw cashews
2 tablespoons melted coconut oil
3 tablespoons pure maple syrup
1 teaspoon pure vanilla extract

Nutty caramel

1½ cups medjool dates (not dried dates), pitted (approx. 16 dates)
3 tablespoons smooth peanut butter
1 teaspoon pure vanilla extract
¼ cup melted coconut oil
½ cup raw cashews
pinch of sea salt
¾ cup unsalted peanuts

Chocolate topping

¼ cup coconut oil
¼ cup raw cacao powder
2 tablespoons pure maple syrup

This would have to be one of my favourite raw treat recipes. I've tried many snickers slices on my travels, so when it came to creating my own mouth-watering version I knew exactly how I wanted it and after only a few attempts I created this insanely addictive slice. It's a wholesome, vegan take on the popular peanut, caramel and chocolate confectionary; an absolute family favourite that never lasts very long in our home.

Line a small baking dish with baking paper.

For the base, place the ingredients in a large food processor and blend into a moist biscuit base. Tip the mixture into the prepared dish and press down firmly to pack evenly. Place in the freezer for at least 20 minutes to set.

For the nutty caramel, place the dates, peanut butter, vanilla, coconut oil, cashews and sea salt in the food processor and blend into a smooth caramel paste. Remove the base from the freezer, spoon the caramel onto the base and spread evenly—you may need to use a spatula. Scatter over the peanuts, and lightly press them into the caramel layer. Return to the freezer for 1–2 hours to set.

For the chocolate topping, heat a small saucepan over medium heat. Add the ingredients and stir until the coconut oil is melted and the ingredients are combined. Remove from the heat. Remove the slice from the freezer and pour over the chocolate layer. Return to the freezer for 1 hour to set.

To serve, remove from the dish and slice into 12–15 pieces.

Store in a sealed container in the fridge or freezer.

NOTE: This slice is best served straight from the freezer.

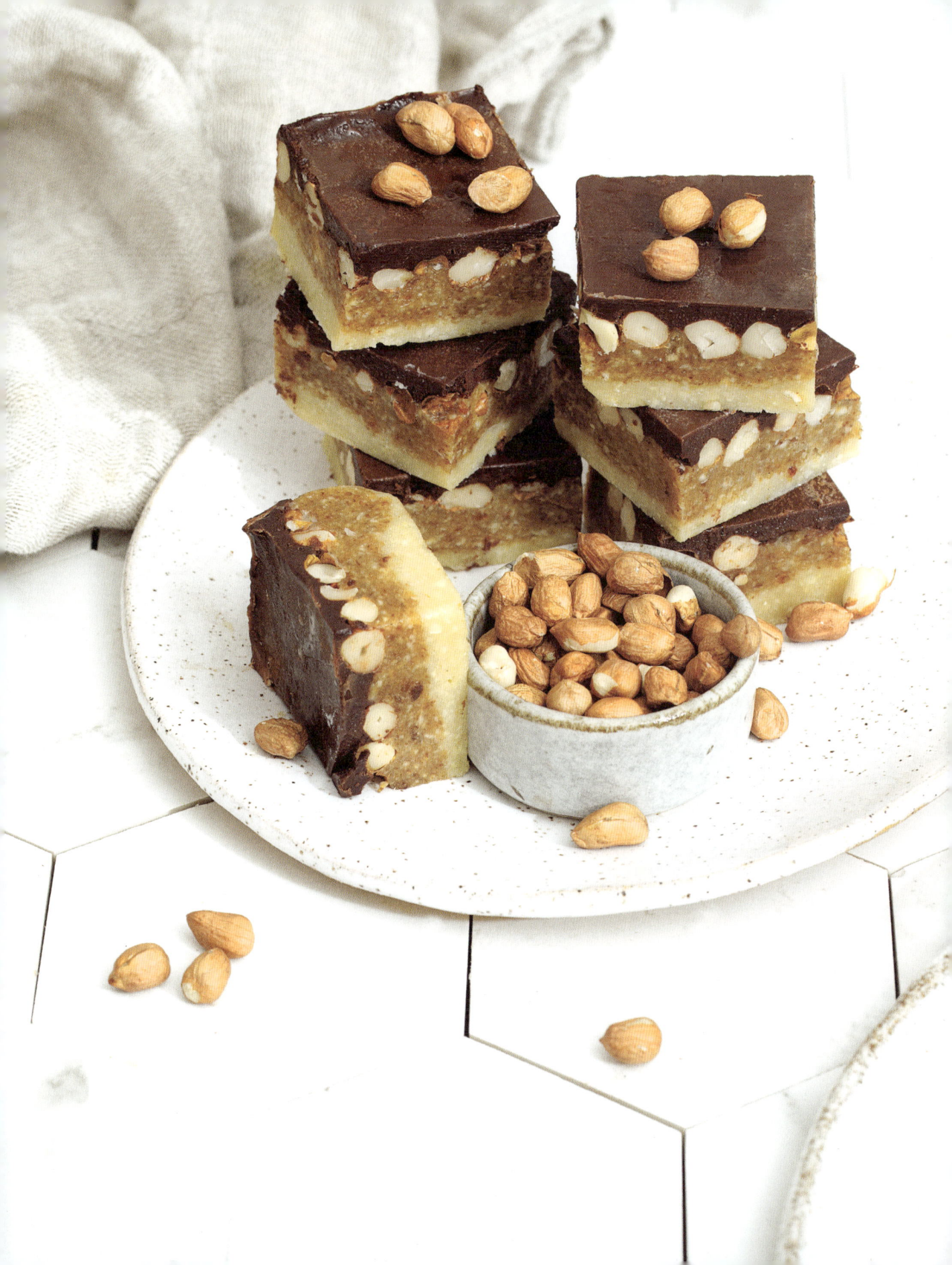

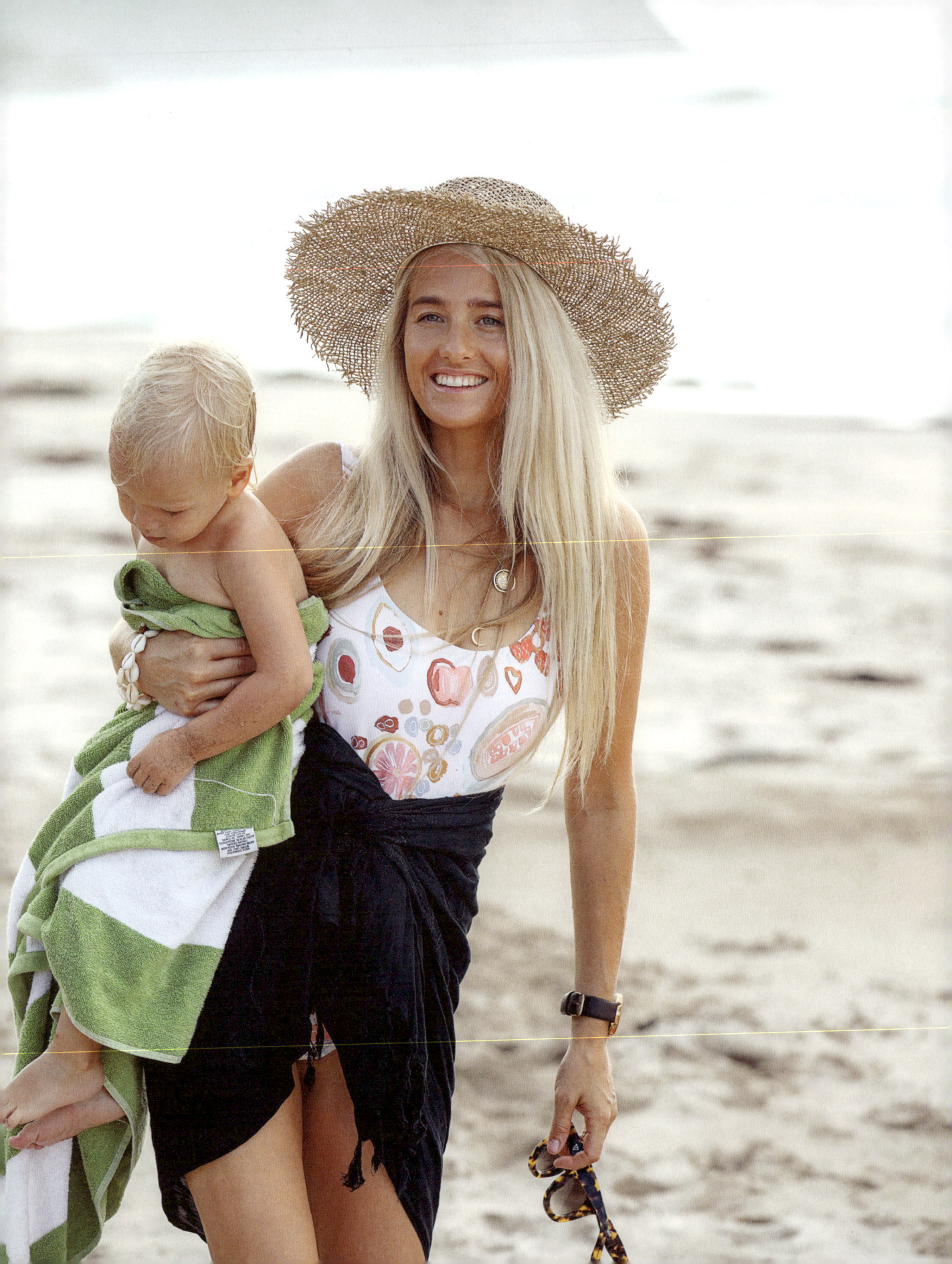

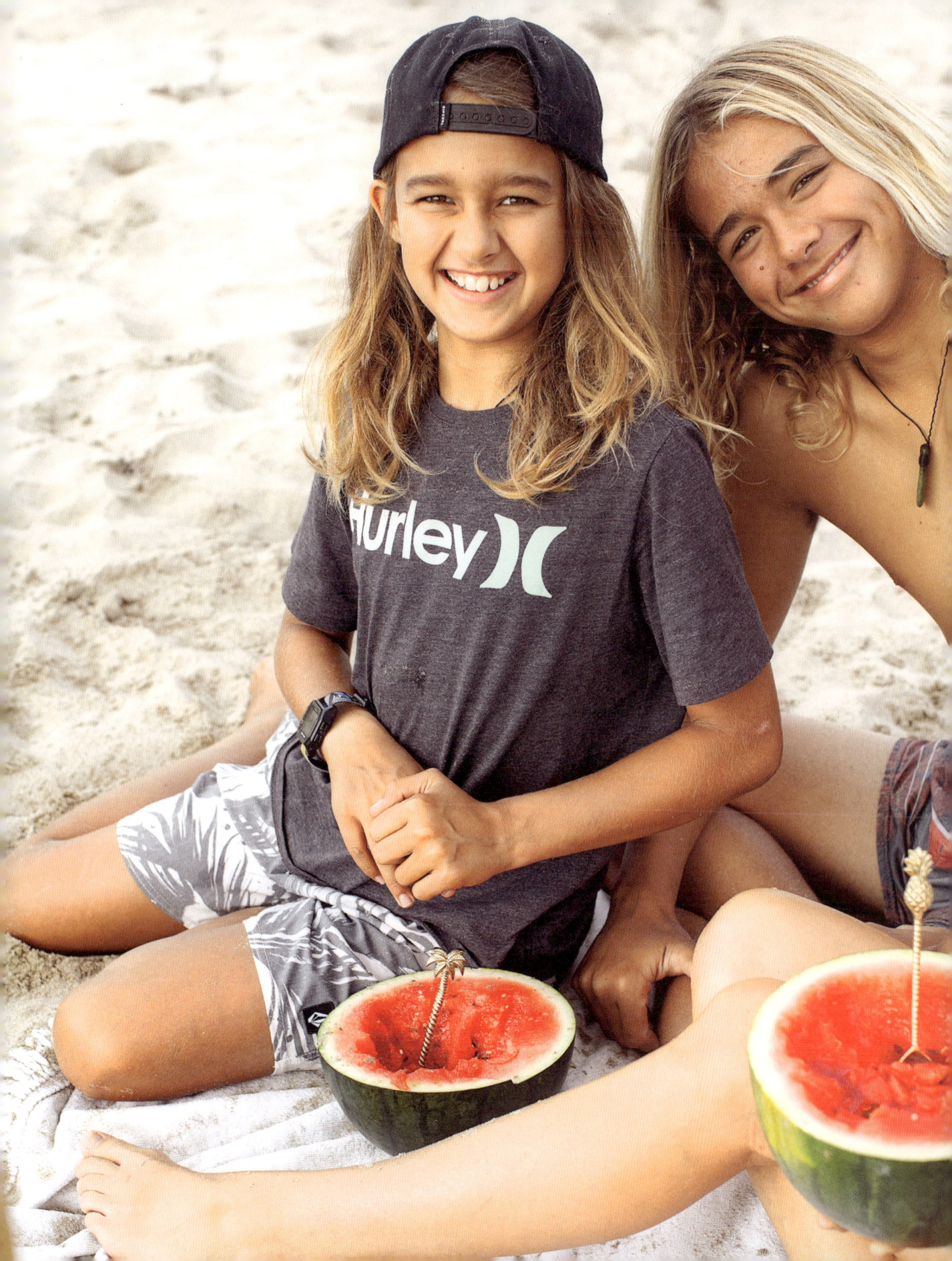

FRUIT and NUT CHOCOLATE

MAKES 15 SQUARES

½ cup coconut oil
½ cup raw cacao powder
⅓ cup pure maple syrup
½ cup desiccated coconut
½ cup raisins
½ cup nuts, crushed (almonds, peanuts, walnuts)

If you're after a quick chocolate fix, I highly recommend this recipe. It takes all of 5 minutes to prepare and is one of my favourite chocolatey treats. The coconut gives it a 'coconut rough' feel, while the nuts and raisins add that crunchy and chewy texture. I like to use crushed peanuts or almonds.

Line a small dish with baking paper.

Heat a small saucepan over medium heat. Add the coconut oil, cacao powder and maple syrup, and stir until the coconut oil is melted and the ingredients are combined. Remove from the heat.

Place the coconut, raisins and nuts in a large bowl. Pour over the chocolate mixture and stir to combine. Ensure all the ingredients are coated.

Tip the mixture into the prepared dish and spread out evenly. Place in the freezer to set for at least 3 hours.

Remove and slice into 15 squares.

Serve immediately, or store in a sealed container in the freezer.

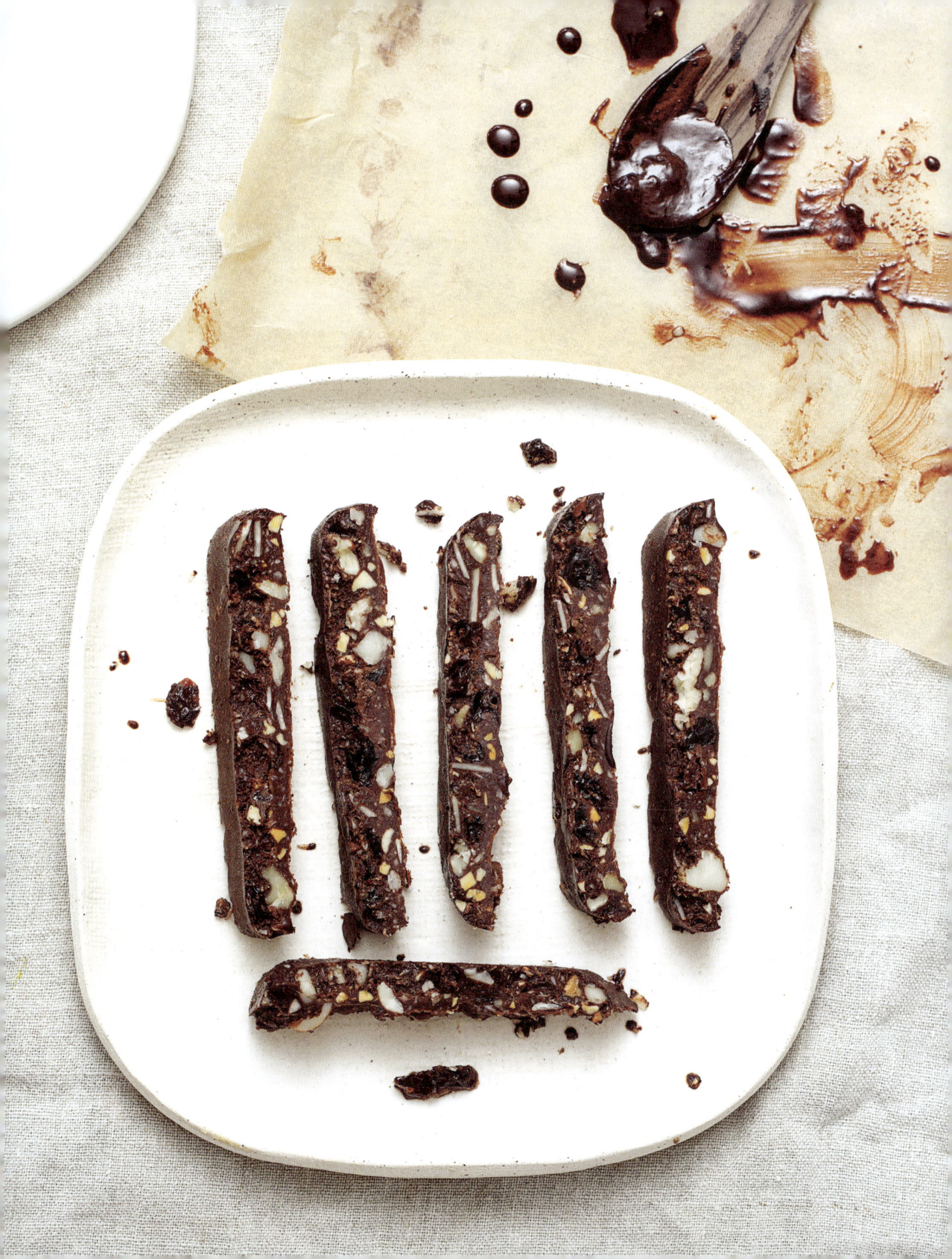

GOOEY CARAMEL BROWNIE SLICE

MAKES 20 PIECES

Brownie base
1¾ cups walnuts
1½ cups medjool dates (not dried dates), pitted (approx. 16 dates)
2 tablespoons coconut sugar
¼ cup cacao powder
1 teaspoon pure vanilla extract
pinch of sea salt

Caramel
1 cup macadamias
1 cup medjool dates (not dried dates), pitted
½ cup pure maple syrup
2 teaspoons pure vanilla extract

Chocolate layer
⅓ cup melted coconut oil
⅓ cup raw cacao powder
2 tablespoons pure maple syrup

If you enjoy a good chocolate brownie and have a weakness for gooey caramel, you will love the two combined in this delightfully rich slice. This was one of the first slices I experimented with; one we still love to make from time to time. This recipe makes a large slice and can be served straight from the freezer as it doesn't completely freeze.

Line a small–medium baking dish with baking paper.

For the base, place the ingredients in a large food processor and blend into a fine crumb. Tip the mixture into the dish and press down firmly to pack evenly.

For the caramel, place the macadamias in the food processor and blend until finely broken down. Add the remaining ingredients and blend until you have a smooth caramel paste. Spoon onto the base and spread evenly—you may need to use a spatula. Place in the freezer to set for 1 hour.

For the chocolate layer, heat a small saucepan over medium heat. Add the coconut oil, cacao powder and maple syrup and stir until the coconut oil is melted and the ingredients are combined. Remove the base from the freezer and pour over the chocolate layer. Return to the freezer for 1 hour to set.

To serve, remove from the dish and slice into 12–15 pieces.

Store in a sealed container in either the fridge or the freezer.

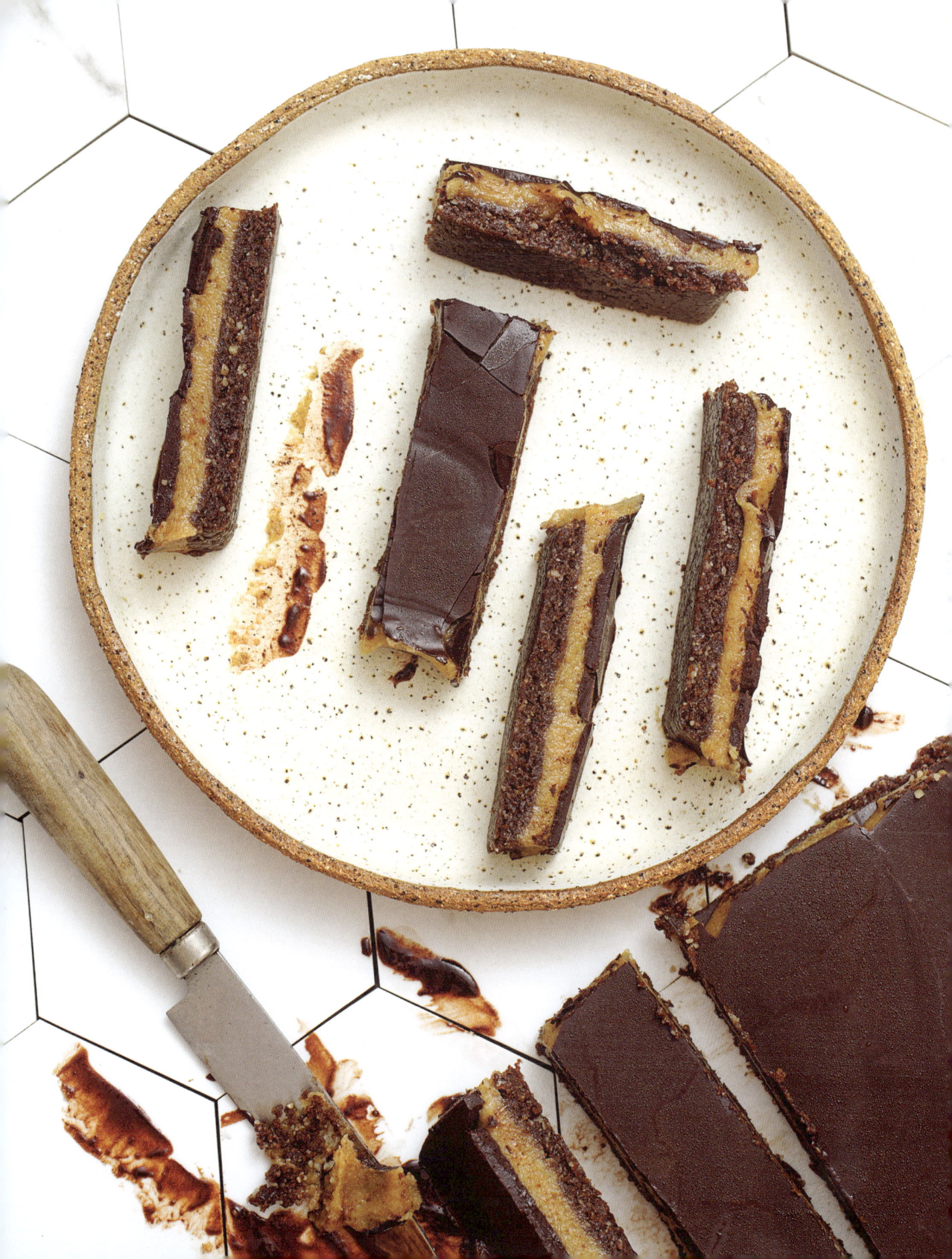

RASPBERRY BOUNTY BARS

MAKES 12 BARS

Bounty base

2¼ cups desiccated coconut
½ cup coconut flour or almond meal
¼ cup pure maple syrup
3 tablespoons coconut oil, melted
½ cup coconut cream (see Recipe Notes page 47)
1 teaspoon pure vanilla extract
½ cup fresh raspberries

Chocolate coating

3 tablespoons coconut oil
3 tablespoons raw cacao powder
1½ tablespoons pure maple syrup

Get the children involved in making these lush bounty bars. They are super fun and easy to whip up, and result in the most beautiful chocolate-coated coconut bars with a sweet raspberry twist. They can also be shaped into bite-sized balls—you'll get twice as many.

Line a large baking dish (or two small ones) with baking paper.

For the base, place the ingredients in a large food processor and blend into a creamy mixture.

Form the mixture into 12 balls, then mould into small bars. The mixture will be very soft and moist from the raspberries, but should still be firm enough to hold a shape. Carefully place each bar into the baking dish as you go, then place them into the freezer to set for 2 hours.

For the chocolate layer, heat a small saucepan over medium heat. Add the coconut oil, cacao powder and maple syrup, and stir until the coconut oil is melted and the ingredients are combined.

Remove the bars from the freezer and dip each bar into the chocolate, then place onto a cooling rack (if you have one) to allow them to drip. Repeat the chocolate dipping 2–3 times, in the same order. Place the bars back into the freezer to completely set for at least 30 minutes.

Serve immediately, or store in a sealed container in the fridge or freezer.

NOTE: Add a sprinkle of freeze-dried raspberry or beetroot powder for a more vibrant raspberry colour.

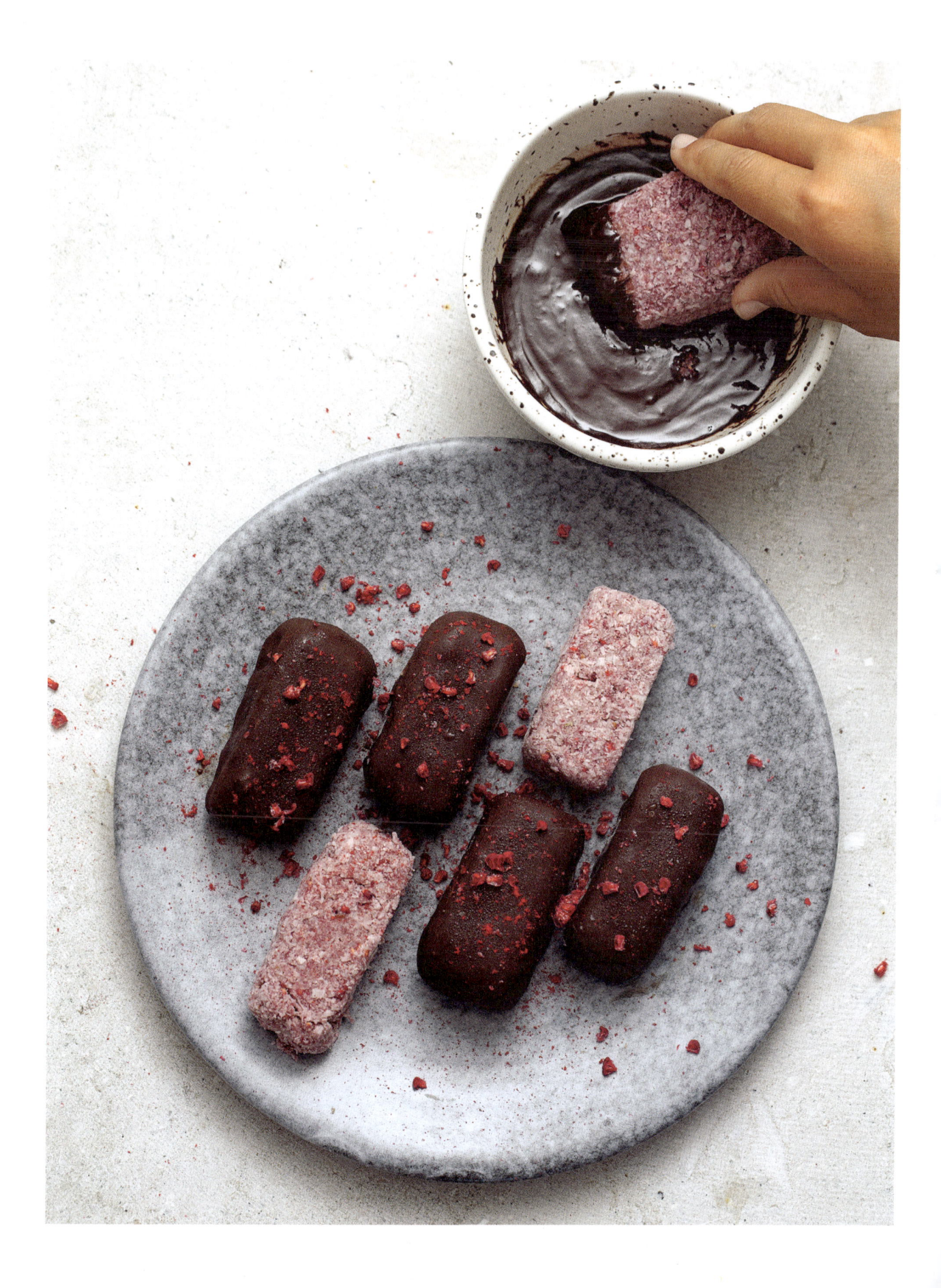

BLUEBERRY CHEESECAKE

MAKES 1 CAKE

Base
- ⅔ cup almond meal
- 1 cup raw cashews
- 2 tablespoons melted coconut oil
- 3 tablespoons pure maple syrup
- 1 teaspoon pure vanilla extract

Filling
- 2 cups raw cashews, presoaked (see Recipe Notes page 47)
- ¾ cup coconut cream (see Recipe Notes page 47)
- 3 tablespoons melted coconut oil
- ¼ cup pure maple syrup
- ¼ cup lemon juice
- 2 teaspoons pure vanilla extract
- ¼ cup blueberries (fresh or frozen)

Topping
- 2 cups blueberries (fresh or frozen)
- 2 tablespoons chia seeds
- 2 tablespoons pure maple syrup

To serve (optional)
- fresh blueberries (or freeze-dried berries)

This is an easy make-ahead dessert for a dinner party. The cashew-based centre creates the perfect alternative to dairy, eggs and refined sugar. This truly is a dreamy cake, topped with a beautifully sweet blueberry layer, and even more wonderful finished with a juicy serving of fresh blueberries or freeze-dried berries.

Line the bottom of a 20 cm–24 cm (8 in–9½ in) springform cake tin with baking paper. Lightly grease the sides with coconut oil.

For the base, place the ingredients in a large food processor and blend into a moist biscuit base. Tip the mixture into the prepared cake tin and press down firmly to pack evenly. Place in the freezer for at least 20 minutes to set while you make the filling.

For the filling, place the ingredients in a blender and blend until smooth and creamy. Take the base out of the freezer, and spread the mixture evenly over it. Place in the freezer for 2 hours, until the cake is firm.

For the topping, place all the ingredients in a blender and blend until smooth. Transfer to a small bowl and place in the fridge while the cake sets.

Remove the cake from the freezer and spread over the topping. Return to the freezer for 1 hour to set.

To serve, remove from the cake tin and top with the fresh blueberries, if using. Slice and serve.

Store in an airtight container in the fridge for up to 1 week, or in the freezer for up to 1 month.

NOTE: This cake is best enjoyed chilled (not frozen).

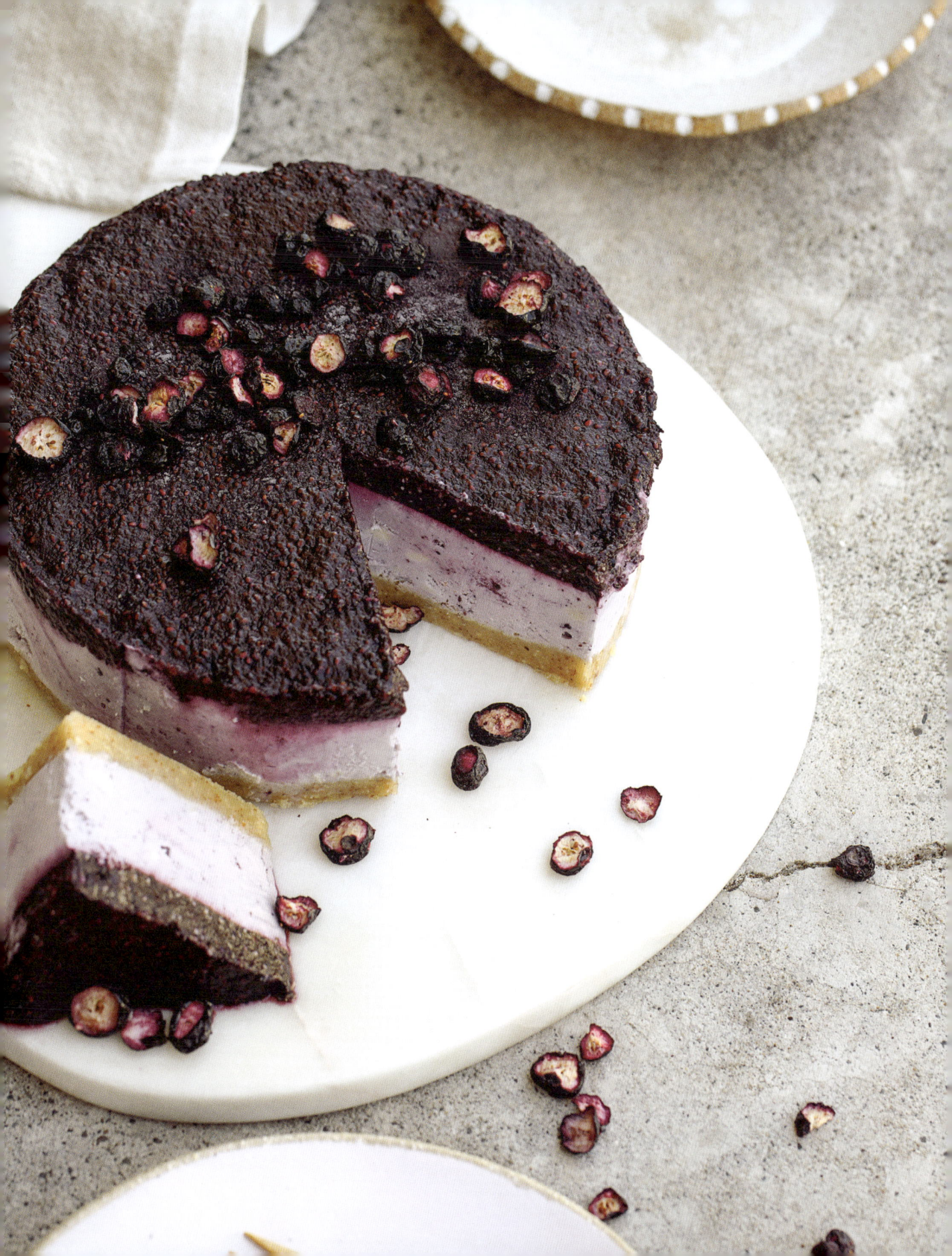

HEMP CHOCOLATE SHAKES

SERVES 2

4 frozen ripe bananas
1½ cups coconut water
3 tablespoons hempseeds
2 tablespoons cacao powder
1 tablespoon pure maple syrup

Toppings (optional)
vegan ice cream
melted or grated vegan chocolate
cacao nibs
coconut flakes

These creamy thick-shakes are my main source of a wholesome chocolate fix; they're often my go-to treat in the afternoons. The key to these shakes is to ensure the bananas are ripe and spotty. This makes them super-sweet, while the hempseeds provide the creaminess. If you want to serve the shakes as a dessert, jazz them up by adding a splash of melted vegan chocolate to the glass. Once set, pour the thick-shake in and finish with a sprinkle of cacao nibs and coconut flakes or a dollop of vegan vanilla ice cream.

Place all the ingredients in a blender and blend until smooth and creamy.

Pour into 2 large glasses (or jars) and enjoy immediately with the toppings of your choice.

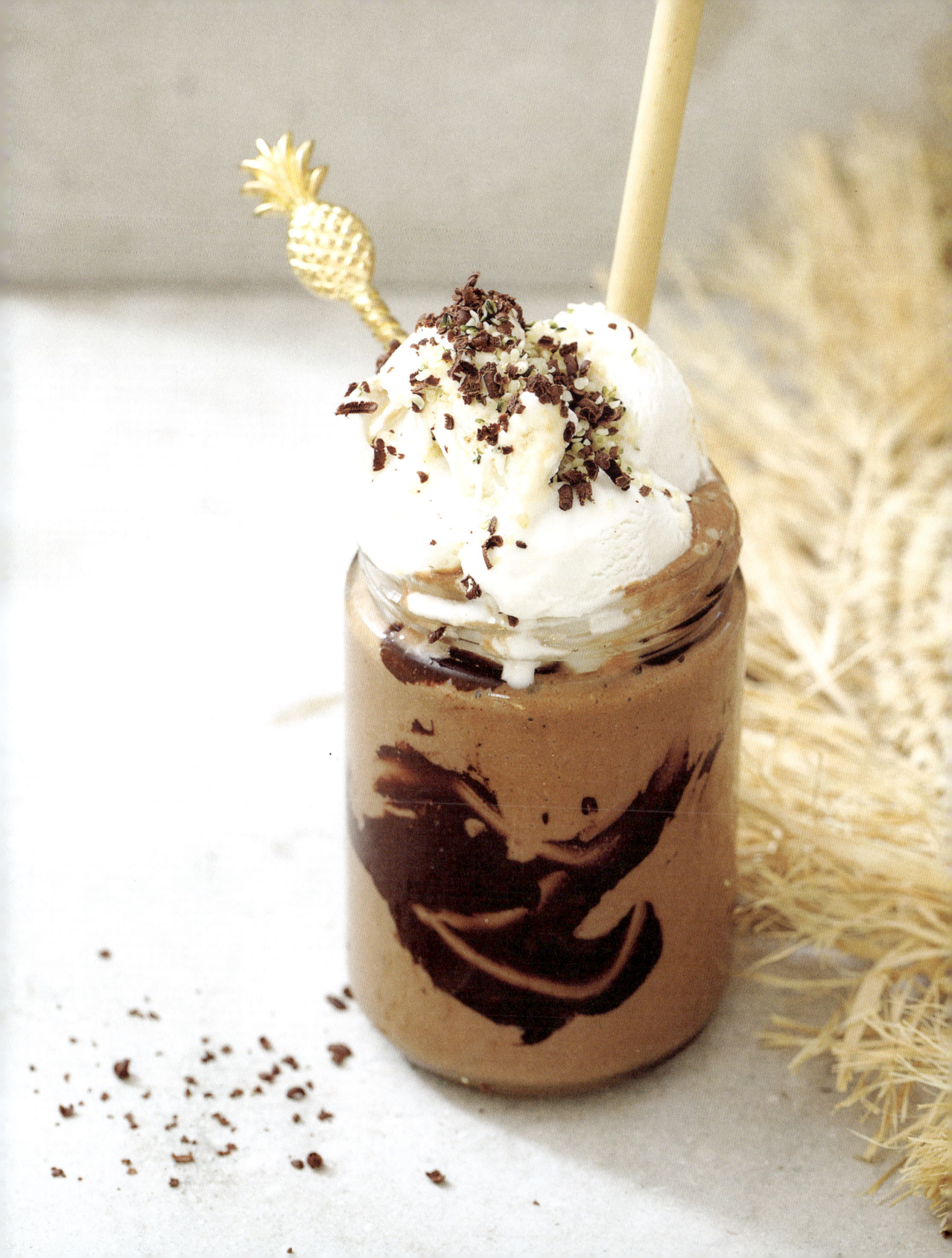

HIMALAYAN ALMOND CRACKLE CLUSTERS

MAKES 15–20 CLUSTERS

⅓ cup coconut oil
¼ cup raw cacao powder
¼ cup pure maple syrup
2 cups raw almonds
1½ cups brown rice puffs
1 teaspoon pure vanilla extract
Himalayan salt

Keep a batch of these clusters in the freezer for a wholesome chocolate fix. I like to use almonds in this recipe, but you can use any of your favourite nuts or even a variety of different nuts. Once they're set, I find it easier to snap them into pieces rather than slicing them with a knife.

Line a 20 cm x 30 cm (8 in x 12 in) dish with baking paper.

Heat a small saucepan over medium heat. Add the coconut oil, cacao powder and maple syrup, and stir until the coconut oil is melted and the ingredients are combined. Remove from the heat.

Place the almonds, rice puffs, vanilla and a good sprinkle of Himalayan salt in a large bowl. Pour over the chocolate mixture and stir until all the ingredients are well coated in the chocolate.

Tip the mixture into the prepared dish and spread out evenly. Lightly sprinkle with Himalayan salt. Place in the freezer to set for at least 2 hours.

Remove from the freezer and either slice or snap into clusters. A few almonds may naturally come loose in the process.

Serve immediately, or store in a sealed container in the freezer.

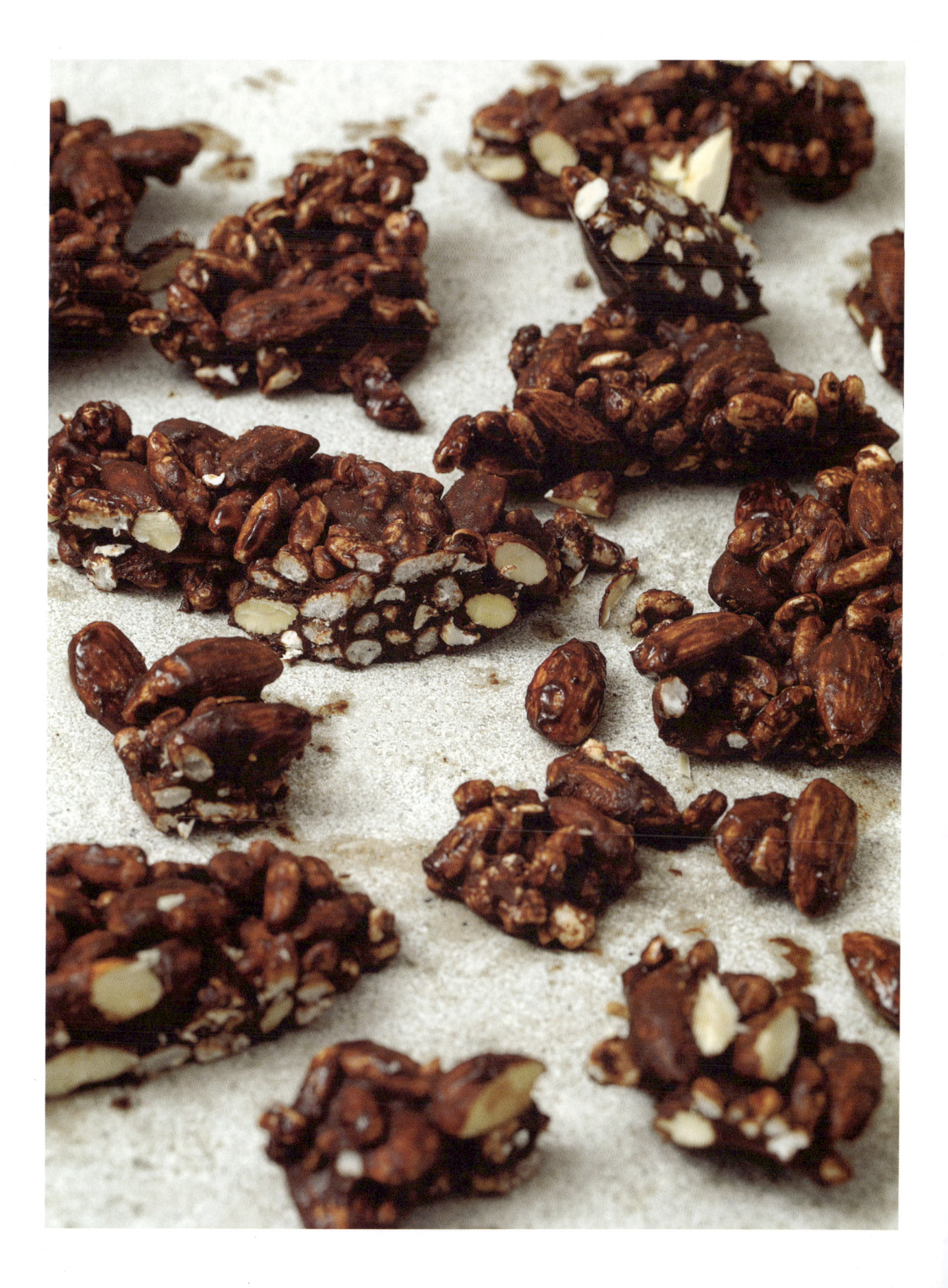

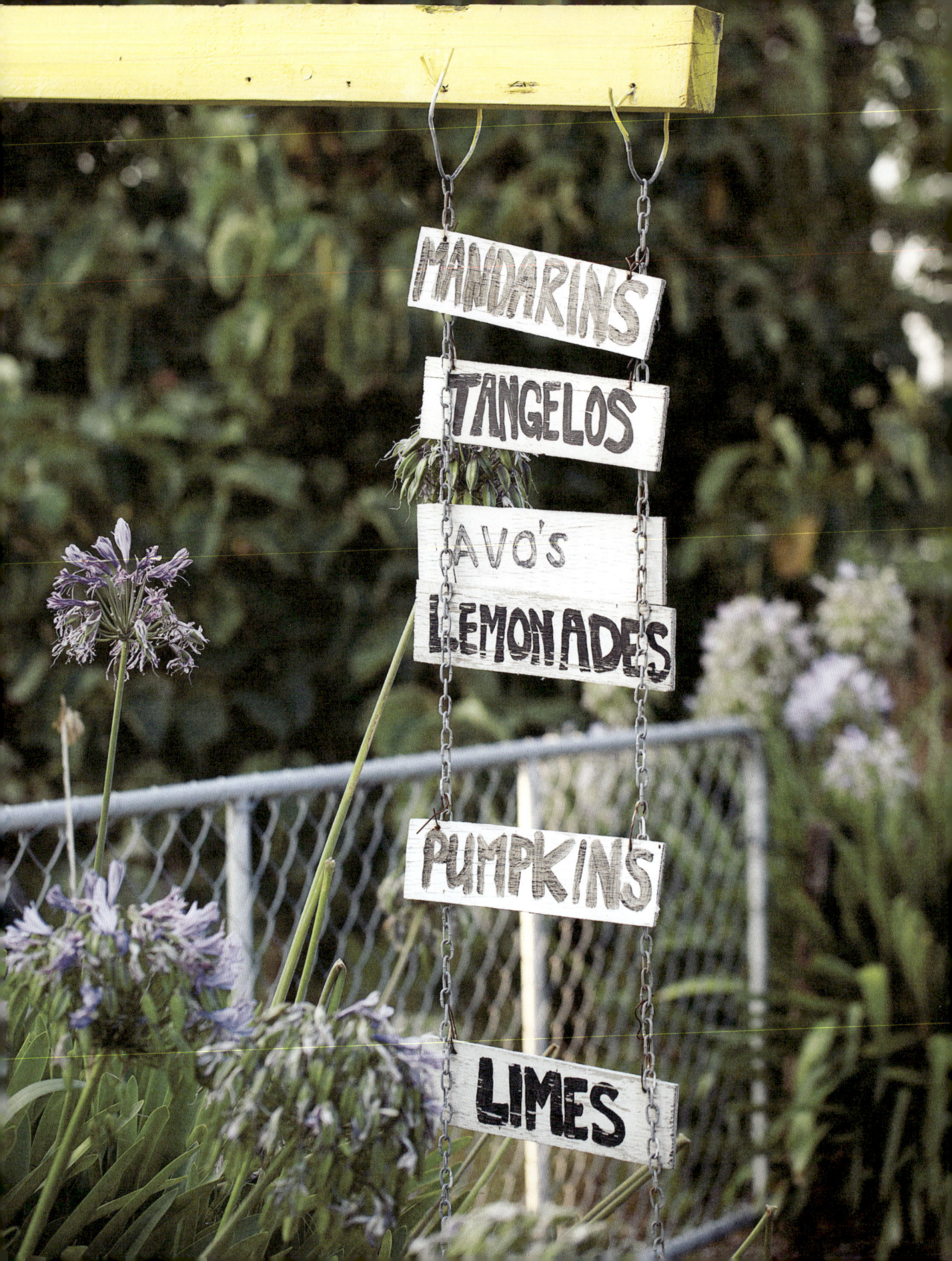

MANDARINS
TANGELOS
AVO'S
LEMONADES
PUMPKINS
LIMES

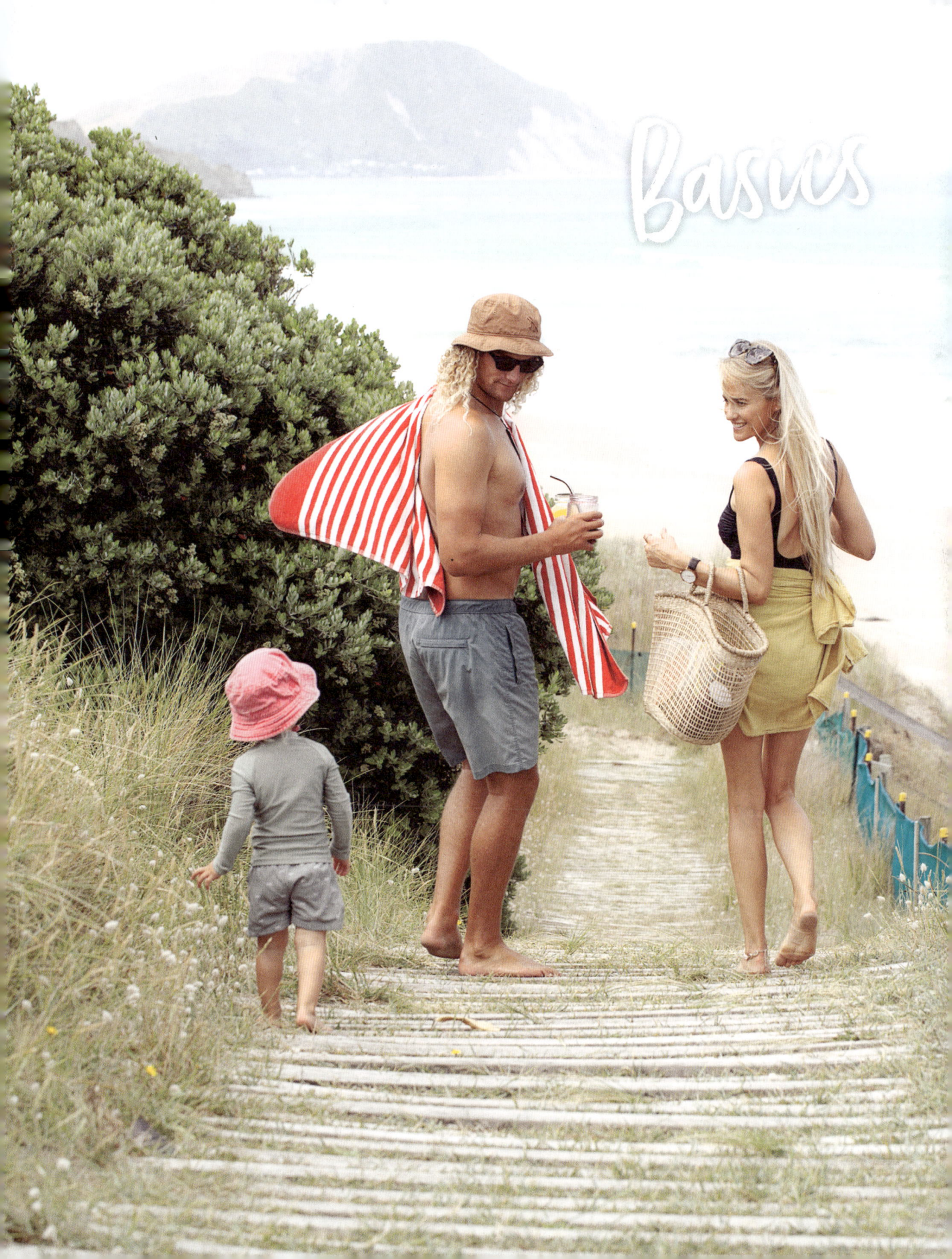

Basics

Basics

A beautiful meal begins with the basics, and this chapter provides you with just that. From creamy aïoli to vegan cheese sauce, nutritious hemp milk to easy chickpea tacos, these are the kitchen staples you'll need to create a wide range of plant-based and gluten-free meals without any additives.

There's almost always a plant-based substitute for anything, and I hope these recipes will show you how to recreate some of your own favourite dishes. There's something extra special about creating a wholesome meal from scratch, especially knowing exactly what's going into your food.

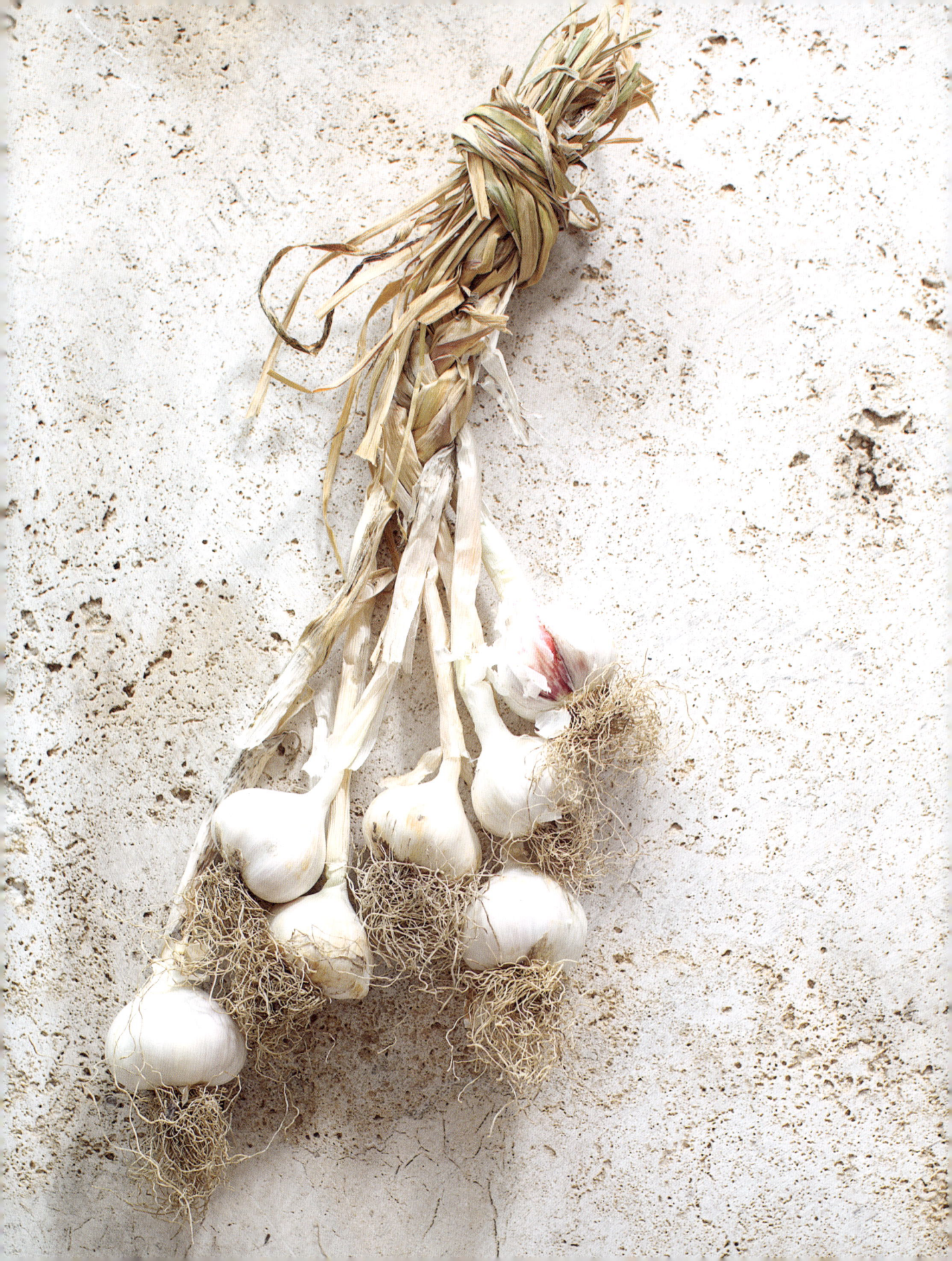

Dressings and Sauces

AÏOLI

MAKES ABOUT 1 CUP

This thick, creamy, cashew-based aïoli makes the perfect plant-based kitchen staple; a great addition to just about anything. Try it slathered on sandwiches, salads, roast vegetables, crackers or as a dip or dressing with almost any of the savoury recipes in this book.

1 cup raw cashews, presoaked (see Recipe Notes page 47)
2 cloves garlic, chopped
1 tablespoon mustard
1 tablespoon apple cider vinegar
1 tablespoon lemon juice
1 teaspoon pure maple syrup
⅛ teaspoon white pepper
⅓ cup rice milk (or any other plant milk)

Place all the ingredients in a blender and blend for about 10–15 seconds, until thick and creamy.

Store in a sealed jar in the fridge for up to 5 days.

MINT AÏOLI

MAKES ABOUT 1 CUP

A refreshing, minty take on the classic aïoli. It's perfect as a salad dressing or paired with any main to add a mild, minty flavour. Try it drizzled over my Roast Butternut, Red Quinoa, Rocket and Cranberry Salad (see page 152).

⅔ cup raw cashews, presoaked (see Recipe Notes page 47)
⅓ packed cup fresh mint leaves
3 tablespoons lemon juice
1 small clove garlic, diced
1 tablespoon pure maple syrup
½ cup water

Place all the ingredients in a blender and blend for about 10–15 seconds, until thick and creamy.

Store in a sealed jar in the fridge for up to 5 days.

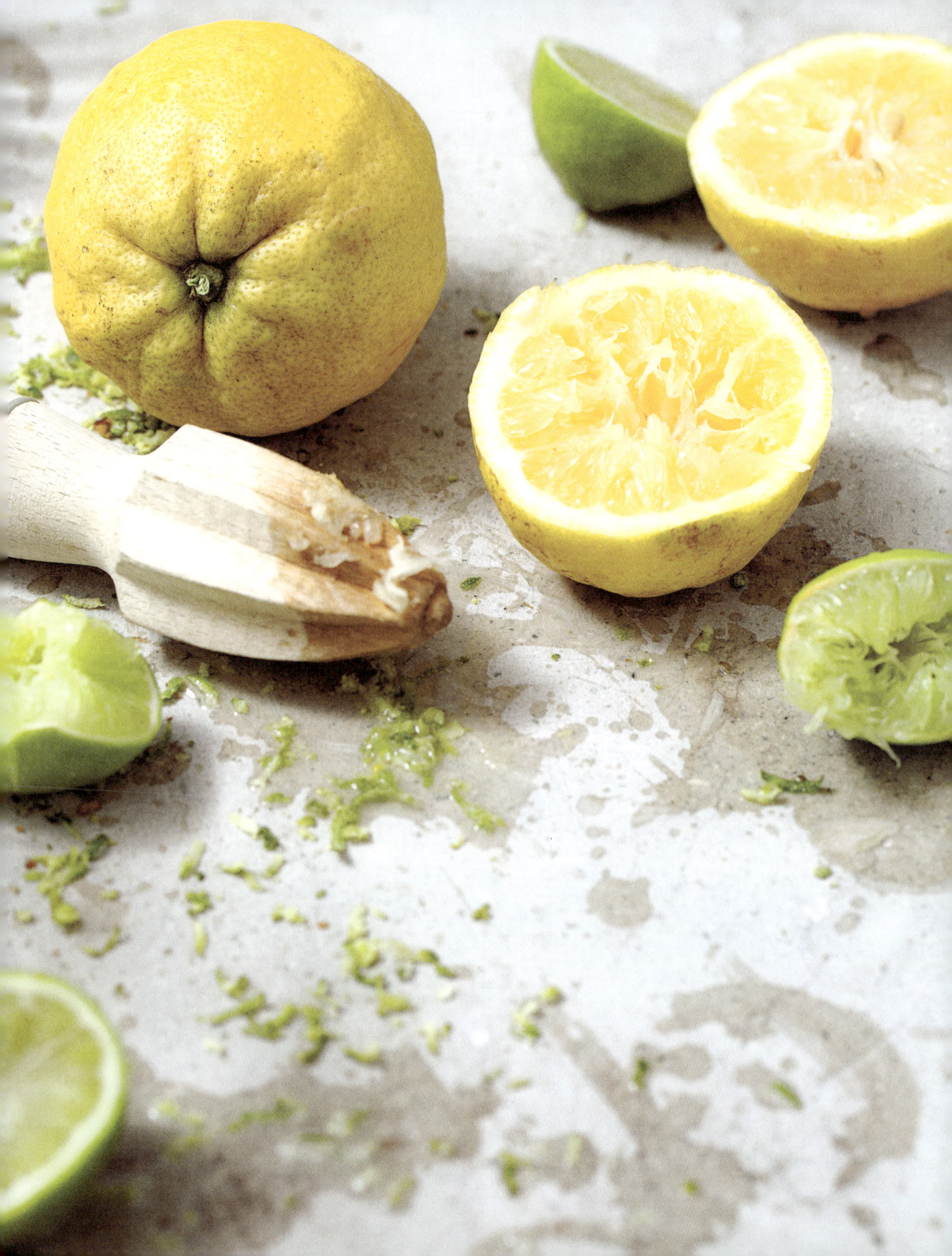

CAESAR SALAD DRESSING

MAKES ABOUT 1 CUP

This is a simple plant-based take on the traditional Caesar salad dressing. The capers give it so much flavour, while the nutritional yeast adds a savoury touch. It's a thick and creamy dressing, perfect poured over potatoes and fresh greens, and is ideal for adding a creamy flavour booster to any salad. Try it on my Creamy Kale Caesar Salad (see page 128) or Potato Wedges, Sweetcorn and Cos Lettuce Salad (see page 150).

1 cup raw cashews, presoaked (see Recipe Notes page 47)
1½ tablespoons nutritional yeast
1½ tablespoons capers
2 tablespoons lemon juice
2 teaspoons pure maple syrup
1 teaspoon apple cider vinegar
1 clove garlic
½ cup water

Place all the ingredients in a blender and blend for about 10–15 seconds, until smooth.

Store in a sealed jar in the fridge for up to 5 days.

RANCH DRESSING OR DIP

MAKES ABOUT 1 CUP

This flavourful dressing is perfect drizzled over fresh greens or paired with roast vegetables. It has a thick and creamy consistency, which also makes it fabulous served as a dip with vege sticks. For a tasty bite to eat, try it dolloped over Caraway Potato and Chickpea Mingle (see page 204).

1 cup raw cashews, presoaked (see Recipe Notes page 47)
½ cup rice milk (or any other plant milk)
1½ tablespoons nutritional yeast
2 teaspoons wholegrain mustard
1 tablespoon lemon juice
2 teaspoons pure maple syrup
2 teaspoons apple cider vinegar
1 clove garlic
2 teaspoons dried or fresh dill
½ teaspoon onion powder
⅛ teaspoon white pepper

Place all the ingredients in a blender and blend for about 10–15 seconds, until smooth. Add more liquid to achieve your desired consistency.

Store in a sealed jar in the fridge for up to 5 days.

VEGAN SOUR CREAM

MAKES ABOUT 2 CUPS

With a creamy, mild and slightly tangy flavour, a dollop of this vegan sour cream is amazing with any dish. It makes the perfect addition to muffins, fritters, salads, Mexican food, spicy food, curries, soups . . . and the list goes on.

1½ cups raw cashews, presoaked (see Recipe Notes page 47)
¾ cup filtered water
3 tablespoons fresh lemon juice
2 teaspoons apple cider vinegar
1 small clove garlic, finely chopped

Place all the ingredients in a blender and blend for about 10–15 seconds, until smooth. Place in the fridge for about 1 hour to firm up.

Store in a sealed jar in the fridge for up to 1 week.

NOTE: For a substitution for the cashews, use 1 cup of coconut yoghurt and remove the water from the recipe.

CASHEW CHEESE SAUCE

MAKES ABOUT 2 CUPS

This is my number-one, go-to cheese sauce. It's creamy, rich, flavourful and makes any meal taste truly moreish, creating the perfect cheesy base for pies, pastas, vege bakes, lasagne and so much more. The miso paste and nutritional yeast give it a savoury, cheesy flavour, while the cashews make it super-creamy. Try it in my Creamy Sunflower and Vegetable Tart (see page 186) or Moreish Potato and Chive Bake (see page 176).

1 cup raw cashews, presoaked (see Recipe Notes page 47)
½ cup nutritional yeast
1 cup rice milk
2 tablespoons lemon juice
2 small cloves garlic
1 tablespoon wholegrain mustard
1 tablespoon white miso paste

Place all the ingredients in a blender and blend for about 10–15 seconds, until smooth.

Store in a sealed jar in the fridge for up to 5 days.

NOTE: Sneak some greens in by adding a cup or so of spinach to create a tasty green pasta sauce.

NACHO CHEESE SAUCE

MAKES ABOUT 4 CUPS

This is the best and most flavourful nacho cheese sauce ever—you wouldn't even know it was vegan. I highly recommend it served with just about anything. Try it drizzled over nachos or steamed veges, as a pasta sauce or as a dip for vege sticks. It makes a large batch that will freeze well, so you'll always have it on hand to create an easy dinner.

2 cups peeled, cubed white potatoes (approx. 2 small potatoes)
1½ cups peeled and sliced carrots (approx. 2 small–medium carrots)
1 white onion, diced
3 cloves garlic, diced
2 cups water
½ cup raw cashews
2 tablespoons wholegrain mustard
½ cup nutritional yeast
2 tablespoons lemon juice
½ teaspoon salt
fresh coriander leaves, to serve

Place the potatoes, carrots, onion, garlic and water in a saucepan, cover, and bring to a boil. Cook for about 10–15 minutes, until the veges are fork tender.

Remove from the heat and transfer all the ingredients, including the cooking water, into a blender along with the cashews, mustard, nutritional yeast, lemon juice and salt. Blend until smooth.

Pour into a bowl and top with fresh coriander to serve.

NOTE: Store any remaining sauce in an airtight container in the fridge for up to 5 days, or in the freezer for up to 3 months.

RAW SWEET CHILLI SAUCE

MAKES ABOUT 1¼ CUPS

Sweet chilli sauce has long been one of my favourite sauces to add a little sweet spice to any meal, especially roast vegetables. I always struggle to find one without additives or an overload of refined sugar. Here's an awesome, healthy alternative, sweetened naturally by medjool dates.

1 red chilli (approx. 4 cm / 1½ in)
2 red capsicums, trimmed, halved and deseeded
1 cm (½ in) piece of fresh ginger, peeled
4 large medjool dates, pitted
¼ cup lime juice
sea salt, to taste

Place all the ingredients in a blender and blend for about 10–15 seconds, until mostly smooth.

Store in a sealed glass jar in the fridge for up to 3 weeks.

NOTE: To make this into a dip, simply add ½ cup raw cashews to the blender.

Basics

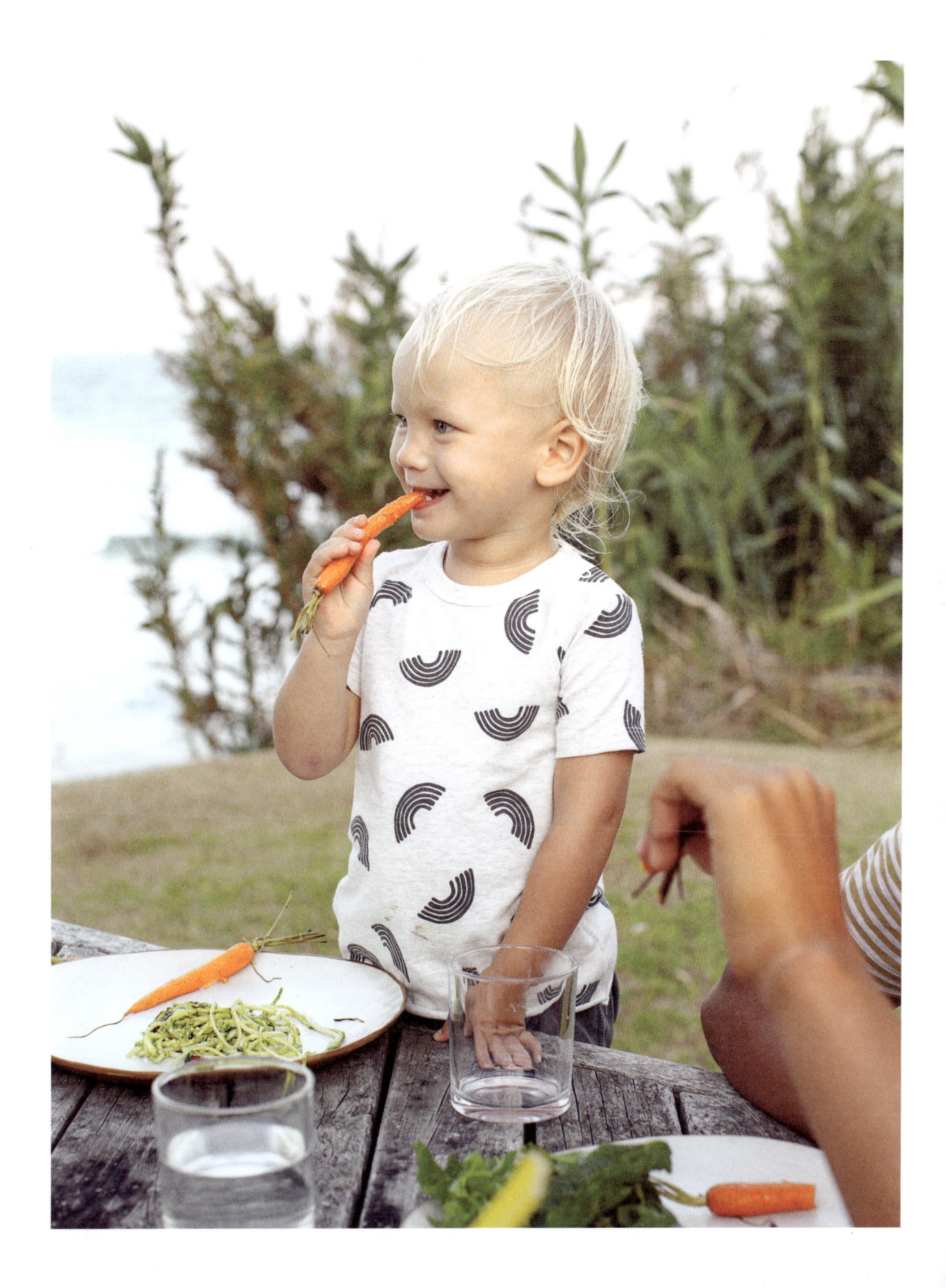

Flavour Boosters

HEMP AND CASHEW PARMESAN
MAKES ABOUT 1 CUP

This is the perfect flavour booster. It resembles Parmesan cheese so perfectly and not only adds amazing flavour to many dishes, but is also incredibly nutritious, boasting protein, magnesium and vitamin B$_{12}$. This is another awesome plant-based staple that I'll often sprinkle over pastas, salads, pizzas or roast vegetables.

½ cup raw cashews
¼ cup hempseeds
¼ cup nutritional yeast
½ teaspoon garlic powder
½ teaspoon onion powder
¼ teaspoon sea salt

Place all the ingredients in a food processor and blend for about 10 seconds, until the cashews are broken down and resemble finely grated Parmesan cheese.

Store in a sealed glass jar in the fridge for up to 3 weeks.

DUKKHA
MAKES ABOUT 1½ CUPS

Dukkha is seriously addictive. It's a fantastic fusion of herbs, nuts, seeds and spices that add a beautiful Middle Eastern touch to any meal. Originating from Egypt, it adds the most wonderfully crunchy texture and flavour. It's commonly used with soups, dips and bread, but my favourite way to enjoy it is sprinkled over salads.

½ cup hazelnuts
¼ cup almonds
2 tablespoons sesame seeds
2 tablespoons sunflower seeds
1 tablespoon cumin seeds
1 tablespoon coriander seeds
½ teaspoon fennel seeds
⅛ teaspoon ground allspice
1 teaspoon sea salt
¼ teaspoon ground pepper
dried herbs such as oregano, thyme or mixed herbs (optional)

Place all the ingredients in a food processor and blitz for about 10 seconds, until the nuts are broken down.

Store in a sealed jar or container in the fridge for up to 4 weeks.

ALMOND BARBECUE TOPPERS

MAKES ABOUT 1 CUP

A fresh batch of these tasty little beauties won't last long. The smoked paprika combined with the tamari creates a cheesy, smoky and salty barbecue flavour. They make for an ideal crunchy topper on salads, pastas, soups, veges or even eaten by the handful as a snack.

1 cup raw sliced almonds
½ teaspoon olive oil
1½ tablespoons tamari
1½ tablespoons smoked paprika

Place all the ingredients in a small bowl and mix to coat the almonds in the mixture.

Heat a small frying pan over medium-high heat. Add the almond mix and cook, mixing frequently, for about 4 minutes, until the almonds are crispy and fragrant.

Once completely cooled, store in a sealed jar for up to 7 days.

NOTE: For a bacon-style topper, replace the sliced almonds with coconut chips.

RAW RELISH

MAKES ABOUT 1½ CUPS

I love this simple sweetcorn relish. It's sweet, juicy and slightly tangy, with a warm, earthy flavour from the cumin seeds. Serve it as a salsa over fritters, wedges, Buddha bowls, salads, roast potatoes and Mexican food.

about 2½ cups fresh sweetcorn kernels
½ red capsicum, deseeded
¼ cup red onion, diced
1 large clove garlic, diced
1½ tablespoons apple cider vinegar
1 teaspoon mustard powder
2 teaspoons cumin seeds
1 teaspoon pure maple syrup
½ teaspoon sea salt

Place all the ingredients in a food processor and blend for about 10 seconds, until it resembles a chunky relish. Be careful not to over-blend, as it will turn into liquid.

Store in a sealed jar in the fridge for up to 5–7 days.

NOTE: Two large corn cobs should give you enough corn kernels.

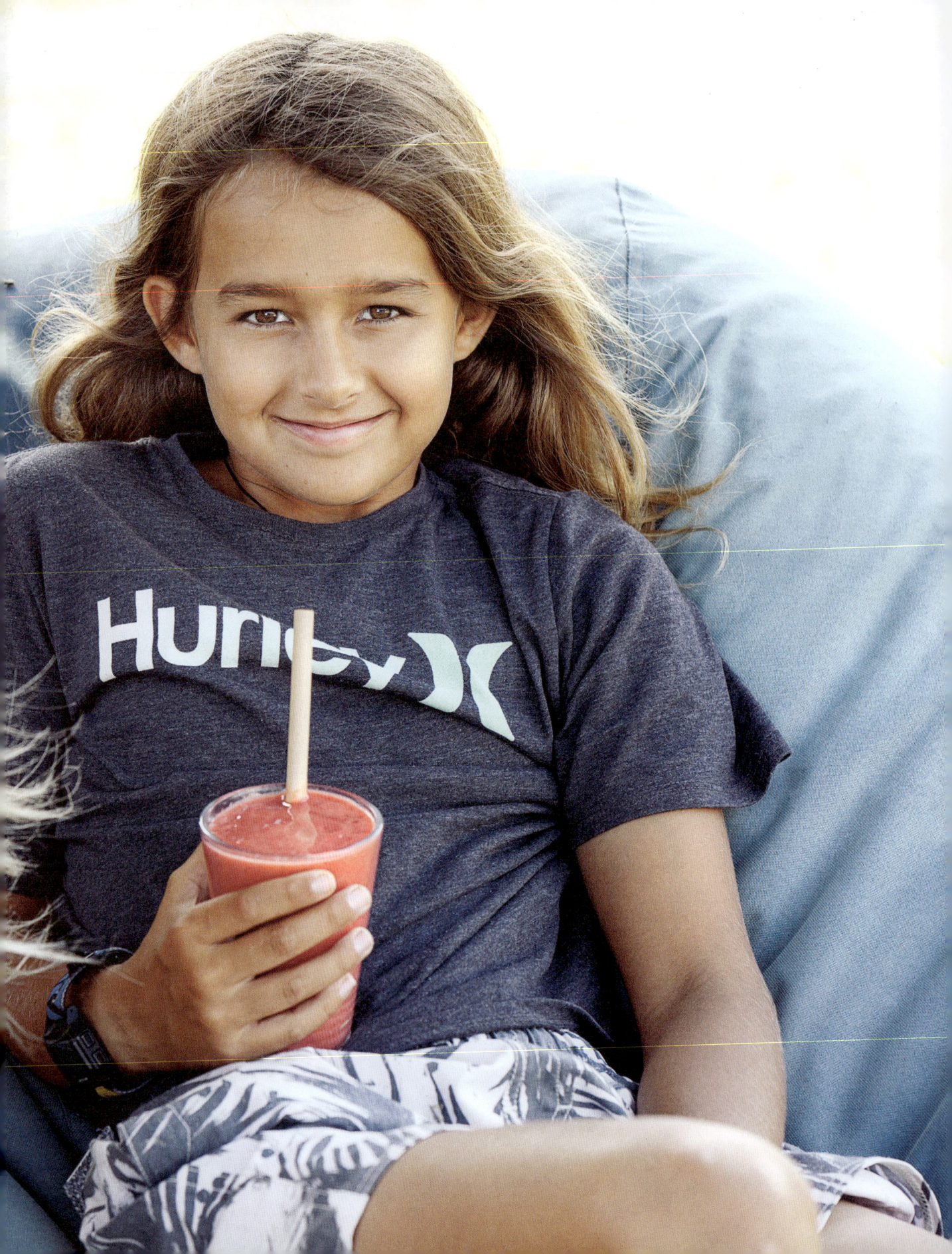

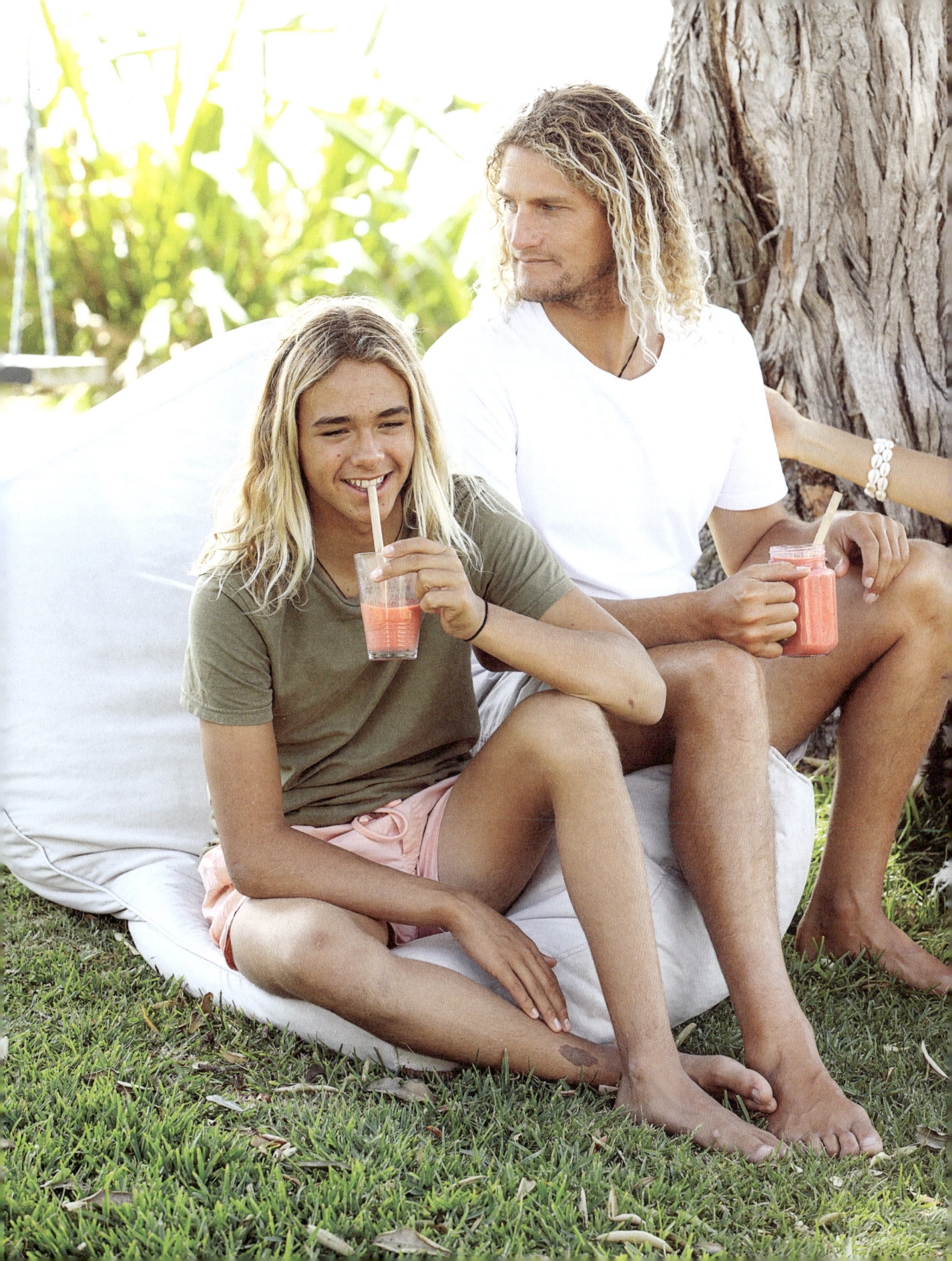

Sweeteners and Spreads

DATE SYRUP

MAKES ABOUT 2 CUPS

Date syrup is a fantastic sweetener with many health benefits. It's an ideal alternative to sugar, and can be used much like pure maple syrup, molasses, brown rice syrup or agave nectar in smoothies, dressings, marinades, raw treats and baking.

1 cup Medjool dates
1½ cups water
1 teaspoon lemon juice (optional)

Place all the ingredients in a blender and blend for about 15 seconds, or until smooth.

Store in a sealed glass jar in the fridge for up to 3 weeks.

CARAMEL SAUCE

MAKES ABOUT ¾–1 CUP

This gooey caramel sauce is absolutely divine and makes a guilt-free dessert topping, without the overload of refined sugar or additives.

1 cup medjool dates, pitted
⅓ cup pure maple syrup
½ cup full-fat coconut milk
1 teaspoon pure vanilla extract
pinch of sea salt

Place all the ingredients in a high-speed blender and blend for about 30 seconds, or until very smooth and creamy. Add more coconut milk for a thinner consistency.

Store in a sealed jar in the fridge for up to 7 days.

RAW RASPBERRY CHIA JAM

MAKES ABOUT 1 CUP

This is a healthy, low-sugar alternative to regular jam, sweetened naturally by the maple and raspberries, creating a beautifully healthy condiment. When chia seeds are combined with liquid, they produce a gelatinous texture that helps things to set, so they are perfect for making jam and also work a treat as an egg replacement. Try this beautiful jam on all of your favourite things.

1 cup fresh raspberries
1 tablespoon water
1 tablespoon lemon juice
1 tablespoon chia seeds
1 tablespoon pure maple syrup

In a small bowl, mash the raspberries with a fork. Add the water, lemon juice, chia seeds and maple syrup, and stir thoroughly to combine.

Let sit in the fridge for at least 1 hour before serving, to allow the jam to set.

Store in a sealed jar in the fridge for up to 2 weeks.

CACAO HAZELNUT SPREAD

MAKES ABOUT 1½ CUPS

This creamy hazelnut spread is a much healthier version of the classic store-bought ones. It's perfect as a toast topper, in a smoothie bowl or try it dolloped into a pitted medjool date, sprinkled with crushed peanuts, then placed in the freezer for the perfect chewy, nutty chocolate treat.

1 cup hazelnuts
3 tablespoons cacao powder
½ cup pure maple syrup
¾ cup canned coconut milk
½ teaspoon pure vanilla extract

Preheat the oven to 180°C (350°F) fan bake. Line a baking tray with baking paper.

Place the hazelnuts on the tray and spread out evenly in a single layer. Bake, tossing once or twice, for about 8 minutes, until fragrant. Watch closely for the last few minutes to avoid burning.

Remove and place in a blender along with the remaining ingredients. Blend until smooth.

Transfer to a sealed jar and place in the fridge to thicken for about 1 hour.

Store in the fridge for 2 weeks.

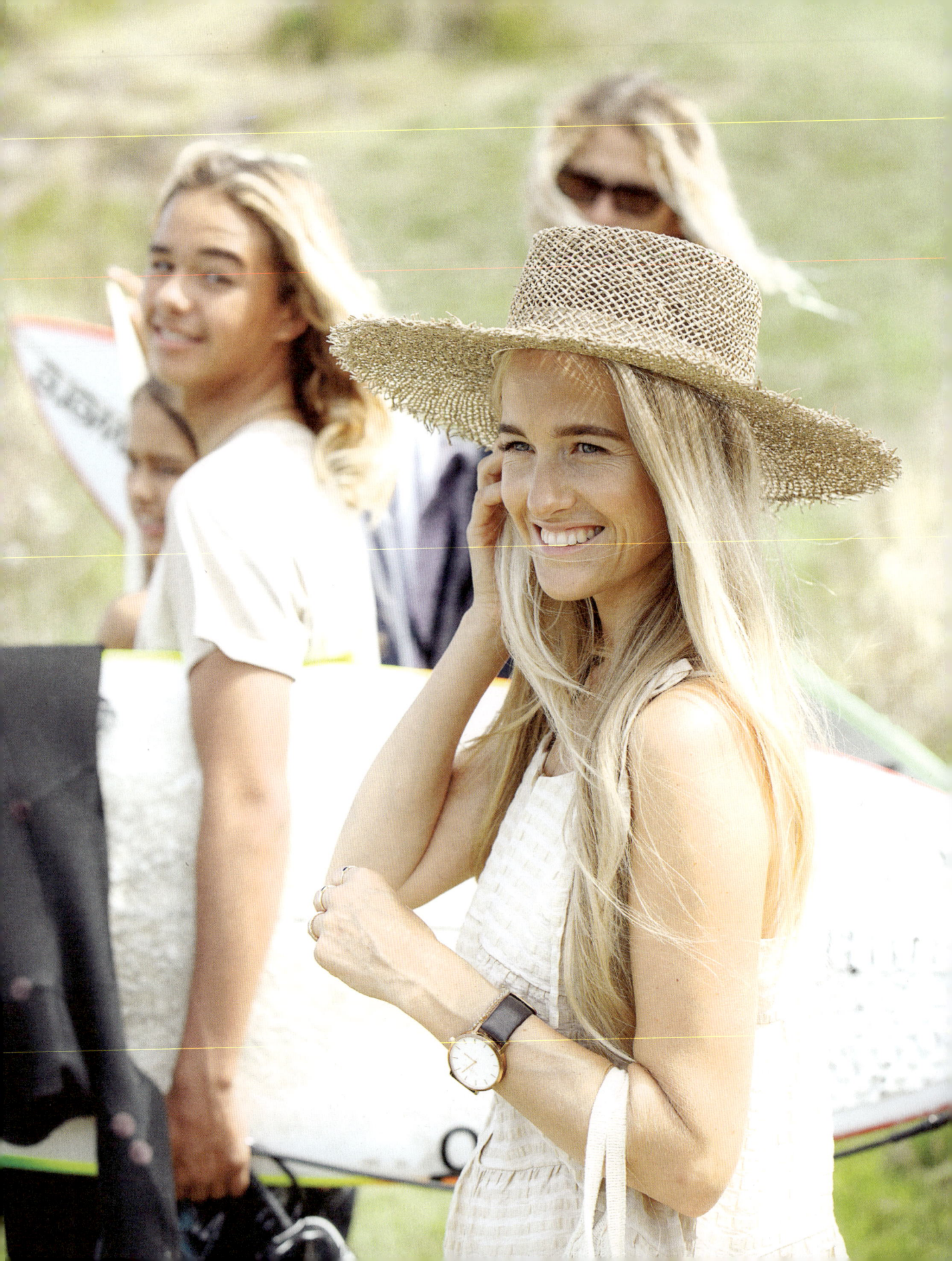

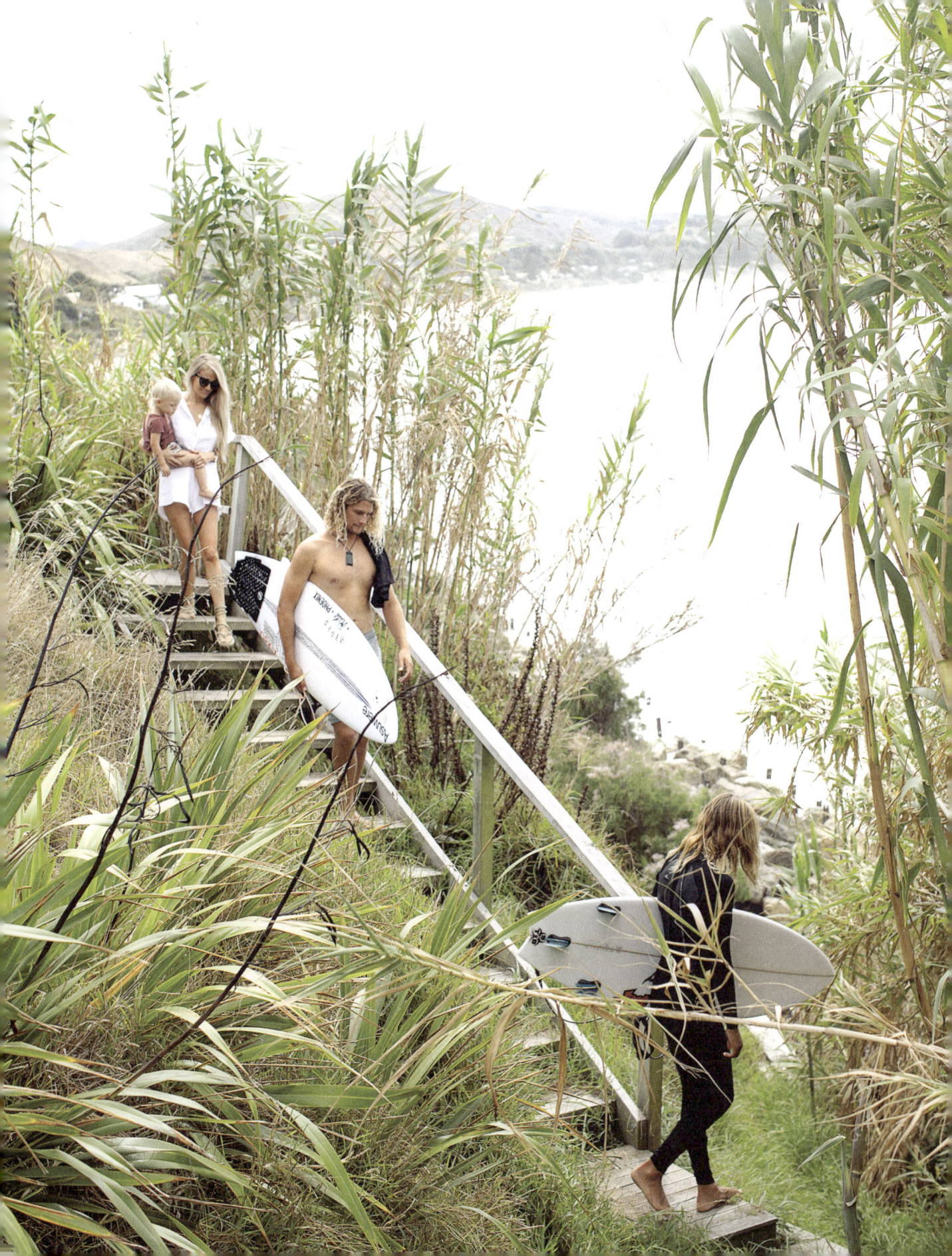

Vegan Milk

HEMP MILK

MAKES 1.5 LITRES (52 FL OZ)

Hemp milk would have to be one of the quickest and healthiest plant milks to make, which is why it's my absolute favourite. This silky nut-like blend is packed with a long list of nutrients, including protein, essential fatty acids, phosphorus, magnesium and iron. It's amazing as a drink or try it with my Wholesome Cacao Pops (see page 84), fresh fruit or as a creamy addition to smoothies, dips and dressings.

1 cup hempseeds
6 medjool dates, pitted
1.5 litres (52 fl oz) filtered water

Place all the ingredients in a 2-litre (70-fl oz) capacity blender and blend for about 10–15 seconds, until smooth and creamy.

Store in a sealed jug or bottle in the fridge for 3–5 days.

ALMOND MILK

MAKES 1 LITRE (35 FL OZ)

Almonds are a great source of vitamin E, magnesium and copper, making this creamy milk a great alternative to cow's milk. This recipe is so easy to make, and unlike many store-bought versions it contains no added sugar, salt or oil.

1 cup almonds, soaked in water for at least 6 hours
1 litre (35 fl oz) filtered water
1 teaspoon pure vanilla extract (optional)
2 medjool dates, pitted (optional)

Rinse and drain the almonds.

Place the almonds and water in a blender and blend for about 2–3 minutes on high speed, until the mixture has a white, creamy consistency.

Place a piece of muslin cloth over a clean jug—at least 1 litre (35 fl oz) capacity—and pour over the almond milk. Wring out the cloth to remove any extra milk. Transfer to a clean, sealable bottle.

Store in the fridge for up to 5 days, or freeze for up to 1 month.

Wraps, Tacos and Pastry

GARLIC CHICKPEA FLATBREAD

SERVE 4–8 AS A SIDE

This soft, herby bread makes the perfect accompaniment to soups, curries, dips and salad, with the most beautiful herb and garlic aromas. Try it with my Roast Cauliflower, Capsicum and Chickpea Yellow Curry (see page 164) for a beautiful warming meal.

1 cup chickpea flour (besan)
1 teaspoon garlic powder
½ teaspoon onion powder
¼ teaspoon sea salt
1 teaspoon olive oil
¾ cup water
½ teaspoon caraway seeds
1 large clove garlic, grated

Preheat the oven to 180°C (350°F) fan bake. Line a baking tray with baking paper.

Whisk together the chickpea flour, garlic powder, onion powder, sea salt, olive oil and water until all the clumps are blended.

Pour the batter onto the prepared tray and sprinkle over the caraway seeds and fresh garlic. Bake for 20–25 minutes, until golden with crispy edges.

EASY CHICKPEA TACOS

MAKES 6 TACOS

These are so easy to whip up and are gluten-free, free of nasty additives and won't break up while you're filling them. Tacos can form the basis of a fun, tasty and wholesome spread with endless filling options; try them with my Balsamic Cajun Jackfruit (see page 200).

1 cup chickpea flour (besan)
½ cup tapioca flour
1 cup water
½ teaspoon sea salt
1 teaspoon onion powder
oil for cooking

In a large bowl, combine all the ingredients and mix until combined into a smooth batter.

Heat a dash of oil in a large non-stick frying pan over medium heat.

Pour about 3 tablespoons of the batter into the pan. Holding the handle, swirl the pan around to form the batter into a circle.

Cook for about 1 minute, or until bubbles begin to form. Flip and cook for another minute on the other side. Remove and set aside. Repeat the steps with the remaining batter.

Store in an airtight container in the fridge for 3–5 days.

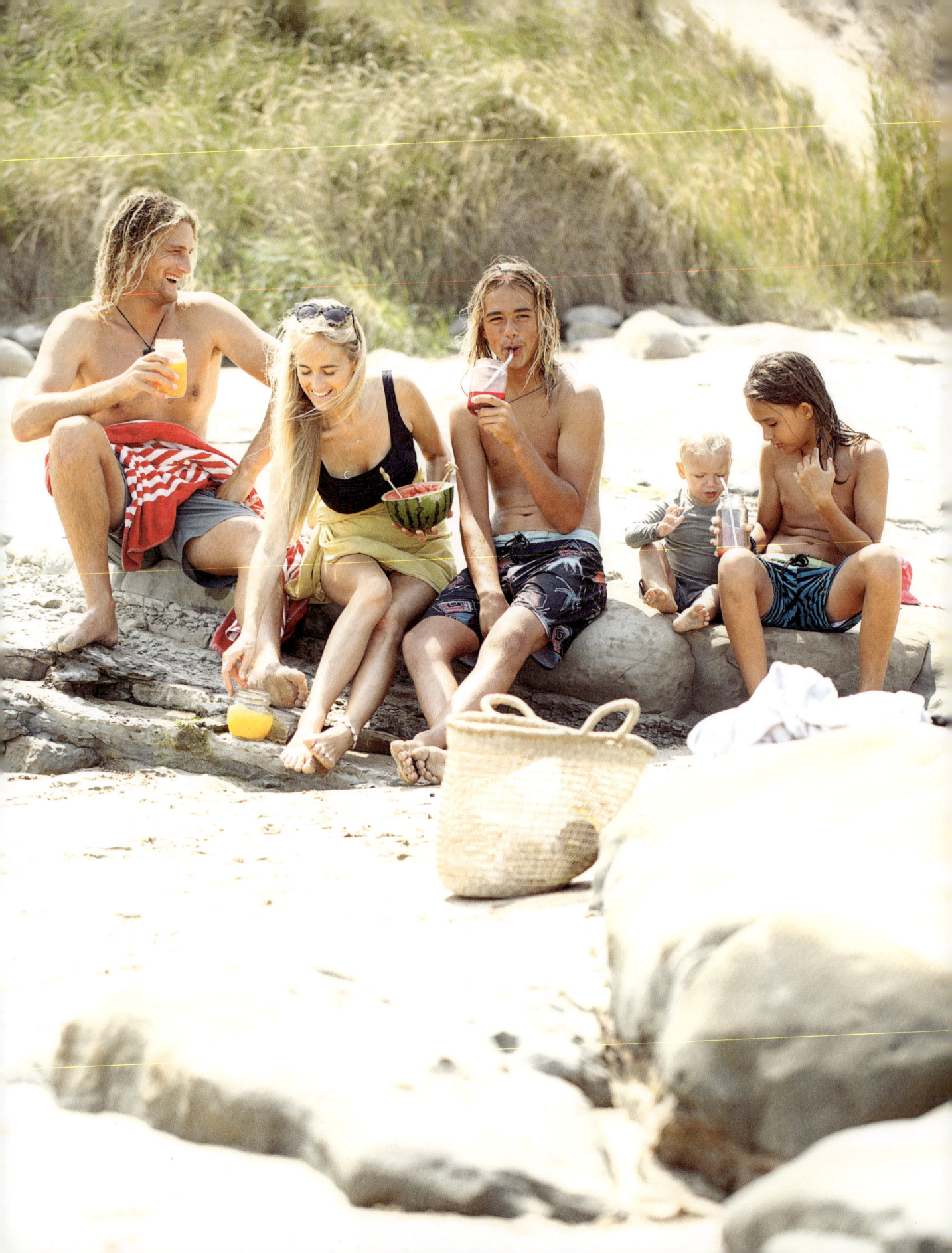

EASY BUCKWHEAT WRAPS

MAKES 4 LARGE OR 6 SMALL WRAPS

I'm one of those people who avidly reads the back of any packaged food to ensure the ingredients are 100 per cent natural. I've noticed that wraps, in particular, are full of many additives and preservatives, which is why I wanted to include these gluten-free, 100 per cent natural buckwheat wraps in the book. They keep well in the fridge and don't rip when you're filling and eating them. Fill them with salad for lunch boxes, use them in Mexican dishes such as burritos and enchiladas, or try them filled with shredded red cabbage and fresh greens topped with my Sesame Baked Falafel Bites with Tzatziki Dip (see page 224) for a Mediterranean-style meal.

1¼ cups buckwheat flour
1½ cups water
¼ cup tapioca flour
½ teaspoon sea salt
1 teaspoon oil, plus extra for cooking

In a large bowl, combine all the ingredients and mix until combined into a smooth batter.

Heat a dash of oil in a large non-stick frying pan over medium heat.

Pour ⅓ cup (or ½ cup if making larger wraps) of the mixture into the pan. Holding the handle, swirl the pan around to form the batter into a circle.

Cook for 1–2 minutes, or until bubbles begin to form. Flip and cook for another 1–2 minutes on the other side. Remove and set aside. Repeat the steps with the remaining batter.

Store in an airtight container in the fridge for 3–5 days.

BUCKWHEAT AND CHIA PASTRY

MAKES ENOUGH PASTRY FOR ONE 20 CM (8 IN) PIE

This makes the perfect gluten-free pastry to use in all of your favourite dishes. It's easy to make, requires minimal ingredients and has a light, mild flavour. I've followed various gluten-free recipes in the past that didn't turn out as they should have, so I experimented a lot with this pastry to ensure it was just right. You could use flax eggs instead of chia eggs by simply replacing the chia seeds with ground flaxseed (linseed).

2 tablespoons chia seeds
6 tablespoons water
1¼ cups buckwheat flour
⅓ cup tapioca flour
2 tablespoons coconut oil
2 tablespoons water
pinch of sea salt

Prepare the chia eggs by placing the chia seeds and water in a small bowl, whisking to combine and letting sit for 5–10 minutes. This will allow the mixture to thicken and form a gel.

In a large bowl, combine the buckwheat flour, tapioca flour, coconut oil, water, salt and chia eggs. Mix with a wooden spoon until a thick dough is formed.

Place the dough on a clean, floured surface and knead for about 30 seconds, until you have a well-combined ball of dough. If the dough is too sticky, simply add a light sprinkle of buckwheat flour and knead again.

On a floured surface, roll out the dough, enough to cover a 20 cm (8 in) round pie dish. It should be about 2 mm (¹⁄₁₆ in) thick. Carefully peel off the pastry and place it onto a greased pie dish, trimming off any excess pastry from around the edges of the dish.

If you are baking the pie for 40–45 minutes, there is no need to blind bake this pastry.

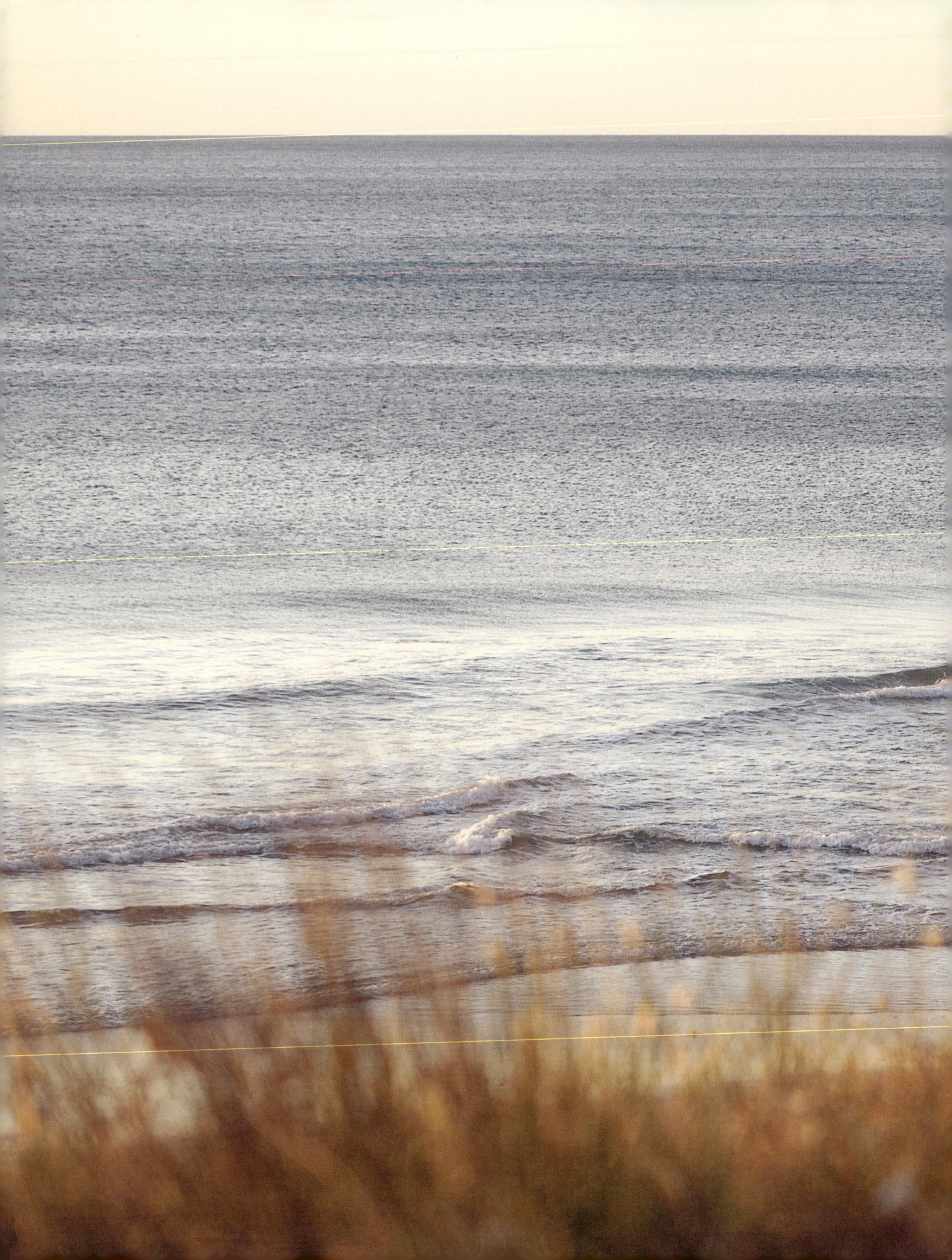

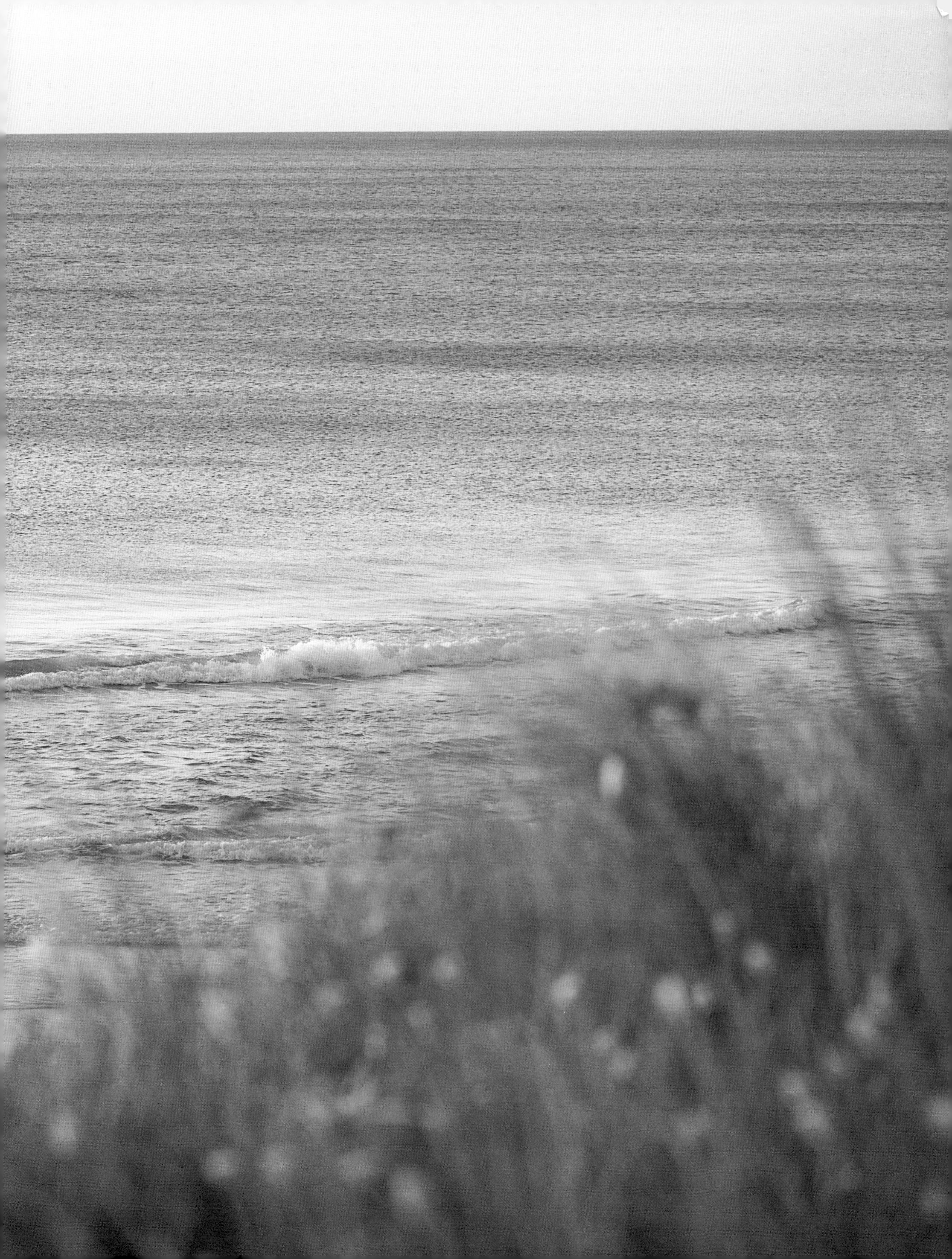

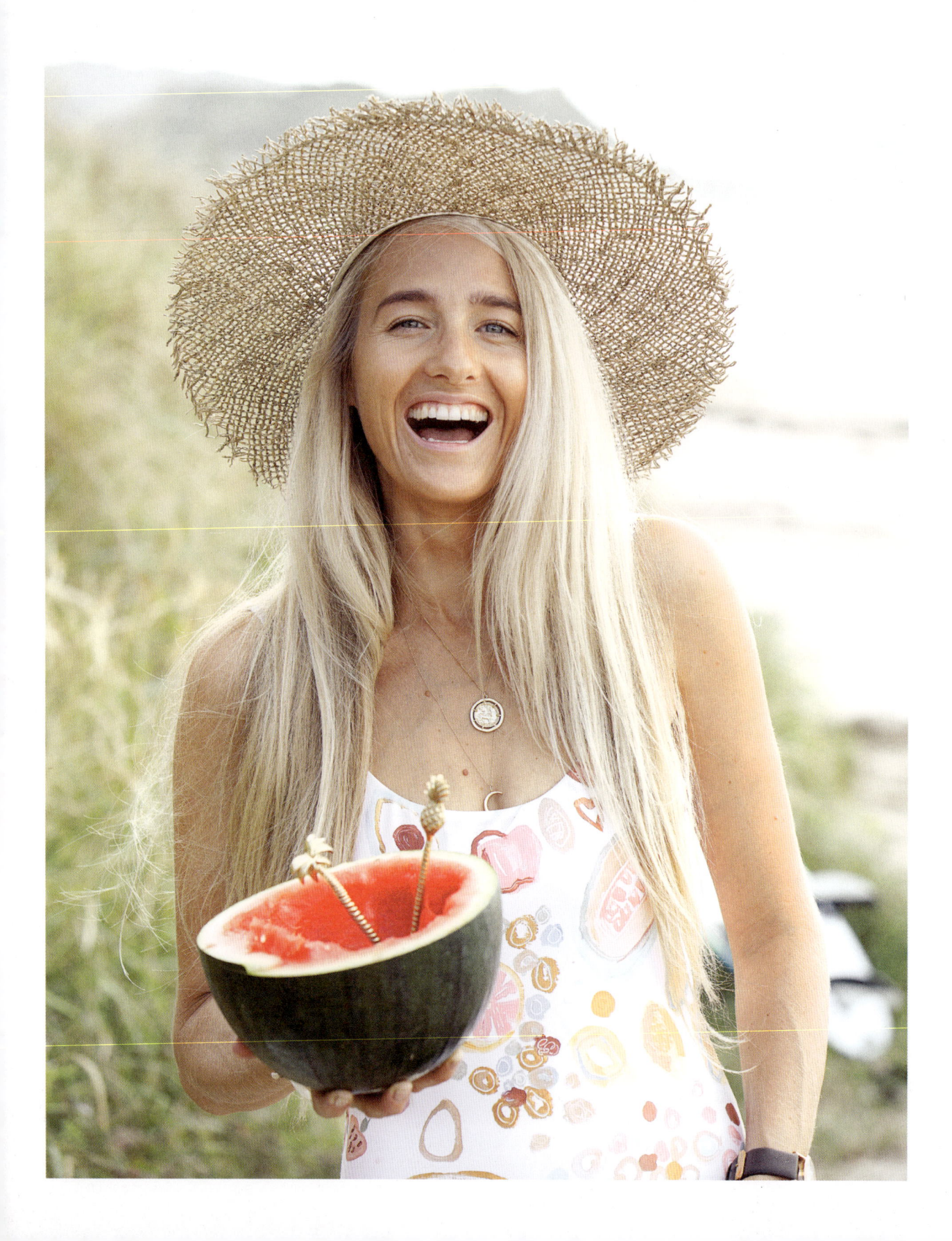

Thank You

Wow! Creating this book has definitely been my biggest challenge yet! I am so grateful for the opportunity to share my love of a plant-based lifestyle. I couldn't have done it without the help of these amazing people.

Firstly, Jenny Hellen. Thank you so much for seeing the potential in this book and giving me this incredible opportunity to make a dream come true! Your advice and encouragement throughout the entire process gave me the confidence to really bring this book to life. Leonie Freeman and Leanne McGregor, you are so lovely and such a dream to work with—thank you for being so patient and making the editing process such a breeze. And to the rest of the team at Allen & Unwin—a big thank you!

My gorgeous boys, Eli, Milo and Jai—we did it! Thank you for your endless patience as I worked away. You are such a big part of Raw and Free and continue to inspire me along this journey. Rich, thank you for always believing in me, encouraging me and supporting me in everything I do! It means more to me than you will ever know.

Mum, a mountain of gratitude for the endless kitchen clean ups, supermarket runs and for being the best team leader throughout our shooting weeks—honestly, you were a true superstar and I couldn't have done it without you!

My beautiful sister, Elly. Your love, support and encouragement means the world to me. Thank you for your positive feedback throughout each stage of this book, and for helping me immensely during your time home from London.

My brother-in-law, Jack, thank you for your amazing advice and encouragement right from the very beginning of this project.

My best friend, Nicole, thank you for testing so many of my recipes, gathering endless amounts of greens and herbs and for being the best kitchen hand I could have ever asked for. You are such a legend!

My photographer, Lottie Hedley. I can't thank you enough for the magic you brought to this book. You understood my vision for it and went above and beyond to capture so many beautiful images! This book truly wouldn't be what it is without your love, passion and dedication.

Kate Barraclough, you designed this so beautifully—thank you for your input and hard work. Síana Clifford, many thanks for your thorough editing, it made the process run so smoothly.

Hayley, thank you for creating such a beautiful, vibrant fruit platter that fits so perfectly into this book. Rosanne Calabrese—your extensive knowledge of the body is a true gift to us all. Thank you for your quote and checking over a few of my words. Sally Cameron, I'm so thankful for your helpful advice prior to shooting and for allowing us the use of your amazing props. To everyone else involved, those who helped with the cover shoot, props or collected herbs from their gardens—thank you, thank you, thank you! My friends and family—please know I'm so grateful for your encouragement, love and support.

And lastly, my wonderful Raw and Free followers. I am so grateful for your continuous support—it truly means the world to me!

Index

Aïoli 276
Alkalising Refresher smoothie 52
All-Day Brekkie Buddha Bowl with Balsamic Yoghurt Mushrooms 100
almonds
  Almond Barbecue Toppers 283
  Dukkha 282
  Green Lentil, Kale, Caper, Mint and Hemp Salad with Crushed Almonds 114
  Himalayan Almond Crackle Clusters 270
  Italian Herb Cracker Rounds 230
  Roast Cauliflower Trees, Curried Yoghurt, Parsley and Toasted Almond Flakes 124
  Rosemary and Thyme Hasselbacks with the Best Ever Creamy Coleslaw 182
  Superfood Granola Bars 232
apple cider vinegar 42
apples
  Apple Slaw 200
  Fruity Nut Bowl with Poppyseed Yoghurt 86
  Green Goodness juice 70
  Revitalise Juice 70
  Sweet Celery Juice 70
avocados
  All-Day Brekkie Buddha Bowl with Balsamic Yoghurt Mushrooms 100
  Avocado, Lemon and Pistachio Fruity Whip 66
  Balsamic Cajun Jackfruit Tacos with Apple Slaw 200
  Black Bean Mexican Bowls with Kūmara and Vegan Sour Cream 188
  Brown Lentil, Beetroot and Avocado Salad with Orange Vinaigrette and Sumac Tahini 134
  Buckwheat, Mesclun, Roast Hazelnuts and Avocado with Apricot and Ginger Dressing 112
  Butter Bean, Lime and Avocado Smash 98

  Citrus Chilli Carrots, Avocado and Pine Nuts 144
  Everyday Superfood Salad with Sweet Lemon Tahini Drizzle 154
  Key Lime Mousse Tart 254
  Mexi Mushrooms and Smashed Avocado with Chipotle Yoghurt Drizzle 138
  Rainbow Wraps and Cucumber Rolls with Thai Lime and Coconut Dipping Sauce 214
Balsamic Cajun Jackfruit Tacos with Apple Slaw 200
bananas
  Avocado, Lemon and Pistachio Fruity Whip 66
  Berry Bliss smoothie 52
  Fruity Nut Bowl with Poppyseed Yoghurt 86
  Green Glow smoothie 52
  Hemp Chocolate Shakes 268
  Mango Madness Bowl with Granola, Coconut and Fresh Fruit 58
  Pineapple Paradise smoothie 54
  Raspberry and Mango Fruity Whip 64
  Raw Banana Bread Bliss Balls 236
  Spirulina Energiser 52
  Sunrise Açaí Bowl with Fresh Granola, Cacao Nibs and Fresh Fruit 56
  Sweet Strawberry Fields with Fresh Strawberries and Coconut 60
  Tropical Love smoothie 54
  Tropical Passion Fruit Fruity Whip 66
  Zesty Strawberry smoothie 54
Banoffee Fudge Bites 250
basil
  Basil Pesto and Zucchini Pasta Salad with Almond Barbecue Toppers 146
  Basil Pesto Potato Top Pie 184
  Hemp, Spinach and Basil Pesto 222
beans, canned

Basil Pesto Potato Top Pie 184
Black Bean Mexican Bowls with Kūmara and Vegan Sour Cream 188
Butter Bean, Lime and Avocado Smash 98
beans, green
  Lemongrass, Lime and Coconut Thai Curry with Crispy Potatoes 172
  Peanut Satay Potato Salad with Raw Greens and Black Sesame 130
  Spiced Sorghum, Goji Berries, Pistachios, Green Beans and Lemony Yoghurt 118
beetroot
  Beetroot, Orange, Walnut and Quinoa Patties, with Lime, Dill and Yoghurt Dressing 202
  Brown Lentil, Beetroot and Avocado Salad with Orange Vinaigrette and Sumac Tahini 134
  Everyday Superfood Salad with Sweet Lemon Tahini Drizzle 154
  Raw Cleansing Beetroot, Carrot and Walnut Salad 116
  Revitalise Juice 70
  Revitalising Raw Beetroot Hummus 220
Black Bean Mexican Bowls with Kūmara and Vegan Sour Cream 188
Black Rice, Pomegranate and Mesclun with Lemon Poppyseed Dressing 126
bliss balls 236–38
blueberries
  Blueberry Cheesecake 266
  Fruity Nut Bowl with Poppyseed Yoghurt 86
  Sunrise Açaí Bowl with Fresh Granola, Cacao Nibs and Fresh Fruit 56
broccoli
  Dukkha-baked Kūmara, Raw Broccoli and Pine Nut Salad with Sumac Tahini Drizzle 194
  Moreish Potato and Chive Bake 176

Raw Broccoli and Sunflower Seed Salad with Creamy Cashew Dressing 122
broccolini
   Lemongrass, Lime and Coconut Thai Curry with Crispy Potatoes 172
   Teriyaki Rainbow Quinoa 174
Brown Lentil, Beetroot and Avocado Salad with Orange Vinaigrette and Sumac Tahini 134
Brown Rice Asian Noodle Salad with Sesame Lime Dressing 156
Buckwheat and Chia Pastry 293
Buckwheat, Mesclun, Roast Hazelnuts and Avocado with Apricot and Ginger Dressing 112
Butter Bean, Lime and Avocado Smash 98

cabbage
   Apple Slaw 200
   Brown Rice Asian Noodle Salad with Sesame Lime Dressing 156
   Everyday Superfood Salad with Sweet Lemon Tahini Drizzle 154
   Rainbow Wraps and Cucumber Rolls with Thai Lime and Coconut Dipping Sauce 214
   Raw Rainbow Thai Salad with Thai Basil and Lime Dressing 132
   Rosemary and Thyme Hasselbacks with the Best Ever Creamy Coleslaw 182
   Sesame Peanutty Pumpkin with Sweet Miso Asian Slaw 192
cacao powder 46
   Cacao Hazelnut Spread 287
   Choc Coconut Quinoa Puff Snack Squares 234
   Fruit and Nut Chocolate 260
   Gooey Caramel Brownie Slice 262
   Hemp Chocolate Shakes 268
   Linseed and Cacao Bircher with Raspberry Jam 90
   Raspberry Bounty Bars 264
   Wholesome Cacao Pops 84
Caesar Salad Dressing 278
capsicums
   Basil Pesto Potato Top Pie 184
   Eggplant, Jackfruit and Black Sesame in Lime-infused Almond Gravy 168
   Greek Black Rice-stuffed Capsicums with Caper and Parsley Yoghurt 196
   Indian Jackfruit Makhani 162
   Lemongrass, Lime and Coconut Thai Curry with Crispy Potatoes 172
   Mini Herb and Fennel Frittatas 94
   Paprika Alfredo Pasta with Hemp and Cashew Parmesan 180
   Pumpkin, Kūmara and Capsicum Dip 216
   Rainbow Wraps and Cucumber Rolls with Thai Lime and Coconut Dipping Sauce 214
   Raw Rainbow Thai Salad with Thai Basil and Lime Dressing 132
   Raw Sweet Chilli Sauce 280
   Roast Cauliflower, Capsicum and Chickpea Yellow Curry 164
   Teriyaki Rainbow Quinoa 174
Caramel Sauce 286
Caraway Potato and Chickpea Mingle with Garden Greens and Ranch Dressing 204
carrots
   Apple Slaw 200
   Carrot, Coconut, Cumin, Orange and Black Quinoa Salad 142
   Cauliflower Kofta Balls with Mint Aïoli 206
   Citrus Chilli Carrots, Avocado and Pine Nuts 144
   Citrus Turmeric Juice 70
   Creamy Sunflower and Vegetable Tart 186
   Everyday Superfood Salad with Sweet Lemon Tahini Drizzle 154
   Indian Jackfruit Makhani 162
   Italian Lentil Bolognaise with Raw Zucchini Noodles 166
   Nacho Cheese Sauce 280
   Quick 'N' Easy Carrot Fritters 102
   Rainbow Wraps and Cucumber Rolls with Thai Lime and Coconut Dipping Sauce 214
   Raw Cleansing Beetroot, Carrot and Walnut Salad 116
   Raw Rainbow Thai Salad with Thai Basil and Lime Dressing 132
   Raw Wholesome Carrot Cake with Lemon Frosting 248
   Revitalise Juice 70
   Rosemary and Thyme Hasselbacks with the Best Ever Creamy Coleslaw 182
cashews 42–43
   Aïoli 276
   Blueberry Cheesecake 266
   Caesar Salad Dressing 278
   Cashew Cheese Sauce 279
   Creamy Cashew Dressing 122
   Creamy Cashew Tahini Dressing 182
   Creamy Lemon and Ginger Dressing 140
   Easy Tropicana Cookies 240
   Hemp and Cashew Parmesan 282
   Indulgent Ginger Slice 252
   Lemon and Poppyseed Bliss Balls 236
   Lemon Frosting 248
   Lime, Herb and Chilli Cashews 228
   Mint Aïoli 276
   Paprika Alfredo Pasta with Hemp and Cashew Parmesan 180
   Ranch Dressing or Dip 278
   Raw Rainbow Thai Salad with Thai Basil and Lime Dressing 132
   Teriyaki Rainbow Quinoa 174
   The Ultimate Snickers Slice 256
   Vegan Sour Cream 279
cauliflower
   Cauliflower Kofta Balls with Mint Aïoli 206
   Cheesy Kale, Pesto and Pine Nut Pizza 198
   Middle Eastern Raw Cauliflower Tabouli with Sweet Roast Chickpeas 108
   Moreish Potato and Chive Bake 176
   Roast Cauliflower, Capsicum and Chickpea Yellow Curry 164
   Roast Cauliflower Trees, Curried Yoghurt, Parsley and Toasted Almond Flakes 124
celery
   Green Goodness juice 70
   Sweet Celery Juice 70
Cheesy Kale, Pesto and Pine Nut Pizza 198
Chewy 'N' Nutty Vanilla Maple Granola 82
chia seeds 43
   Blueberry Cheesecake 266
   Buckwheat and Chia Pastry 293
   Mango, Hemp and Chia Yoghurt 80
   Raw Raspberry Chia Jam 287
   Superfood Granola Bars 232

Very Berry Antioxidant Chia
  Pudding 76
chickpeas
  Caraway Potato and Chickpea
    Mingle with Garden Greens and
    Ranch Dressing 204
  Creamy Kale Caesar Salad with
    Chickpea Croutons and Hemp and
    Cashew Parmesan 128
  Middle Eastern Raw Cauliflower
    Tabouli with Sweet Roast
    Chickpeas 108
  Revitalising Raw Beetroot
    Hummus 220
  Roast Cauliflower, Capsicum and
    Chickpea Yellow Curry 164
  Sesame Baked Falafel Bites with
    Tzatziki Dip 224
Choc Coconut Quinoa Puff Snack
  Squares 234
Citrus Chilli Carrots, Avocado and
  Pine Nuts 144
Citrus Turmeric Juice 70
coconut 43
  bliss balls 236
  Carrot, Coconut, Cumin, Orange
    and Black Quinoa Salad 142
  Chewy 'N' Nutty Vanilla Maple
    Granola 82
  Choc Coconut Quinoa Puff Snack
    Squares 234
  Easy Tropicana Cookies 240
  Fruit and Nut Chocolate 260
  Key Lime Mousse Tart 254
  Raspberry Bounty Bars 264
  Raw Wholesome Carrot Cake with
    Lemon Frosting 248
  Raw Zesty Hemp 'Nola 78
  Wholesome Cacao Pops 84
  Wild Rice Salad with Lemongrass,
    Turmeric and Coconut
    Dressing 110
coconut yoghurt
  All-Day Brekkie Buddha Bowl with
    Balsamic Yoghurt Mushrooms 100
  Apple Slaw 200
  Caper and Parsley Yoghurt 196
  Chipotle Yoghurt Drizzle 138
  Fruity Nut Bowl with Poppyseed
    Yoghurt 86
  Key Lime Mousse Tart 254
  Lime, Dill and Yoghurt Dressing 202
  Roast Cauliflower Trees, Curried

  Yoghurt, Parsley and Toasted
    Almond Flakes 124
  Spiced Sorghum, Goji Berries,
    Pistachios, Green Beans and
    Lemony Yoghurt 118
  Creamy Kale Caesar Salad with
    Chickpea Croutons and Hemp and
    Cashew Parmesan 128
  Creamy Sunflower and Vegetable
    Tart 186
cucumber
  Peanut Satay Potato Salad with Raw
    Greens and Black Sesame 130
  Rainbow Wraps and Cucumber
    Rolls with Thai Lime and Coconut
    Dipping Sauce 214
  Tzatziki Dip 224
  Wild Rice Salad with Lemongrass,
    Turmeric and Coconut
    Dressing 110

dressings
  Aïoli 276
  Apricot and Ginger Dressing 112
  Caesar Salad Dressing 278
  Chipotle Yoghurt Drizzle 138
  Creamy Cashew Dressing 122
  Creamy Cashew Tahini Dressing 182
  Creamy Lemon and Ginger
    Dressing 140
  Lemon Poppyseed Dressing 126
  Lemongrass, Turmeric and Coconut
    Dressing 110
  Lime, Dill and Yoghurt Dressing 202
  Mint Aïoli 276
  Orange Vinaigrette 134
  Ranch Dressing or Dip 278
  Sesame Lime Dressing 156
  Sumac Tahini Drizzle 134
  Sweet Lemon Tahini Drizzle 154
  Sweet Miso Dressing 192
  Thai Basil and Lime Dressing 132
Dukkha 282
Dukkha-baked Kūmara, Raw Broccoli
  and Pine Nut Salad with Sumac
  Tahini Drizzle 194

Easy Buckwheat Wraps 293
Easy Chickpea Tacos 291
Easy Tropicana Cookies 240
Eggplant, Coriander and Balsamic
  Dip 218
Eggplant, Jackfruit and Black Sesame

  in Lime-infused Almond Gravy 168
  Everyday Superfood Salad with Sweet
    Lemon Tahini Drizzle 154

figs, dried
  Raw Zesty Hemp 'Nola 78
  Walnut, Pear and Fig Loaf 92
  Fruit and Nut Chocolate 260
  Fruity Nut Bowl with Poppyseed
    Yoghurt 86

Garlic Chickpea Flatbread 291
goji berries
  Spiced Sorghum, Goji Berries,
    Pistachios, Green Beans and
    Lemony Yoghurt 118
  Superfood Granola Bars 232
Gooey Caramel Brownie Slice 262
Greek Black Rice-stuffed Capsicums
  with Caper and Parsley Yoghurt 196
Green Glow smoothie 52
Green Goodness juice 70
Green Lentil, Kale, Caper, Mint
  and Hemp Salad with Crushed
  Almonds 114

hazelnuts
  Buckwheat, Mesclun, Roast
    Hazelnuts and Avocado with
    Apricot and Ginger Dressing 112
  Cacao Hazelnut Spread 287
  Dukkha 282
  Heavenly Hazelnut smoothie 54
hempseeds 44
  Everyday Superfood Salad with
    Sweet Lemon Tahini Drizzle 154
  Green Lentil, Kale, Caper, Mint
    and Hemp Salad with Crushed
    Almonds 114
  Hemp and Cashew Parmesan 282
  Hemp Chocolate Shakes 268
  Hemp Milk 290
  Hemp, Spinach and Basil Pesto 222
  Mango, Hemp and Chia Yoghurt 80
  Raw Zesty Hemp 'Nola 78
  Superfood Granola Bars 232
Herby Sunflower Seed Hummus 220
Himalayan Almond Crackle
  Clusters 270
hummus
  Herby Sunflower Seed Hummus 220
  Revitalising Raw Beetroot
    Hummus 220

Indian Jackfruit Makhani 162
Indulgent Ginger Slice 252
Italian Herb Cracker Rounds 230
Italian Lentil Bolognaise with Raw
   Zucchini Noodles 166

jackfruit 44
   Balsamic Cajun Jackfruit Tacos with
      Apple Slaw 200
   Eggplant, Jackfruit and Black
      Sesame in Lime-infused Almond
      Gravy 168
   Indian Jackfruit Makhani 162

kale
   Cheesy Kale, Pesto and Pine Nut
      Pizza 198
   Creamy Kale Caesar Salad with
      Chickpea Croutons and Hemp and
      Cashew Parmesan 128
   Everyday Superfood Salad with
      Sweet Lemon Tahini Drizzle 154
   Green Lentil, Kale, Caper, Mint
      and Hemp Salad with Crushed
      Almonds 114
   Italian Herb Cracker Rounds 230
Key Lime Mousse Tart 254
kūmara
   Black Bean Mexican Bowls
      with Kūmara and Vegan Sour
      Cream 188
   Creamy Sunflower and Vegetable
      Tart 186
   Dukkha-baked Kūmara, Raw
      Broccoli and Pine Nut Salad with
      Sumac Tahini Drizzle 194
   Moroccan Millet and Roast Kūmara
      Salad in Creamy Lemon and
      Ginger Dressing 140
   Pumpkin, Kūmara and Capsicum
      Dip 216

Lemongrass, Lime and Coconut Thai
   Curry with Crispy Potatoes 172
Lemongrass, Turmeric and Coconut
   Dressing 110
lemons
   Avocado, Lemon and Pistachio
      Fruity Whip 66
   Citrus Chilli Carrots, Avocado and
      Pine Nuts 144
   Citrus Turmeric Juice 70
   Creamy Lemon and Ginger
      Dressing 140
   Lemon and Poppyseed Bliss
      Balls 236
   Lemon Frosting 248
   Lemon Poppyseed Dressing 126
   Raspberry Lemonade Slushie 242
   Sweet Lemon Tahini Drizzle 154
   Vitamin C Blast juice 70
lentils
   Brown Lentil, Beetroot and Avocado
      Salad with Orange Vinaigrette and
      Sumac Tahini 134
   Green Lentil, Kale, Caper, Mint
      and Hemp Salad with Crushed
      Almonds 114
   Italian Lentil Bolognaise with Raw
      Zucchini Noodles 166
limes
   Butter Bean, Lime and Avocado
      Smash 98
   Eggplant, Jackfruit and Black
      Sesame in Lime-infused Almond
      Gravy 168
   Key Lime Mousse Tart 254
   Lemongrass, Lime and Coconut Thai
      Curry with Crispy Potatoes 172
   Lime, Dill and Yoghurt Dressing 202
   Lime, Herb and Chilli Cashews 228
   Sesame Lime Dressing 156
   Thai Basil and Lime Dressing 132
   Thai Lime and Coconut Dipping
      Sauce 214
linseed
   Italian Herb Cracker Rounds 230
   Linseed and Cacao Bircher with
      Raspberry Jam 90

macadamias
   Gooey Caramel Brownie Slice 262
   Macadamia Salted Caramel Bliss
      Balls 236
mangos
   Green Glow smoothie 52
   Mango, Hemp and Chia Yoghurt 80
   Mango Madness Bowl with Granola,
      Coconut and Fresh Fruit 58
   Raspberry and Mango Fruity
      Whip 64
   Tropical Love smoothie 54
   Tropical Passion Fruit Fruity
      Whip 66
   Zesty Strawberry smoothie 54
medjool dates 44–45

Caramel Sauce 286
Chewy 'N' Nutty Vanilla Maple
   Granola 82
Choc Coconut Quinoa Puff Snack
   Squares 234
Gooey Caramel Brownie Slice 262
Key Lime Mousse Tart 254
Peanut, Raisin and Cacao Bliss
   Balls 236, 238
Raw Wholesome Carrot Cake with
   Lemon Frosting 248
Raw Zesty Hemp 'Nola 78
Superfood Granola Bars 232
The Ultimate Snickers Slice 256
Mexi Mushrooms and Smashed
   Avocado with Chipotle Yoghurt
   Drizzle 138
Middle Eastern Raw Cauliflower
   Tabouli with Sweet Roast
   Chickpeas 108
millet
   Millet and Quinoa Loaf 96
   Moroccan Millet and Roast Kūmara
      Salad in Creamy Lemon and
      Ginger Dressing 140
Mini Herb and Fennel Frittatas 94
Mint Aïoli 276
Moreish Potato and Chive Bake 176
Moroccan Millet and Roast Kūmara
   Salad in Creamy Lemon and Ginger
   Dressing 140
mushrooms
   All-Day Brekkie Buddha Bowl with
      Balsamic Yoghurt Mushrooms 100
   Basil Pesto Potato Top Pie 184
   Cheesy Kale, Pesto and Pine Nut
      Pizza 198
   Creamy Sunflower and Vegetable
      Tart 186
   Eggplant, Jackfruit and Black
      Sesame in Lime-infused Almond
      Gravy 168
   Italian Lentil Bolognaise with Raw
      Zucchini Noodles 166
   Mexi Mushrooms and Smashed
      Avocado with Chipotle Yoghurt
      Drizzle 138
   Mini Herb and Fennel Frittatas 94
   Teriyaki Rainbow Quinoa 174

Nacho Cheese Sauce 280

oats
  Easy Tropicana Cookies 240
  Linseed and Cacao Bircher with Raspberry Jam 90
  Millet and Quinoa Loaf 96
  Raw Zesty Hemp 'Nola 78
  Superfood Granola Bars 232
oranges
  Beetroot, Orange, Walnut and Quinoa Patties, with Lime, Dill and Yoghurt Dressing 202
  Carrot, Coconut, Cumin, Orange and Black Quinoa Salad 142
  Citrus Chilli Carrots, Avocado and Pine Nuts 144
  Citrus Turmeric Juice 70
  Orange Vinaigrette 134
  Pineapple, Orange and Passion Fruit Slushie 242
  Revitalise Juice 70
  Tropical Love smoothie 54
  Vitamin C Blast juice 70

Paprika Alfredo Pasta with Hemp and Cashew Parmesan 180
passion fruit
  Pineapple, Orange and Passion Fruit Slushie 242
  Tropical Passion Fruit Fruity Whip 66
pasta
  Basil Pesto and Zucchini Pasta Salad with Almond Barbecue Toppers 146
  Paprika Alfredo Pasta with Hemp and Cashew Parmesan 180
peanuts
  Peanut, Raisin and Cacao Bliss Balls 236
  Peanut Satay Potato Salad with Raw Greens and Black Sesame 130
  The Ultimate Snickers Slice 256
pears
  Green Goodness juice 70
  Walnut, Pear and Fig Loaf 92
pineapple
  Easy Tropicana Cookies 240
  Pineapple, Orange and Passion Fruit Slushie 242
  Pineapple Paradise smoothie 54
  Tropical Love smoothie 54
  Vitamin C Blast juice 70
pistachios

Avocado, Lemon and Pistachio Fruity Whip 66
Black Rice, Pomegranate and Mesclun with Lemon Poppyseed Dressing 126
Greek Black Rice-stuffed Capsicums with Caper and Parsley Yoghurt 196
Spiced Sorghum, Goji Berries, Pistachios, Green Beans and Lemony Yoghurt 118
potatoes
  Basil Pesto Potato Top Pie 184
  Caraway Potato and Chickpea Mingle with Garden Greens and Ranch Dressing 204
  Cauliflower Kofta Balls with Mint Aïoli 206
  Lemongrass, Lime and Coconut Thai Curry with Crispy Potatoes 172
  Moreish Potato and Chive Bake 176
  Nacho Cheese Sauce 280
  Peanut Satay Potato Salad with Raw Greens and Black Sesame 130
  Potato Wedges, Sweetcorn and Cos Lettuce Salad in Creamy Caesar Dressing 150
  Rosemary and Thyme Hasselbacks with the Best Ever Creamy Coleslaw 182
pumpkin
  Creamy Sunflower and Vegetable Tart 186
  Pumpkin, Kūmara and Capsicum Dip 216
  Roast Butternut, Red Quinoa, Rocket and Cranberry Salad with Mint Aïoli 152
  Sesame Peanutty Pumpkin with Sweet Miso Asian Slaw 192

Quick 'N' Easy Carrot Fritters 102
quinoa 46
  All-Day Brekkie Buddha Bowl with Balsamic Yoghurt Mushrooms 100
  Beetroot, Orange, Walnut and Quinoa Patties, with Lime, Dill and Yoghurt Dressing 202
  Carrot, Coconut, Cumin, Orange and Black Quinoa Salad 142
  Choc Coconut Quinoa Puff Snack Squares 234
  Millet and Quinoa Loaf 96

Roast Butternut, Red Quinoa, Rocket and Cranberry Salad with Mint Aïoli 152
Teriyaki Rainbow Quinoa 174

Rainbow Wraps and Cucumber Rolls with Thai Lime and Coconut Dipping Sauce 214
Ranch Dressing or Dip 278
raspberries
  Raspberry and Mango Fruity Whip 64
  Raspberry Bounty Bars 264
  Raspberry Lemonade Slushie 242
  Raw Raspberry Chia Jam 287
  Very Berry Antioxidant Chia Pudding 76
Raw Banana Bread Bliss Balls 236
Raw Broccoli and Sunflower Seed Salad with Creamy Cashew Dressing 122
Raw Cleansing Beetroot, Carrot and Walnut Salad 116
Raw Rainbow Thai Salad with Thai Basil and Lime Dressing 132
Raw Relish 283
Raw Sweet Chilli Sauce 280
Raw Wholesome Carrot Cake with Lemon Frosting 248
Raw Zesty Hemp 'Nola 78
Revitalise Juice 70
Revitalising Raw Beetroot Hummus 220
rice
  Black Rice, Pomegranate and Mesclun with Lemon Poppyseed Dressing 126
  Greek Black Rice-stuffed Capsicums with Caper and Parsley Yoghurt 196
  Wild Rice Salad with Lemongrass, Turmeric and Coconut Dressing 110
rice puffs
  Himalayan Almond Crackle Clusters 270
  Wholesome Cacao Pops 84
Roast Butternut, Red Quinoa, Rocket and Cranberry Salad with Mint Aïoli 152
Roast Cauliflower, Capsicum and Chickpea Yellow Curry 164
Roast Cauliflower Trees, Curried

Yoghurt, Parsley and Toasted Almond Flakes 124
Rosemary and Thyme Hasselbacks with the Best Ever Creamy Coleslaw 182

sesame seeds
　Brown Rice Asian Noodle Salad with Sesame Lime Dressing 156
　Dukkha 282
　Eggplant, Jackfruit and Black Sesame in Lime-infused Almond Gravy 168
　Rainbow Wraps and Cucumber Rolls with Thai Lime and Coconut Dipping Sauce 214
　Raw Rainbow Thai Salad with Thai Basil and Lime Dressing 132
　Sesame Baked Falafel Bites with Tzatziki Dip 224
　Wild Rice Salad with Lemongrass, Turmeric and Coconut Dressing 110
　Sesame Peanutty Pumpkin with Sweet Miso Asian Slaw 192

spinach
　Alkalising Refresher smoothie 52
　All-Day Brekkie Buddha Bowl with Balsamic Yoghurt Mushrooms 100
　Caraway Potato and Chickpea Mingle with Garden Greens and Ranch Dressing 204
　Citrus Chilli Carrots, Avocado and Pine Nuts 144
　Creamy Sunflower and Vegetable Tart 186
　Everyday Superfood Salad with Sweet Lemon Tahini Drizzle 154
　Green Glow smoothie 52
　Green Goodness juice 70
　Hemp, Spinach and Basil Pesto 222
　Lemongrass, Turmeric and Coconut Dressing 110
　Mini Herb and Fennel Frittatas 94
　Paprika Alfredo Pasta with Hemp and Cashew Parmesan 180
　Spirulina Energiser 52
Spirulina Energiser smoothie 52

strawberries
　Sweet Strawberry Fields with Fresh Strawberries and Coconut 60
　Zesty Strawberry smoothie 54

sunflower seeds
　Creamy Sunflower and Vegetable Tart 186
　Dukkha 282
　Herby Sunflower Seed Hummus 220
　Raw Broccoli and Sunflower Seed Salad with Creamy Cashew Dressing 122
　Sunrise Açaí Bowl with Fresh Granola, Cacao Nibs and Fresh Fruit 56
　Superfood Granola Bars 232
　Sweet Strawberry Fields with Fresh Strawberries and Coconut 60

sweetcorn
　Black Bean Mexican Bowls with Kūmara and Vegan Sour Cream 188
　Potato Wedges, Sweetcorn and Cos Lettuce Salad in Creamy Caesar Dressing 150
　Raw Relish 283

tacos
　Balsamic Cajun Jackfruit Tacos with Apple Slaw 200
　Easy Chickpea Tacos 291

tahini 46–47
　Brown Lentil, Beetroot and Avocado Salad with Orange Vinaigrette and Sumac Tahini 134
　Creamy Cashew Tahini Dressing 182
　Eggplant, Coriander and Balsamic Dip 218
　Pumpkin, Kūmara and Capsicum Dip 216
　Revitalising Raw Beetroot Hummus 220
　Sumac Tahini Drizzle 134
　Sweet Lemon Tahini Drizzle 154
Teriyaki Rainbow Quinoa 174

tomatoes
　All-Day Brekkie Buddha Bowl with Balsamic Yoghurt Mushrooms 100
　Black Bean Mexican Bowls with Kūmara and Vegan Sour Cream 188
　Buckwheat, Mesclun, Roast Hazelnuts and Avocado with Apricot and Ginger Dressing 112
　Cheesy Kale, Pesto and Pine Nut Pizza 198
　Tropical Love smoothie 54
　Tropical Passion Fruit Fruity Whip 66

The Ultimate Snickers Slice 256
Vegan Sour Cream 279
Very Berry Antioxidant Chia Pudding 76
Vitamin C Blast juice 70

walnuts
　Beetroot, Orange, Walnut and Quinoa Patties, with Lime, Dill and Yoghurt Dressing 202
　Gooey Caramel Brownie Slice 262
　Raw Cleansing Beetroot, Carrot and Walnut Salad 116
　Raw Wholesome Carrot Cake with Lemon Frosting 248
　Walnut, Pear and Fig Loaf 92
　Watermelon and Mint juice 70
　Wholesome Cacao Pops 84
　Wild Rice Salad with Lemongrass, Turmeric and Coconut Dressing 110

wraps
　Easy Buckwheat Wraps 293
　Rainbow Wraps and Cucumber Rolls with Thai Lime and Coconut Dipping Sauce 214

Zesty Strawberry smoothie 54

zucchini
　Basil Pesto and Zucchini Pasta Salad with Almond Barbecue Toppers 146
　Basil Pesto Potato Top Pie 184
　Italian Lentil Bolognaise with Raw Zucchini Noodles 166
　Lemongrass, Lime and Coconut Thai Curry with Crispy Potatoes 172
　Raw Rainbow Thai Salad with Thai Basil and Lime Dressing 132

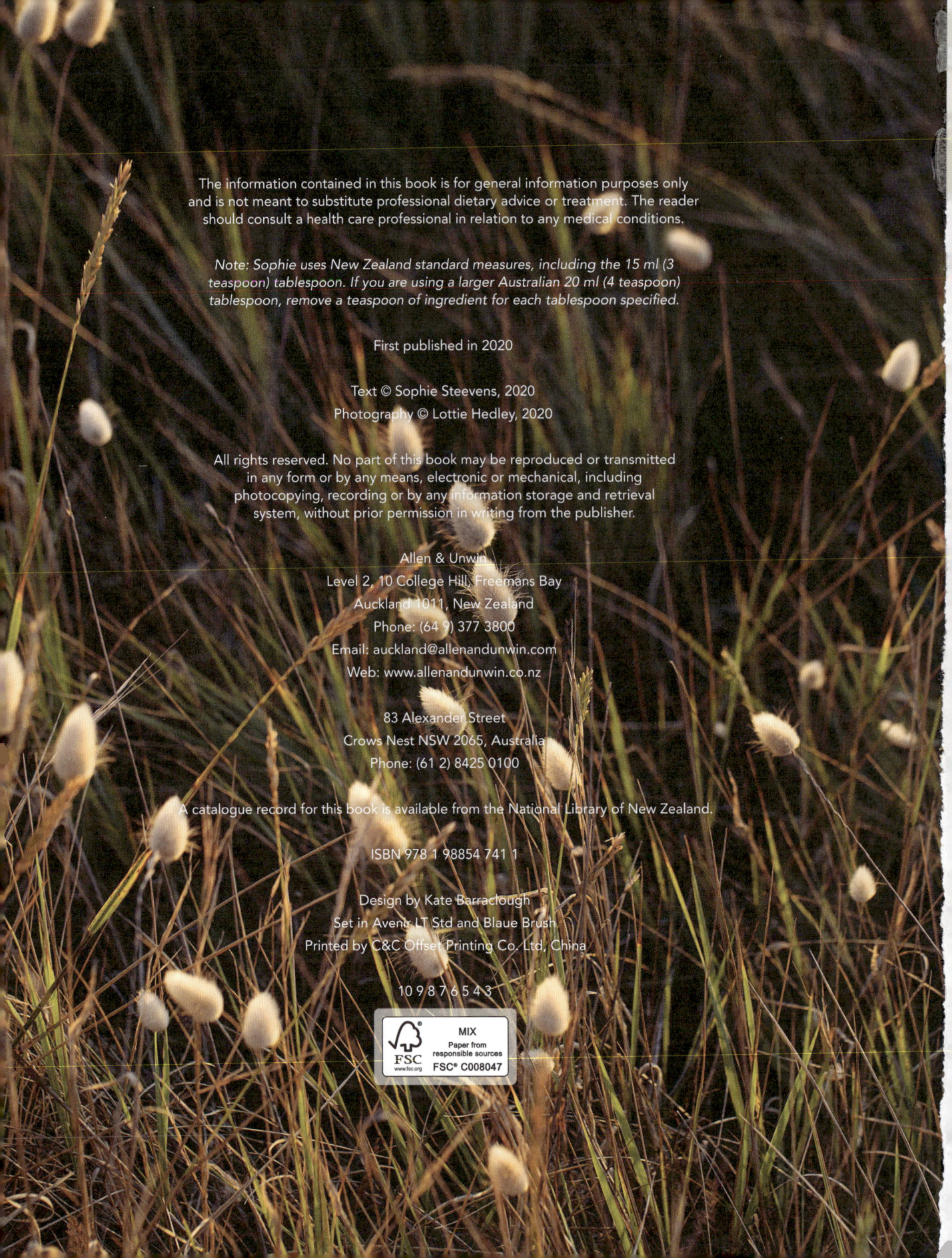

The information contained in this book is for general information purposes only and is not meant to substitute professional dietary advice or treatment. The reader should consult a health care professional in relation to any medical conditions.

Note: Sophie uses New Zealand standard measures, including the 15 ml (3 teaspoon) tablespoon. If you are using a larger Australian 20 ml (4 teaspoon) tablespoon, remove a teaspoon of ingredient for each tablespoon specified.

First published in 2020

Text © Sophie Steevens, 2020
Photography © Lottie Hedley, 2020

All rights reserved. No part of this book may be reproduced or transmitted in any form or by any means, electronic or mechanical, including photocopying, recording or by any information storage and retrieval system, without prior permission in writing from the publisher.

Allen & Unwin
Level 2, 10 College Hill, Freemans Bay
Auckland 1011, New Zealand
Phone: (64 9) 377 3800
Email: auckland@allenandunwin.com
Web: www.allenandunwin.co.nz

83 Alexander Street
Crows Nest NSW 2065, Australia
Phone: (61 2) 8425 0100

A catalogue record for this book is available from the National Library of New Zealand.

ISBN 978 1 98854 741 1

Design by Kate Barraclough
Set in Avenir LT Std and Blaue Brush
Printed by C&C Offset Printing Co. Ltd, China

10 9 8 7 6 5 4 3

MIX
Paper from responsible sources
FSC® C008047